Access Your Online Resources

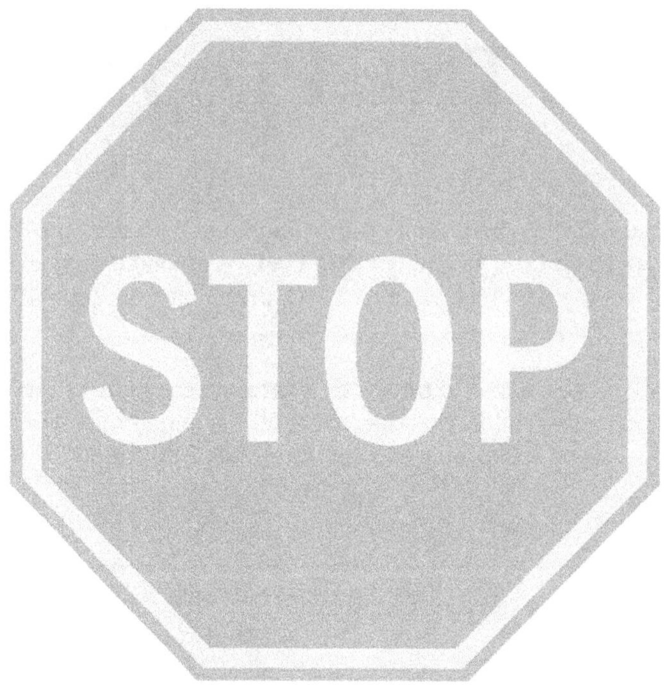

Don't miss out on the Online Resources included with your purchase!

Your purchase of this product unlocks access to our Online Resources page. Elevate your study experience with our **interactive practice test interface**, along with all of the additional resources that we couldn't include in this book.

Flip to the Online Resources section at the end of this book to find the link and a QR code to get started!

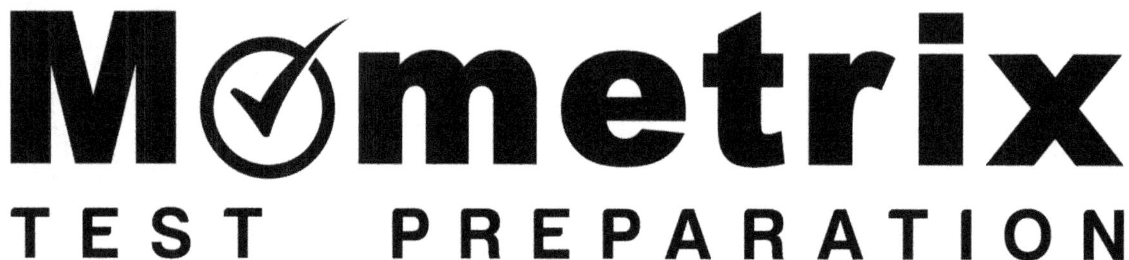

VTNE®

Secrets

Study Guide

Your Key to Exam Success

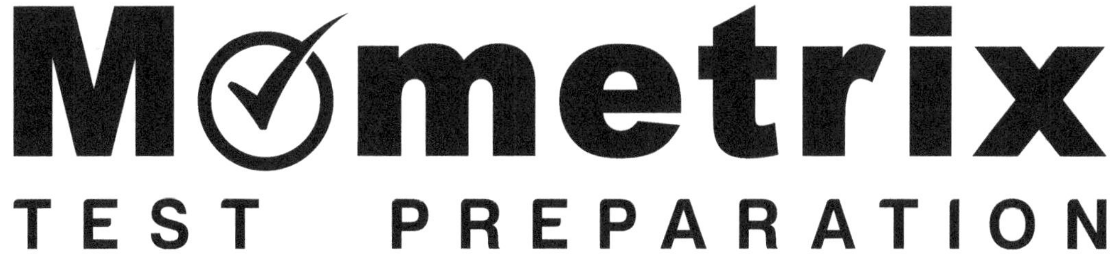

Written and edited by the Mometrix Veterinary Certification Test Team

Paperback
ISBN 13: 978-1-61073-014-3
ISBN 10: 1-61073-014-3

Ebook
ISBN 13: 978-1-62120-461-9
ISBN 10: 1-62120-461-8

Hardback
ISBN 13: 978-1-5167-0567-2
ISBN 10: 1-5167-0567-X

DEAR FUTURE EXAM SUCCESS STORY

First of all, **THANK YOU** for purchasing Mometrix study materials!

Second, congratulations! You are one of the few determined test-takers who are committed to doing whatever it takes to excel on your exam. **You have come to the right place.** We developed these study materials with one goal in mind: to deliver you the information you need in a format that's concise and easy to use.

In addition to optimizing your guide for the content of the test, we've outlined our recommended steps for breaking down the preparation process into small, attainable goals so you can make sure you stay on track.

We've also analyzed the entire test-taking process, identifying the most common pitfalls and showing how you can overcome them and be ready for any curveball the test throws you.

Standardized testing is one of the biggest obstacles on your road to success, which only increases the importance of doing well in the high-pressure, high-stakes environment of test day. Your results on this test could have a significant impact on your future, and this guide provides the information and practical advice to help you achieve your full potential on test day.

Your success is our success

We would love to hear from you! If you would like to share the story of your exam success or if you have any questions or comments in regard to our products, please contact us at **800-673-8175** or **support@mometrix.com**.

Thanks again for your business and we wish you continued success!

Sincerely,
The Mometrix Test Preparation Team

Need more help? Check out our flashcards at:
http://MometrixFlashcards.com/VTNE

TABLE OF CONTENTS

Introduction

Thank you for purchasing this resource! You have made the choice to prepare yourself for a test that could have a huge impact on your future, and this guide is designed to help you be fully ready for test day. Obviously, it's important to have a solid understanding of the test material, but you also need to be prepared for the unique environment and stressors of the test, so that you can perform to the best of your abilities.

For this purpose, the first section that appears in this guide is the **Secret Keys**. We've devoted countless hours to meticulously researching what works and what doesn't, and we've boiled down our findings to the five most impactful steps you can take to improve your performance on the test. We start at the beginning with study planning and move through the preparation process, all the way to the testing strategies that will help you get the most out of what you know when you're finally sitting in front of the test.

We recommend that you start preparing for your test as far in advance as possible. However, if you've bought this guide as a last-minute study resource and only have a few days before your test, we recommend that you skip over the first two Secret Keys since they address a long-term study plan.

If you struggle with **test anxiety**, we strongly encourage you to check out our recommendations for how you can overcome it. Test anxiety is a formidable foe, but it can be beaten, and we want to make sure you have the tools you need to defeat it.

Secret Key #1 – Plan Big, Study Small

There's a lot riding on your performance. If you want to ace this test, you're going to need to keep your skills sharp and the material fresh in your mind. You need a plan that lets you review everything you need to know while still fitting in your schedule. We'll break this strategy down into three categories.

Information Organization

Start with the information you already have: the official test outline. From this, you can make a complete list of all the concepts you need to cover before the test. Organize these concepts into groups that can be studied together, and create a list of any related vocabulary you need to learn so you can brush up on any difficult terms. You'll want to keep this vocabulary list handy once you actually start studying since you may need to add to it along the way.

Time Management

Once you have your set of study concepts, decide how to spread them out over the time you have left before the test. Break your study plan into small, clear goals so you have a manageable task for each day and know exactly what you're doing. Then just focus on one small step at a time. When you manage your time this way, you don't need to spend hours at a time studying. Studying a small block of content for a short period each day helps you retain information better and avoid stressing over how much you have left to do. You can relax knowing that you have a plan to cover everything in time. In order for this strategy to be effective though, you have to start studying early and stick to your schedule. Avoid the exhaustion and futility that comes from last-minute cramming!

Study Environment

The environment you study in has a big impact on your learning. Studying in a coffee shop, while probably more enjoyable, is not likely to be as fruitful as studying in a quiet room. It's important to keep distractions to a minimum. You're only planning to study for a short block of time, so make the most of it. Don't pause to check your phone or get up to find a snack. It's also important to **avoid multitasking**. Research has consistently shown that multitasking will make your studying dramatically less effective. Your study area should also be comfortable and well-lit so you don't have the distraction of straining your eyes or sitting on an uncomfortable chair.

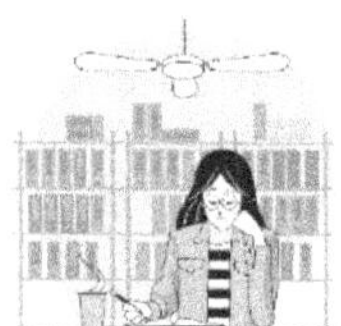

The time of day you study is also important. You want to be rested and alert. Don't wait until just before bedtime. Study when you'll be most likely to comprehend and remember. Even better, if you know what time of day your test will be, set that time aside for study. That way your brain will be used to working on that subject at that specific time and you'll have a better chance of recalling information.

Finally, it can be helpful to team up with others who are studying for the same test. Your actual studying should be done in as isolated an environment as possible, but the work of organizing the information and setting up the study plan can be divided up. In between study sessions, you can discuss with your teammates the concepts that you're all studying and quiz each other on the details. Just be sure that your teammates are as serious about the test as you are. If you find that your study time is being replaced with social time, you might need to find a new team.

Secret Key #2 – Make Your Studying Count

You're devoting a lot of time and effort to preparing for this test, so you want to be absolutely certain it will pay off. This means doing more than just reading the content and hoping you can remember it on test day. It's important to make every minute of study count. There are two main areas you can focus on to make your studying count.

Retention

It doesn't matter how much time you study if you can't remember the material. You need to make sure you are retaining the concepts. To check your retention of the information you're learning, try recalling it at later times with minimal prompting. Try carrying around flashcards and glance at one or two from time to time or ask a friend who's also studying for the test to quiz you.

To enhance your retention, look for ways to put the information into practice so that you can apply it rather than simply recalling it. If you're using the information in practical ways, it will be much easier to remember. Similarly, it helps to solidify a concept in your mind if you're not only reading it to yourself but also explaining it to someone else. Ask a friend to let you teach them about a concept you're a little shaky on (or speak aloud to an imaginary audience if necessary). As you try to summarize, define, give examples, and answer your friend's questions, you'll understand the concepts better and they will stay with you longer. Finally, step back for a big picture view and ask yourself how each piece of information fits with the whole subject. When you link the different concepts together and see them working together as a whole, it's easier to remember the individual components.

Finally, practice showing your work on any multi-step problems, even if you're just studying. Writing out each step you take to solve a problem will help solidify the process in your mind, and you'll be more likely to remember it during the test.

Modality

Modality simply refers to the means or method by which you study. Choosing a study modality that fits your own individual learning style is crucial. No two people learn best in exactly the same way, so it's important to know your strengths and use them to your advantage.

For example, if you learn best by visualization, focus on visualizing a concept in your mind and draw an image or a diagram. Try color-coding your notes, illustrating them, or creating symbols that will trigger your mind to recall a learned concept. If you learn best by hearing or discussing information, find a study partner who learns the same way or read aloud to yourself. Think about how to put the information in your own words. Imagine that you are giving a lecture on the topic and record yourself so you can listen to it later.

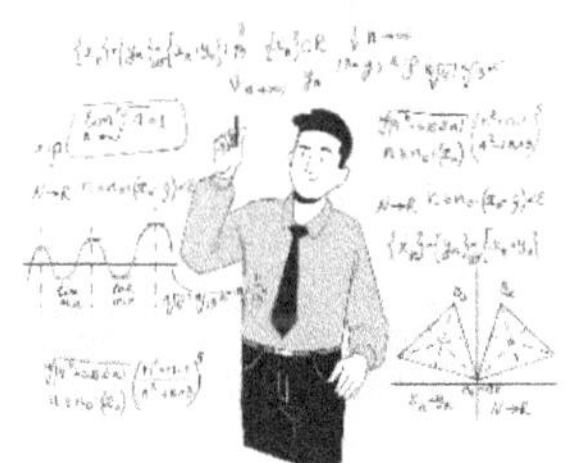

For any learning style, flashcards can be helpful. Organize the information so you can take advantage of spare moments to review. Underline key words or phrases. Use different colors for different categories. Mnemonic devices (such as creating a short list in which every item starts with the same letter) can also help with retention. Find what works best for you and use it to store the information in your mind most effectively and easily.

Secret Key #3 – Practice the Right Way

Your success on test day depends not only on how many hours you put into preparing, but also on whether you prepared the right way. It's good to check along the way to see if your studying is paying off. One of the most effective ways to do this is by taking practice tests to evaluate your progress. Practice tests are useful because they show exactly where you need to improve. Every time you take a practice test, pay special attention to these three groups of questions:

- The questions you got wrong
- The questions you had to guess on, even if you guessed right
- The questions you found difficult or slow to work through

This will show you exactly what your weak areas are, and where you need to devote more study time. Ask yourself why each of these questions gave you trouble. Was it because you didn't understand the material? Was it because you didn't remember the vocabulary? Do you need more repetitions on this type of question to build speed and confidence? Dig into those questions and figure out how you can strengthen your weak areas as you go back to review the material.

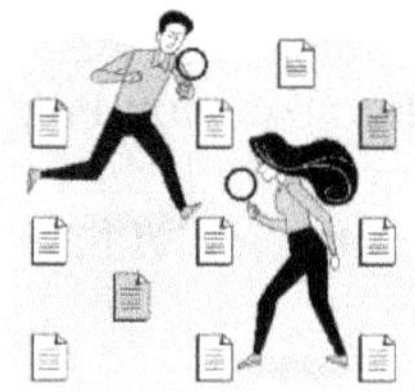

Additionally, many practice tests have a section explaining the answer choices. It can be tempting to read the explanation and think that you now have a good understanding of the concept. However, an explanation likely only covers part of the question's broader context. Even if the explanation makes perfect sense, **go back and investigate** every concept related to the question until you're positive you have a thorough understanding.

As you go along, keep in mind that the practice test is just that: practice. Memorizing these questions and answers will not be very helpful on the actual test because it is unlikely to have any of the same exact questions. If you only know the right answers to the sample questions, you won't be prepared for the real thing. **Study the concepts** until you understand them fully, and then you'll be able to answer any question that shows up on the test.

It's important to wait on the practice tests until you're ready. If you take a test on your first day of study, you may be overwhelmed by the amount of material covered and how much you need to learn. Work up to it gradually.

On test day, you'll need to be prepared for answering questions, managing your time, and using the test-taking strategies you've learned. It's a lot to balance, like a mental marathon that will have a big impact on your future. Like training for a marathon, you'll need to start slowly and work your way up. When test day arrives, you'll be ready.

Start with the strategies you've read in the first two Secret Keys—plan your course and study in the way that works best for you. If you have time, consider using multiple study resources to get different approaches to the same concepts. It can be helpful to see difficult concepts from more than one angle. Then find a good source for practice tests. Many times, the test website will suggest potential study resources or provide sample tests.

Practice Test Strategy

If you're able to find at least three practice tests, we recommend this strategy:

Untimed and Open-Book Practice

Take the first test with no time constraints and with your notes and study guide handy. Take your time and focus on applying the strategies you've learned.

Timed and Open-Book Practice

Take the second practice test open-book as well, but set a timer and practice pacing yourself to finish in time.

Timed and Closed-Book Practice

Take any other practice tests as if it were test day. Set a timer and put away your study materials. Sit at a table or desk in a quiet room, imagine yourself at the testing center, and answer questions as quickly and accurately as possible.

Keep repeating timed and closed-book tests on a regular basis until you run out of practice tests or it's time for the actual test. Your mind will be ready for the schedule and stress of test day, and you'll be able to focus on recalling the material you've learned.

Secret Key #4 – Pace Yourself

Once you're fully prepared for the material on the test, your biggest challenge on test day will be managing your time. Just knowing that the clock is ticking can make you panic even if you have plenty of time left. Work on pacing yourself so you can build confidence against the time constraints of the exam. Pacing is a difficult skill to master, especially in a high-pressure environment, so **practice is vital**.

Set time expectations for your pace based on how much time is available. For example, if a section has 60 questions and the time limit is 30 minutes, you know you have to average 30 seconds or less per question in order to answer them all. Although 30 seconds is the hard limit, set 25 seconds per question as your goal, so you reserve extra time to spend on harder questions. When you budget extra time for the harder questions, you no longer have any reason to stress when those questions take longer to answer.

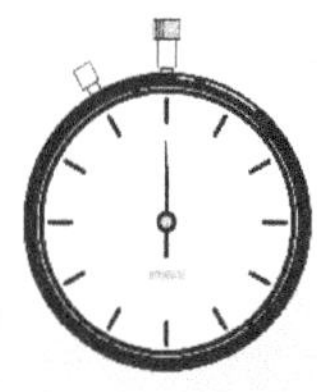

Don't let this time expectation distract you from working through the test at a calm, steady pace, but keep it in mind so you don't spend too much time on any one question. Recognize that taking extra time on one question you don't understand may keep you from answering two that you do understand later in the test. If your time limit for a question is up and you're still not sure of the answer, mark it and move on, and come back to it later if the time and the test format allow. If the testing format doesn't allow you to return to earlier questions, just make an educated guess; then put it out of your mind and move on.

On the easier questions, be careful not to rush. It may seem wise to hurry through them so you have more time for the challenging ones, but it's not worth missing one if you know the concept and just didn't take the time to read the question fully. Work efficiently but make sure you understand the question and have looked at all of the answer choices, since more than one may seem right at first.

Even if you're paying attention to the time, you may find yourself a little behind at some point. You should speed up to get back on track, but do so wisely. Don't panic; just take a few seconds less on each question until you're caught up. Don't guess without thinking, but do look through the answer choices and eliminate any you know are wrong. If you can get down to two choices, it is often worthwhile to guess from those. Once you've chosen an answer, move on and don't dwell on any that you skipped or had to hurry through. If a question was taking too long, chances are it was one of the harder ones, so you weren't as likely to get it right anyway.

On the other hand, if you find yourself getting ahead of schedule, it may be beneficial to slow down a little. The more quickly you work, the more likely you are to make a careless mistake that will affect your score. You've budgeted time for each question, so don't be afraid to spend that time. Practice an efficient but careful pace to get the most out of the time you have.

Secret Key #5 – Have a Plan for Guessing

When you're taking the test, you may find yourself stuck on a question. Some of the answer choices seem better than others, but you don't see the one answer choice that is obviously correct. What do you do?

The scenario described above is very common, yet most test takers have not effectively prepared for it. Developing and practicing a plan for guessing may be one of the single most effective uses of your time as you get ready for the exam.

In developing your plan for guessing, there are three questions to address:

- When should you start the guessing process?
- How should you narrow down the choices?
- Which answer should you choose?

When to Start the Guessing Process

Unless your plan for guessing is to select C every time (which, despite its merits, is not what we recommend), you need to leave yourself enough time to apply your answer elimination strategies. Since you have a limited amount of time for each question, that means that if you're going to give yourself the best shot at guessing correctly, you have to decide quickly whether or not you will guess.

Of course, the best-case scenario is that you don't have to guess at all, so first, see if you can answer the question based on your knowledge of the subject and basic reasoning skills. Focus on the key words in the question and try to jog your memory of related topics. Give yourself a chance to bring the knowledge to mind, but once you realize that you don't have (or you can't access) the knowledge you need to answer the question, it's time to start the guessing process.

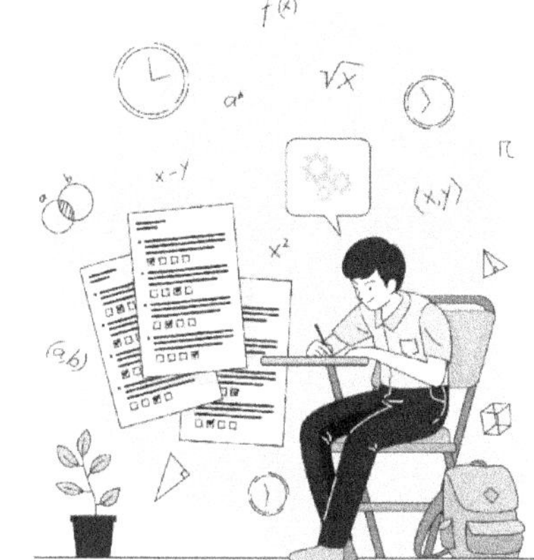

It's almost always better to start the guessing process too early than too late. It only takes a few seconds to remember something and answer the question from knowledge. Carefully eliminating wrong answer choices takes longer. Plus, going through the process of eliminating answer choices can actually help jog your memory.

Summary: Start the guessing process as soon as you decide that you can't answer the question based on your knowledge.

How to Narrow Down the Choices

The next chapter in this book (**Test-Taking Strategies**) includes a wide range of strategies for how to approach questions and how to look for answer choices to eliminate. You will definitely want to read those carefully, practice them, and figure out which ones work best for you. Here though, we're going to address a mindset rather than a particular strategy.

Your odds of guessing an answer correctly depend on how many options you are choosing from.

Number of options left	5	4	3	2	1
Odds of guessing correctly	20%	25%	33%	50%	100%

You can see from this chart just how valuable it is to be able to eliminate incorrect answers and make an educated guess, but there are two things that many test takers do that cause them to miss out on the benefits of guessing:

- Accidentally eliminating the correct answer
- Selecting an answer based on an impression

We'll look at the first one here, and the second one in the next section.

To avoid accidentally eliminating the correct answer, we recommend a thought exercise called **the $5 challenge**. In this challenge, you only eliminate an answer choice from contention if you are willing to bet $5 on it being wrong. Why $5? Five dollars is a small but not insignificant amount of money. It's an amount you could afford to lose but wouldn't want to throw away. And while losing $5 once might not hurt too much, doing it twenty times will set you back $100. In the same way, each small decision you make—eliminating a choice here, guessing on a question there—won't by itself impact your score very much, but when you put them all together, they can make a big difference. By holding each answer choice elimination decision to a higher standard, you can reduce the risk of accidentally eliminating the correct answer.

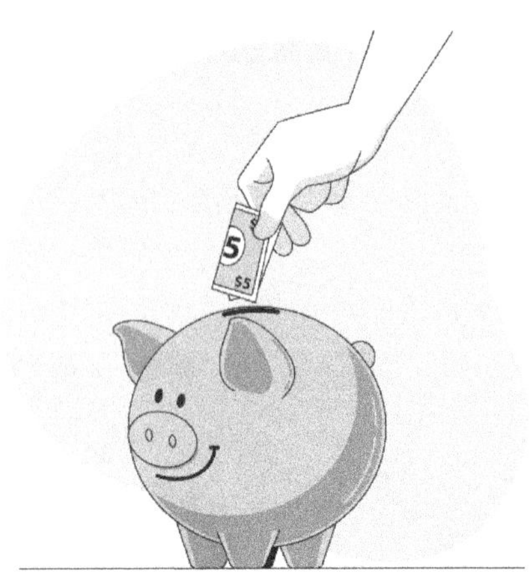

The $5 challenge can also be applied in a positive sense: If you are willing to bet $5 that an answer choice *is* correct, go ahead and mark it as correct.

Summary: Only eliminate an answer choice if you are willing to bet $5 that it is wrong.

Which Answer to Choose

You're taking the test. You've run into a hard question and decided you'll have to guess. You've eliminated all the answer choices you're willing to bet $5 on. Now you have to pick an answer. Why do we even need to talk about this? Why can't you just pick whichever one you feel like when the time comes?

The answer to these questions is that if you don't come into the test with a plan, you'll rely on your impression to select an answer choice, and if you do that, you risk falling into a trap. The test writers know that everyone who takes their test will be guessing on some of the questions, so they intentionally write wrong answer choices to seem plausible. You still have to pick an answer though, and if the wrong answer choices are designed to look right, how can you ever be sure that you're not falling for their trap? The best solution we've found to this dilemma is to take the decision out of your hands entirely. Here is the process we recommend:

Once you've eliminated any choices that you are confident (willing to bet $5) are wrong, select the first remaining choice as your answer.

Whether you choose to select the first remaining choice, the second, or the last, the important thing is that you use some preselected standard. Using this approach guarantees that you will not be enticed into selecting an answer choice that looks right, because you are not basing your decision on how the answer choices look.

A. This is wrong.
B. Also wrong.
C. Maybe?
D. Maybe?

This is not meant to make you question your knowledge. Instead, it is to help you recognize the difference between your knowledge and your impressions. There's a huge difference between thinking an answer is right because of what you know, and thinking an answer is right because it looks or sounds like it should be right.

Summary: To ensure that your selection is appropriately random, make a predetermined selection from among all answer choices you have not eliminated.

Test-Taking Strategies

This section contains a list of test-taking strategies that you may find helpful as you work through the test. By taking what you know and applying logical thought, you can maximize your chances of answering any question correctly!

It is very important to realize that every question is different and every person is different: no single strategy will work on every question, and no single strategy will work for every person. That's why we've included all of them here, so you can try them out and determine which ones work best for different types of questions and which ones work best for you.

Question Strategies

☑ Read Carefully

Read the question and the answer choices carefully. Don't miss the question because you misread the terms. You have plenty of time to read each question thoroughly and make sure you understand what is being asked. Yet a happy medium must be attained, so don't waste too much time. You must read carefully and efficiently.

☑ Contextual Clues

Look for contextual clues. If the question includes a word you are not familiar with, look at the immediate context for some indication of what the word might mean. Contextual clues can often give you all the information you need to decipher the meaning of an unfamiliar word. Even if you can't determine the meaning, you may be able to narrow down the possibilities enough to make a solid guess at the answer to the question.

☑ Prefixes

If you're having trouble with a word in the question or answer choices, try dissecting it. Take advantage of every clue that the word might include. Prefixes can be a huge help. Usually, they allow you to determine a basic meaning. *Pre-* means before, *post-* means after, *pro-* is positive, *de-* is negative. From prefixes, you can get an idea of the general meaning of the word and try to put it into context.

☑ Hedge Words

Watch out for critical hedge words, such as *likely, may, can, often, almost, mostly, usually, generally, rarely,* and *sometimes*. Question writers insert these hedge phrases to cover every possibility. Often an answer choice will be wrong simply because it leaves no room for exception. Be on guard for answer choices that have definitive words such as *exactly* and *always*.

☑ Switchback Words

Stay alert for *switchbacks*. These are the words and phrases frequently used to alert you to shifts in thought. The most common switchback words are *but, although,* and *however*. Others include *nevertheless, on the other hand, even though, while, in spite of, despite,* and *regardless of*. Switchback words are important to catch because they can change the direction of the question or an answer choice.

☑ Face Value

When in doubt, use common sense. Accept the situation in the problem at face value. Don't read too much into it. These problems will not require you to make wild assumptions. If you have to go beyond creativity and warp time or space in order to have an answer choice fit the question, then you should move on and consider the other answer choices. These are normal problems rooted in reality. The applicable relationship or explanation may not be readily apparent, but it is there for you to figure out. Use your common sense to interpret anything that isn't clear.

Answer Choice Strategies

⊘ Answer Selection

The most thorough way to pick an answer choice is to identify and eliminate wrong answers until only one is left, then confirm it is the correct answer. Sometimes an answer choice may immediately seem right, but be careful. The test writers will usually put more than one reasonable answer choice on each question, so take a second to read all of them and make sure that the other choices are not equally obvious. As long as you have time left, it is better to read every answer choice than to pick the first one that looks right without checking the others.

⊘ Answer Choice Families

An answer choice family consists of two (in rare cases, three) answer choices that are very similar in construction and cannot all be true at the same time. If you see two answer choices that are direct opposites or parallels, one of them is usually the correct answer. For instance, if one answer choice says that quantity *x* increases and another either says that quantity *x* decreases (opposite) or says that quantity *y* increases (parallel), then those answer choices would fall into the same family. An answer choice that doesn't match the construction of the answer choice family is more likely to be incorrect. Most questions will not have answer choice families, but when they do appear, you should be prepared to recognize them.

⊘ Eliminate Answers

Eliminate answer choices as soon as you realize they are wrong, but make sure you consider all possibilities. If you are eliminating answer choices and realize that the last one you are left with is also wrong, don't panic. Start over and consider each choice again. There may be something you missed the first time that you will realize on the second pass.

⊘ Avoid Fact Traps

Don't be distracted by an answer choice that is factually true but doesn't answer the question. You are looking for the choice that answers the question. Stay focused on what the question is asking for so you don't accidentally pick an answer that is true but incorrect. Always go back to the question and make sure the answer choice you've selected actually answers the question and is not merely a true statement.

⊘ Extreme Statements

In general, you should avoid answers that put forth extreme actions as standard practice or proclaim controversial ideas as established fact. An answer choice that states the "process should be used in certain situations, if..." is much more likely to be correct than one that states the "process should be discontinued completely." The first is a calm rational statement and doesn't even make a definitive, uncompromising stance, using a hedge word *if* to provide wiggle room, whereas the second choice is far more extreme.

⊘ Benchmark

As you read through the answer choices and you come across one that seems to answer the question well, mentally select that answer choice. This is not your final answer, but it's the one that will help you evaluate the other answer choices. The one that you selected is your benchmark or standard for judging each of the other answer choices. Every other answer choice must be compared to your benchmark. That choice is correct until proven otherwise by another answer choice beating it. If you find a better answer, then that one becomes your new benchmark. Once you've decided that no other choice answers the question as well as your benchmark, you have your final answer.

☑ PREDICT THE ANSWER

Before you even start looking at the answer choices, it is often best to try to predict the answer. When you come up with the answer on your own, it is easier to avoid distractions and traps because you will know exactly what to look for. The right answer choice is unlikely to be word-for-word what you came up with, but it should be a close match. Even if you are confident that you have the right answer, you should still take the time to read each option before moving on.

General Strategies

☑ TOUGH QUESTIONS

If you are stumped on a problem or it appears too hard or too difficult, don't waste time. Move on! Remember though, if you can quickly check for obviously incorrect answer choices, your chances of guessing correctly are greatly improved. Before you completely give up, at least try to knock out a couple of possible answers. Eliminate what you can and then guess at the remaining answer choices before moving on.

☑ CHECK YOUR WORK

Since you will probably not know every term listed and the answer to every question, it is important that you get credit for the ones that you do know. Don't miss any questions through careless mistakes. If at all possible, try to take a second to look back over your answer selection and make sure you've selected the correct answer choice and haven't made a costly careless mistake (such as marking an answer choice that you didn't mean to mark). This quick double check should more than pay for itself in caught mistakes for the time it costs.

☑ PACE YOURSELF

It's easy to be overwhelmed when you're looking at a page full of questions; your mind is confused and full of random thoughts, and the clock is ticking down faster than you would like. Calm down and maintain the pace that you have set for yourself. Especially as you get down to the last few minutes of the test, don't let the small numbers on the clock make you panic. As long as you are on track by monitoring your pace, you are guaranteed to have time for each question.

☑ DON'T RUSH

It is very easy to make errors when you are in a hurry. Maintaining a fast pace in answering questions is pointless if it makes you miss questions that you would have gotten right otherwise. Test writers like to include distracting information and wrong answers that seem right. Taking a little extra time to avoid careless mistakes can make all the difference in your test score. Find a pace that allows you to be confident in the answers that you select.

☑ KEEP MOVING

Panicking will not help you pass the test, so do your best to stay calm and keep moving. Taking deep breaths and going through the answer elimination steps you practiced can help to break through a stress barrier and keep your pace.

Final Notes

The combination of a solid foundation of content knowledge and the confidence that comes from practicing your plan for applying that knowledge is the key to maximizing your performance on test day. As your foundation of content knowledge is built up and strengthened, you'll find that the strategies included in this chapter become more and more effective in helping you quickly sift through the distractions and traps of the test to isolate the correct answer.

Now that you're preparing to move forward into the test content chapters of this book, be sure to keep your goal in mind. As you read, think about how you will be able to apply this information on the test. If you've already seen sample questions for the test and you have an idea of the question format and style, try to come up with questions of your own that you can answer based on what you're reading. This will give you valuable practice applying your knowledge in the same ways you can expect to on test day.

Good luck and good studying!

Six-Week VTNE Study Plan

On the next few pages, we've provided an optional study plan to help you use this study guide to its fullest potential over the course of six weeks. If you have twelve weeks available and want to spread it out more, spend two weeks on each section of the plan.

Below is a quick summary of the subjects covered in each week of the plan.

- Week 1: Pharmacy and Pharmacology & Surgical Nursing
- Week 2: Dentistry & Laboratory Procedures
- Week 3: Animal Care and Nursing & Diagnostic Imaging
- Week 4: Anesthesia & Emergency Medicine and Critical Care
- Week 5: Pain Management/Analgesia & Communication and Veterinary Professional Support Services
- Week 6: Practice Tests

Please note that not all subjects will take the same amount of time to work through.

Three full-length practice tests are included in this study guide. We recommend saving the third practice test and any additional tests for after you've completed the study plan. Take these practice tests timed and without any reference materials a day or two before the real thing as practice runs to get you in the mode of answering questions at a good pace.

Week 1: Pharmacy and Pharmacology & Surgical Nursing

Instructional Content

First, read carefully through the Pharmacy and Pharmacology & Surgical Nursing chapters in this book, checking off your progress as you go:

❑ Classifications of Drugs
❑ Drug Storage, Handling, and Inventory
❑ Calculating Dosage
❑ Drug Administration
❑ Preparing Medication
❑ Surgical Anatomy and Physiology
❑ Surgical Equipment
❑ Surgical Cleanliness
❑ Surgical Preparation
❑ Surgical Procedures
❑ Suture Techniques

As you read, do the following:

- Highlight any sections, terms, or concepts you think are important
- Draw an asterisk (*) next to any areas you are struggling with
- Watch the review videos to gain more understanding of a particular topic
- Take notes in your notebook or in the margins of this book

After you've read through everything, go back and review any sections that you highlighted or that you drew an asterisk next to, referencing your notes along the way.

Week 2: Dentistry & Laboratory Procedures

Instructional Content

First, read carefully through the Dentistry & Laboratory Procedures chapters in this book, checking off your progress as you go:

❑ Dental Anatomy and Physiology
❑ Dental Pathophysiology
❑ Instruments and Equipment
❑ Oral Examinations and Treatment
❑ Dental Radiography
❑ Clinical Hematology
❑ Clinical Biochemistry
❑ Clinical Cytology
❑ Clinical Urinalysis
❑ Clinical Parasitology
❑ Clinical Microbiology
❑ Maintaining Laboratory Equipment and Supplies

As you read, do the following:

- Highlight any sections, terms, or concepts you think are important
- Draw an asterisk (*) next to any areas you are struggling with
- Take notes in your notebook or in the margins of this book

After you've read through everything, go back and review any sections that you highlighted or that you drew an asterisk next to, referencing your notes along the way.

Week 3: Animal Care and Nursing & Diagnostic Imaging

INSTRUCTIONAL CONTENT

First, read carefully through the Animal Care and Nursing & Diagnostic Imaging chapters in this book, checking off your progress as you go:

❏ Animal Terminology
❏ Animal Handling and Restraint
❏ Information and Evaluation
❏ Common Conditions and Treatment
❏ Nursing and Rehabilitation
❏ Clinical Diagnostic Procedures
❏ Producing Diagnostic Imagery
❏ Equipment and Related Materials

As you read, do the following:

- Highlight any sections, terms, or concepts you think are important
- Draw an asterisk (*) next to any areas you are struggling with
- Watch the review videos to gain more understanding of a particular topic
- Take notes in your notebook or in the margins of this book

After you've read through everything, go back and review any sections that you highlighted or that you drew an asterisk next to, referencing your notes along the way.

Week 4: Anesthesia & Emergency Medicine and Critical Care

INSTRUCTIONAL CONTENT

First, read carefully through the Anesthesia & Emergency Medicine and Critical Care chapters in this book, checking off your progress as you go:

❏ Classifications of Anesthetic Drugs
❏ Pre-Procedural
❏ Anesthetic Process and Monitoring
❏ Maintaining, Cleaning, and Preparing Equipment
❏ Triage
❏ Emergency Nursing Procedures

As you read, do the following:

- Highlight any sections, terms, or concepts you think are important
- Draw an asterisk (*) next to any areas you are struggling with
- Take notes in your notebook or in the margins of this book

After you've read through everything, go back and review any sections that you highlighted or that you drew an asterisk next to, referencing your notes along the way.

Week 5: Pain Management/Analgesia & Communication and Veterinary Professional Support Services

Instructional Content

First, read carefully through the Pain Management/Analgesia & Communication and Veterinary Professional Support Services chapters in this book, checking off your progress as you go:

❑ Assessing Pain
❑ Treating Pain
❑ Client Education
❑ Communication
❑ Collecting Patient Information
❑ Euthanasia

As you read, do the following:

- Highlight any sections, terms, or concepts you think are important
- Draw an asterisk (*) next to any areas you are struggling with
- Take notes in your notebook or in the margins of this book

After you've read through everything, go back and review any sections that you highlighted or that you drew an asterisk next to, referencing your notes along the way.

Week 6: Practice Tests

Your success on test day depends not only on how many hours you put into preparing, but also on whether you prepared the right way. It's good to check along the way to see if your studying is paying off. One of the most effective ways to do this is by taking practice tests to evaluate your progress. Practice tests are useful because they show exactly where you need to improve. Every time you take a practice test, pay special attention to these three groups of questions:

- The questions you got wrong
- The questions you had to guess on, even if you guessed right
- The questions you found difficult or slow to work through

This will show you exactly what your weak areas are, and where you need to devote more study time. Ask yourself why each of these questions gave you trouble. Was it because you didn't understand the material? Was it because you didn't remember the vocabulary? Do you need more repetitions on this type of question to build speed and confidence? Dig into those questions and figure out how you can strengthen your weak areas as you go back to review the material.

Practice Test #1

Now that you've read over the instructional content, it's time to take a practice test. Complete Practice Test #1. Take this test with **no time constraints**, and feel free to reference the applicable sections of this guide as you go. Once you've finished, check your answers against the provided answer key. For any questions you answered incorrectly, review the answer rationale, and then **go back and review** the applicable sections of the book. The goal in this stage is to understand why you answered the question incorrectly, and make sure that the next time you see a similar question, you will get it right.

Practice Test #2

Next, complete Practice Test #2. This time, give yourself **3 hours** to complete all of the questions. You should again feel free to reference the guide and your notes, but be mindful of the clock. If you run out of time before you finish all of the questions, mark where you were when time expired, but go ahead and finish taking the practice test. Once you've finished, check your answers against the provided answer key, and as before, review the answer rationale for any that you answered incorrectly and then go back and review the associated instructional content. Your goal is still to increase understanding of the content but also to get used to the time constraints you will face on the test.

As you go along, keep in mind that the practice test is just that: practice. Memorizing these questions and answers will not be very helpful on the actual test because it is unlikely to have any of the same exact questions. If you only know the right answers to the sample questions, you won't be prepared for the real thing. **Study the concepts** until you understand them fully, and then you'll be able to answer any question that shows up on the test.

Pharmacy and Pharmacology

Transform passive reading into active learning! After immersing yourself in this chapter, put your comprehension to the test by taking a quiz. The insights you gained will stay with you longer this way. Scan the QR code to go directly to the chapter quiz interface for this study guide. If you're using a computer, simply visit the online resources page at **mometrix.com/resources719/vtne** and click the Chapter Quizzes link.

Classifications of Drugs

Drugs, Poisons, and Generics

Drugs can cause significant physiological changes within the body and can work to improve the body's ability to function properly. Synonymously known as medicine, drugs can also be prescribed in preventive care, in response to a specific diagnosis, and as a treatment.

Poison is a toxic substance which can produce injury, sickness, or death. Drugs that are not applied in the correct dosage may produce poisonous results. Toxic substances may be given through ingestion, injection, inhalation, or absorption through the skin, or they may be created by chemical processes within the body. Many common substances like water or vitamins can be harmful or poisonous when taken in excess.

Generic is a term used to designate the name of a drug in its basic chemical form. It may or may not hold the same chemical formula as brand-name medications (often depending upon whether or not the patent has expired). The chemical name or generic name of a drug can be used in place of other proprietary or trademark names for the same drug substance.

Therapeutic Index (TI)

The **therapeutic index** or **TI** (also known as the therapeutic ratio) is used to address the relative safety of a drug. The therapeutic index is expressed by the following formula: $TI = LD_{50}/EC_{50}$.

LD_{50} refers to the **lethal dosage** for 50% of a designated population, while EC_{50} refers to the minimum **effective concentration** for 50% of that same population.

Drugs with a higher TI are considered safer than those with a lower TI. Drugs with a lower TI provide a narrower available dosage range between a desired therapeutic effect and toxic or poisonous results. Thus, drugs with a lower TI offer fewer dosage options in treating a given condition before adverse effects may begin to arise. They can also be hazardous to handle and much more difficult to prescribe and manage. Typically, more frequent provider contacts are required, more detailed status reports are needed, and laboratory testing for both therapeutic levels and signs of deleterious secondary effects are more critical.

Allergenics

Histamines are an important part of the body's immune system. They are largely responsible for how the body processes and defends against foreign allergens, such as pollen, dander, or dust. However, the histamine response may cause respiratory difficulties, itching, rashes, **anaphylaxis** (an exaggerated allergic reaction), and other inflammatory responses.

Diphenhydramine (Benadryl) is given to patients in anaphylactic shock. **Anaphylactic shock** is an allergic reaction severe enough to cause the death of the patient. Patients in anaphylactic shock may have symptoms of low blood pressure, itching, swelling, and extreme respiratory problems. In such situations, diphenhydramine should be given intravenously as quickly as possible to offer maximal support.

ANTIHISTAMINES

Antihistamines are drugs which are able to block histamine release or their uptake by specific cell receptors. These drugs can be used to prevent or reduce severe allergic reactions. Common antihistamines include chlorpheniramine, cyproheptadine, diphenhydramine, hydroxyzine, and clemastine. These drugs often produce somnolence, or drowsiness, as an undesirable side effect, and patients may also exhibit symptoms of dry mouth or marked thirst. Some antihistamines have additional treatment purposes, as well. For example, cyproheptadine can enhance feline appetite.

Antihistamines work in one of two ways: by blocking either H_1 receptors or H_2 receptors in the body. The H_1 receptors in the body are responsible for **pruritus** (itching) and also cause inflammatory cells to be drawn to the site. Antihistamines that are H_1 blockers try to beat the histamine to the H_1 receptor sites by antagonizing the histamine instead of blocking histamine release. The H_1-blocking antihistamines are effective for treatment of anaphylaxis because they stop bronchoconstriction and vasodilation, but they are less effective as anti-inflammatories or for allergy treatment because histamine is not the only factor for the body's entire inflammatory response; most allergy cases require a multimodal approach for treatment. The other class of antihistamines is H_2 antagonists, which are used to suppress gastric secretory effects caused by histamine and also have mild anti-inflammatory effects. Benadryl and Claritin are H_1-blocking antihistamines; famotidine is an H_2-blocking antihistamine.

ANTI-INFECTIVE AGENTS

Antimicrobials kill microorganisms or prevent them from multiplying. Antibiotics are used to treat infection caused by bacteria, antifungals are for infection caused by fungi, antivirals are for infection caused by viruses, and antiprotozoals are used for infection caused by protozoa.

Antimicrobial drugs work in many ways, including: 1) hindering cell wall growth, 2) preventing the organism from synthesizing proteins, 3) inhibiting nucleic acid synthesis, 4) inhibiting metabolic pathways in the bacteria that do not exist in the host, and 5) damaging cytoplasmic membranes.

INHIBITION OF MICROBIAL PROTEIN SYNTHESIS

Antimicrobials can be effective in obstructing microbial protein synthesis. This interference is accomplished as the antimicrobial substance is introduced into the microbe and fastens itself to the microbial ribosomes. Ribosomes are submicroscopic clusters of proteins and RNA found within the cytoplasm of cells which are necessary for protein synthesis.

Many **aminoglycosides**, some of which also prevent microbial protein synthesis, are bactericidal in nature. By contrast, other antibiotics such as tetracycline, lincosamide, chloramphenicol, and macrolides, which also use this mechanism, are bacteriostatic agents—they do not kill the bacteria outright (except in high concentrations) but rather inhibit growth and reproduction.

Still other antimicrobial drugs slow down nucleic acid production in an invading organism, causing genetic information transmissions and protein and enzymatic processes and syntheses to be reduced. Thus, bacteriostatic drugs may also be responsible for microbial inability to divide, as they interrupt microbial metabolic activity.

ANTIBIOTICS

Antibiotics are used to stop bacterial infections by either preventing them from growing (bacteriostatic) or by killing the organisms (bactericidal). Though antibiotics do not kill viruses, they can be effective in treating secondary bacterial infections that can occur while a patient is ill from a virus. Antibiotics can be isolated from natural sources or synthetically produced. They are most effective when given clear passage to the site of infection.

Broad spectrum antibiotics are effective against gram-positive and gram-negative bacteria, but overprescribing broad spectrum antibiotics has led to antibiotic-resistant bacteria. **Narrow spectrum antibiotics** are only effective against certain types of bacteria.

Beta-Lactams

Bactericidal **β-lactam antibiotics** inhibit bacterial cell wall synthesis by targeting penicillin-binding proteins and interrupting mucopeptide synthesis. Antibiotics in this class include:

- Penicillins: Narrow spectrum
- Cephalosporins: Narrow spectrum (1st generation) and broad spectrum (2nd–4th generations)
- Carbapenems: Broad spectrum
- Monobactams: Narrow spectrum

Patients with a known allergy to penicillin should not be administered first-generation cephalosporins, which include: cefadroxil, cefazolin, and cephalexin. An example of a second-generation cephalosporin is cefoxitin, while ceftiofur is a third-generation cephalosporin.

β-lactams are used in large animals (ruminants, pigs, horses), poultry, dogs, and cats to treat streptococcal and clostridial infections, among others.

Chloramphenicol

Bacteriostatic, broad-spectrum **chloramphenicol** inhibits protein synthesis. It is illegal to administer it to food animals in the United States, but it can be used in companion animal medicine to treat anaerobic infections, including middle and inner ear infections, serious eye infections, and salmonellosis. Possible side effects include vomiting, diarrhea, and anaphylaxis.

Lincosamides

Lincosamides, such as clindamycin and lincomycin, inhibit protein synthesis. They are effective against most anaerobes and are considered moderate spectrum. Depending on the concentration of medication and characteristics of the infection (species, severity), lincosamides can have bactericidal or bacteriostatic effects. They should not be used in horses.

Fluoroquinolones

Bactericidal **fluoroquinolones** inhibit nucleic acid synthesis, and some are broad spectrum (3rd generation), though most are narrow spectrum. Antibiotics in this class end in the suffix *-floxacin* and include: ciprofloxacin, danofloxacin, orbifloxacin, enrofloxacin, and difloxacin. They can be used in ruminants, pigs, horses, cats, and dogs.

Aminoglycosides

Bactericidal **aminoglycosides** inhibit protein synthesis. They are considered broad spectrum but are not effective against anaerobic bacteria, and their use is limited to treatment of severe infection due to their nephrotoxicity and ototoxicity. They are used orally to treat Enterobacteriaceae infections as well as topically.

Macrolides

Narrow-spectrum **macrolides** inhibit protein synthesis and are bacteriostatic unless administered at high concentrations. Erythromycin is a common macrolide that can be used to treat animals allergic to penicillin.

Tetracyclines

Bacteriostatic, broad-spectrum **tetracyclines** inhibit protein synthesis. Drugs in this class end with the suffix *-cycline* or *-tetracycline* and include: doxycycline, oxytetracycline, and chlortetracycline. They are used to treat local and systemic infections; however, bacterial resistance to this category of drug has significantly increased over time.

ANTIBIOTIC RESISTANCE

Given a sufficient duration of time, antibiotics administered in the proper dosage and concentration can kill or impede the growth of many disease-causing microbes. However, when antibiotics are not given as prescribed, the bacteria may survive to develop a resistance to the drug.

More and more bacteria are becoming resistant to antibiotics commonly given to both humans and animals. Once this resistance has developed, the bacteria are able to survive despite the presence of the antibiotic within the body. Further, the bacteria's offspring will inherit this same resistance. Consequently, animal caregivers should be aware of the need for proper antibiotic administration and complete treatment of all disease-causing microbes.

ANTIFUNGALS

Antifungal drugs work by attempting to exploit distinguishing features between mammalian and fungi cells. This has been challenging as both are eukaryotic, both have DNA organized into chromosomes in a nucleus, and both have similar intracellular organelles. They even have similar biosynthetic processes for DNA replication and protein synthesis. However, one important difference has been noted: While mammalian cell walls contain significant amounts of cholesterol (about 25% of the cell membrane, by weight), fungi cell walls contain primarily ergosterol.

Several antifungal agents have been designed to exploit this difference in sterol content, including the polyenes, azoles, and allylamines. **Polyene antifungals** bind with the sterols in the fungal cell wall, making it permeable. This allows the cellular contents to spill out and ultimately results in the elimination of the cell. The cholesterol found in animal cells is less susceptible to this process, leaving these cells structurally undisturbed. Two kinds of polyene antifungals are nystatin and amphotericin B.

AZOLE ANTIFUNGAL AGENTS

Imidazole and triazole are **azole antifungal drugs** that work by blocking or obstructing an enzyme essential to ergosterol synthesis in the fungal cell wall. Enzymes are complex proteins that act as catalysts to encourage biochemical reactions. The enzyme is not changed chemically through this process, and thus it remains effective throughout the biochemical intervention and available for continued bioactivity. The azole antifungal agents target a lanosterol demethylase enzyme necessary to convert or change lanosterol to ergosterol. In this way fungi are unable to obtain and maintain sufficient ergosterol to sustain cell wall integrity.

By blocking certain kinds of sterol syntheses in the cell, imidazole and triazole cause a depletion of normal sterols and an abnormal accumulation of sterol precursors, resulting in fungal cell toxicity and death. Triazole antifungal drugs are not as toxic or as poisonous as many other drugs used for a similar purpose. Further, the triazoles often produce a more positive result than the imidazoles, thus they may be among the more preferred antifungal drugs available. Two examples of triazoles are fluconazole and itraconazole. Two examples of imidazoles are miconazole and ketoconazole.

VACCINES

Vaccines are biological preparations designed to engage a patient's protective immune response through antibody production in order to prevent disease or lessen disease severity. Successful vaccination or inoculation requires the administration of a subclinical (small, insufficient to cause clinical infection) amount of the target viral matter or **inoculant** to the patient. The inoculation can take the form of an oral dose, an injection, or an inhalation. Injected vaccines can take a few weeks to provide protective immunity. Vaccines given nasally may take only a few days to become effective, but nasally administered vaccines tend to produce fewer antibodies.

Vaccines are an important component of public health as they prevent disease transmission between animals and protect against **zoonotic** disease spread between animals and people.

TYPES OF VACCINES

Vaccines can be classified by the different forms of viral matter they use to induce an immune response. These include:

- **Live vaccines** (also known as modified-live or attenuated vaccines) induce a strong immune response and offer the most protection. They must be stored and handled strictly according to label instructions.
- **Killed vaccines** (or inactivated vaccines) are composed of the killed pathogen and produce a lesser immune response. Initial vaccination usually requires 2 doses, followed by annual revaccination. Killed vaccines are more stable and easier to store and handle.
- **Recombinant vaccines** (or DNA vaccines) consist of certain non-disease-causing components normally produced by the pathogen. The protein gene is removed from the pathogen, transmitted to a different organism, and grown in a laboratory. These proteins are then concentrated into a vaccine. Antibodies created to recognize the proteins by the immune system will also recognize them as a part of the pathogen if it invades the animal. Recombinant vector vaccines are obtained by administering genetically altered organisms from a laboratory through the vaccine to the animal.
- **Toxoid vaccines** are made from attenuated toxins that induce a short-lived humoral immune response.

VACCINE EFFICACY

If a vaccination is effective, it will cause **antibodies** to be produced that recognize the inoculant **antigens**, which are large protein molecules found on the outer surface of disease-causing pathogens. The antigens are responsible for the body's creation of antibodies to fight off the disease. The body's immune system identifies the foreign antigens when an exposure has occurred. With a vaccine, the first exposure occurs at the time of inoculation. The body then synthesizes the proper antibodies to fight the specific antigens encountered.

Later, subsequent contacts with the disease allow the body to fight off the microorganisms with a larger, existing collection of antigen-specific antibodies. The degree of vaccination success and duration of antibody persistence will depend upon certain conditions, including the animal's age, breed, and health; the strength of the animal's immune system; the method of storage of the vaccine; and the inoculation method and type chosen by the veterinarian.

ANAPHYLACTIC REACTION TO VACCINES

Anaphylactic reactions are severe allergic reactions sometimes seen after a vaccination. Anaphylactic reactions can occur after the first vaccine the patient gets or the third—it is impossible to predict—but if the patient has had a previous reaction, they can be given an antihistamine injection prior to the vaccine to prevent a reaction in the future. Anaphylactic reactions normally happen less than 24 hours from vaccination and cause itching, weakness, apnea, sudden onset of diarrhea and vomiting, facial swelling, pale gums, and seizures. If this type of reaction is not treated immediately, it can lead to respiratory failure, heart failure, and shock. Treatment for anaphylaxis includes administration of epinephrine (adrenaline), antihistamines, oxygen therapy, and intravenous (IV) fluids if necessary.

CARDIOVASCULAR DRUGS

There are a multitude of drugs which can be used to effectively treat various symptoms and conditions involving the heart.

Antiarrhythmic drugs can be useful in the restoration of normal electrical activity in the heart. Lidocaine and procainamide are **sodium channel blockers**, as they restrain or limit the flow of the electrolyte sodium (Na^+). Propranolol hydrochloride is a negative inotrope. It can obstruct beta-adrenergic receptors, which might otherwise reduce myocardial contractility.

Myocardial contractility refers to the "pumping" movement of the thick muscular wall of the heart. **Calcium channel blockers** are antiarrhythmics and include verapamil and diltiazem. Antiarrhythmics such as these slow the conduction or transmission of electrical activity in the heart, thereby allowing cardiac functions to more readily normalize.

Finally, **positive inotropes** and **catecholamines** are drugs which are used to make the contractions of the heart stronger. One example of a positive inotrope is digoxin. Digoxin can increase the quantity of calcium accessible to the heart.

Anticoagulants and Thrombolytics

Anticoagulants are given to stop the formation of blood clots. **Thrombolytics** can break up and dissolve blood clots. Blood clots are formed from the process of coagulation by the protein **thrombin**. Thrombin is a blood enzyme which is responsible for increasing the conversion rate of fibrinogen to fibrin. **Fibrin** is a protein which induces the blood to clot. **Antithrombin** is a protein molecule that inactivates several enzymes in the body's coagulation system, including the enzyme thrombin. Thrombin is also stopped by the use of a medication called **heparin** and its various derivatives. However, while heparin inhibits clot formation, it does not actively break up existing clots. Thrombolytics such as t-PA (alteplase Activase), streptokinase (Kabikinase, Streptase), and urokinase (Abbokinase) serve this purpose. Thrombolytics work to activate the production of plasmin. Plasmin is an enzyme which works to separate and disintegrate the strands of fibrin within a blood clot.

Thromboembolism

Patients suffering with thromboembolism may have one or more blood clots in the pulmonary vasculature—the blood vessels involving the lungs. The situation becomes life-threatening if the blood clots totally obstruct the flow of blood in the pulmonary vessels.

The drugs used in the treatment of this disease are **anticoagulants** and **thrombolytics**. However, research indicates that thrombolytics are not fully effective in treating this disease in veterinary patients. Anticoagulants, rather than thrombolytics, are more effective in veterinary patients with thromboembolism. Anticoagulants can be administered to the patient by injection with a syringe. They also work to stop the formation of clots in the blood samples drawn for use in medical tests. Uncoagulated whole blood is often necessary to obtain accurate results in laboratory tests.

Erythropoietin for Treating Anemia

Chemotherapeutics can induce bone marrow suppression, reducing red blood cell production and creating an anemic condition. **Anemia** (low hemoglobin) can also be caused by other conditions. To remedy anemia, patients may be given blood-building products called **hematics** (or hematinics). Three types of hematics include erythropoietin, androgens, and blood substitutes. Patients that take hematics will experience an increase in the oxygen carrying capacity of the blood, as available hemoglobin increases.

Hemoglobin is an oxygen-carrying iron complex required for red blood cells to function properly. The patient that exhibits symptoms of anemia should be given a blood test to determine the volume of hemoglobin that is present (typically measured in grams per deciliter of blood). Patients with anemia will have lower volumes of hemoglobin. Erythropoietin (also called hematopoietin or hemopoietin) is a hormone that regulates the production of red blood cells. Both the kidney and the liver—the latter to a lesser degree—produce this hormone in response to low blood levels. Where hemoglobin levels have fallen precipitously, the patient can be given a synthetic version in the form of an injection to boost red blood cell production and related hemoglobin availability.

Androgens and Blood Substitutes for Treating Anemia

The hormone erythropoietin stimulates the production of red blood cells in the bone marrow. However, if the body does not produce sufficient erythropoietin, red blood cell production will also fall and cause anemia. While the liver does produce erythropoietin, about four-fifths of all erythropoietin is produced by the kidneys. Patients suffering from chronic anemia can be given androgens or anabolic steroids to stimulate the kidney's production of erythropoietin. However, the administration and secondary effects of androgens can be problematic. Therefore, this is not the drug of choice in the care of most patients with anemia.

A useful blood substitute that may be given to patients suffering from anemia is known as Oxyglobin. Oxyglobin is derived from chemically stabilized bovine hemoglobin. This substance gives short-term relief to the patient. Oxyglobin is able to raise and sustain higher oxygen levels in the blood. However, Oxyglobin is only intended for use with animals.

Colloid Solutions

Colloid solutions have large molecules and only compose the plasma compartment of the body. Natural colloids include whole blood and plasma that can be used in patients who are anemic. Synthetic colloids include hetastarch, pentastarch, and dextran. Hetastarch aids in retaining fluids in the intravascular compartment. Patients in shock experience a metabolic disturbance caused by the circulatory system failing to provide adequate perfusion to the body's vital organs. Colloids are used to restore the body's organ perfusion, and colloid solutions are also used in patients with pulmonary contusions and head trauma. A major benefit of colloid use is that resuscitation is achieved at a lower rate than that of crystalloids because colloids stay in the vascular space for a longer time frame than do crystalloids.

Crystalloid Solutions

Crystalloid solutions are fluids that hold electrolyte and nonelectrolyte solutes that move freely around vascular spaces. Crystalloid solutions come in three forms: isotonic, hypertonic, and hypotonic. Isotonic solutions are balanced electrolyte solutions that are equal to the osmolality of the red blood cells (RBCs) and plasma of the patient. Isotonic solutions such as lactated Ringer's, Normosol-R, and Plasma-Lyte are used to support perfusion and volume replacement. Hypertonic solutions have a higher osmolality than the RBCs and plasma, causing fluids to be drawn from the intracellular space into the intravascular space making these solutions useful for those patients who need large amounts of fluids quickly. Hypotonic solutions such as 5% dextrose in water and 0.45% sodium chloride have lower osmolality than the intravascular fluid and draw the fluids into the cells; they are primarily used to correct electrolyte imbalances.

Blood Products

Fresh whole blood is given when an animal exhibits one or more of the following: hemorrhagic shock, anemia, excessive surgical hemorrhage, clotting disorders, non-immune-mediated hemolytic anemia, and sometimes immune-mediated hemolytic anemia.

Crystalloid (an isotonic or hypertonic fluid, such as Lactated Ringer's solution, used as a blood volume expander) is given in combination with packed red blood cells (RBCs) when it becomes necessary to maintain the animal's fluid balance and osmotic pressure. Packed RBCs can be given to the animal that has suffered from hemolytic and nonregenerative anemias. RBCs may be maintained in an "extender" solution such as ADSOL (adenine, glucose, mannitol, and sodium chloride). Packed RBCs stored in ADSOL will naturally have a greater total volume than packed RBCs stored alone. Further, the unit volume of RBCs packed in other preservatives (e.g., Optisol, Nutricel) may vary from that of ADSOL. However, the cell count per unit should be the same regardless of the solution used. When mixing packed RBCs with ADSOL, add the solution to the cells rather than the cells to the solution. This reduces the degree of hemolysis during and after mixing. The shock and burn patient can benefit from a plasma transfusion. This type of transfusion will supply volume replacement when tissue-based fluids are lost in the absence of skin.

Nervous System Drugs

Drugs that impact the nervous system include controlled drugs, including anesthetics, analgesics, tranquilizers and sedatives, anticonvulsants, stimulants, and other psychoactive medications.

Anesthetics

Fully anesthetized animals cannot sense pain, temperature, or pressure. **General anesthesia** serves to bring a patient into a coma-like state of deep unconsciousness, sufficient to produce a loss of all sensation. General anesthetics are administered to the patient as inhalants or injectables. Death can occur if an overdose of some general anesthetics occurs. Local anesthesia merely deprives a patient of sensation in a limited area, and the animal doesn't lose consciousness. Both general and local anesthesia are reversible.

Barbiturates are injectable anesthetics; pentobarbital is a short-acting barbiturate and phenobarbital is a long-acting barbiturate.

Propofol

Propofol is an anesthetic that provides smooth, rapid induction and recovery from anesthesia. Propofol is given intravenously as a hypnotic agent used for sedation in ventilated patients, as well as induction and maintenance of anesthesia (up to 20 minutes). Propofol should be titrated (given to effect) for up to 1 minute or until the patient exhibits signs of onset of anesthesia. Rapid IV injection of propofol can cause apnea, hypotension, and oxygen desaturation. Maintenance of anesthesia with propofol may be used for shorter procedures (20 minutes) or as a transition to inhalant anesthetic. Propofol decreases cardiac output and causes vasodilation and should be used with caution in patients with hypotension (low blood pressure), hypovolemia (a condition in which the blood plasma is too low), or cardiovascular insufficiencies. Propofol is metabolized in the liver and excreted through the urine. Propofol provides a rapid recovery in which the patient is standing in fewer than 20 minutes; however, certain premedications may prolong this recovery.

Dissociative Anesthetics

Dissociative anesthetics are *N*-methyl-D-aspartate (NMDA) antagonists. They work by dissociating the thalamocortical and limbic systems, which produces altered consciousness. They also produce amnesia and provide analgesia. By working as NMDA antagonists, they block the excitatory pathway but don't produce sleepiness, so patients that are anesthetized with dissociative agents (ketamine) don't appear sleepy and often have their eyes open and have increased muscle tone. However, that does not mean that they are not adequately anesthetized. Ketamine provides analgesia by preventing wind-up pain in the dorsal horn of the spinal cord. Ketamine causes increased cranial pressure as well as cerebral oxygen demands, increases cerebral blood flow, lowers the seizure threshold, and increases intraocular pressures. Along with this, ketamine increases sympathetic (fight-or-flight) tone resulting in an increased heart rate and high blood pressure. Ketamine can also cause respiratory depression and cause apneustic breathing (fast breaths followed by holding breaths on inspiration).

Preanesthetic Drug Protocol for an Emergency C-Section

Careful assessment of **preanesthetic drugs** to be used for a C-section (hysterotomy) is important. They should not be able to cross the placental barrier and should be short-acting and metabolized rapidly. Certain drugs that do cross the placental barrier like ketamine, barbiturates, and atropine affect the survival of the offspring and should not be used. Anesthetic protocol should include drugs that aren't metabolized by the liver or excreted by the kidneys because these organs are deficient in the offspring as well. The patient should be preoxygenated prior to surgery, and the procedure should be done as efficiently as possible to move on to resuscitation of the offspring.

Analgesics

Analgesics reduce the perception of pain without much impact on the other sensations.

Opioid or **narcotic analgesics**, **corticosteroids**, and **nonsteroidal anti-inflammatory drugs** are all analgesic and/or anti-inflammatory drugs.

Nonsteroidal anti-inflammatory drugs (NSAIDs) commonly include phenylbutazone, aspirin, ibuprofen, etodolac, and carprofen. Nearly all NSAIDs work to block the prostaglandin production that results from the inflammatory process. However, NSAIDs are not useful in counteracting visceral (organ) pain or the pain associated with broken bones, as they do not produce sufficient analgesic effects.

By contrast, **opioid analgesics** can entirely block all awareness of neural pain impulses and can control more intense pain symptoms, such as those related to visceral pain or broken bones. Morphine, meperidine, oxymorphone, butorphanol, and codeine are all types of opioids.

Many perianesthetics are also **opioids** that work as both analgesics and sedatives. Many sedatives can also be effective as tranquilizers.

Corticosteroids are anti-inflammatory drugs which can also relieve pain. However, it is important to use caution with these drugs, as they can have negative effects on the endocrine and immune systems. The most widely used corticosteroids are dexamethasone and prednisone.

Opioids

Opioids are analgesics (painkillers). Opioids act on the CNS to relieve pain and may produce side effects including mood changes, excitement, and sedation. There are two classes of opioids: pure-mu agonists such as morphine, hydromorphone, fentanyl, and meperidine and partial-mu agonists such as buprenorphine. Pure-mu agonists will provide a more effective analgesia, but they can also cause side effects such as vomiting, respiratory depression, and sedation. Partial-mu agonists, however, bind with the less effective analgesic receptor (k receptor). Butorphanol is neither a pure- nor partial-mu agonist, but rather a mu antagonist that reverses the effects of the pure-mu opioids, leaving the patient with weaker analgesic effects. Butorphanol has a short duration of action and does not provide adequate analgesia for more painful procedures.

Simbadol

Simbadol is an **opioid agonist** and is a controlled substance under Schedule III. Simbadol is a high-concentration buprenorphine (not sustained release) that can be used in cats and has a 24-hour duration of action. Simbadol is routinely administered SQ, but when given IM, its duration of action is reduced to 6 hours. Simbadol is indicated for postoperative pain in cats and is dosed at 0.24 mg/kg. Simbadol should be used with caution in cats with liver disease because it is metabolized through the liver, but it is not excreted in the urine. Simbadol can be administered once daily for up to 3 days for pain control.

NSAIDs

Nonsteroidal anti-inflammatory drugs (NSAIDs) are used to control pain and inflammation as well as reduce swelling. They do this by blocking the production of prostaglandin molecules that promote pain and also provide analgesia by reducing inflammation that triggers the pain sensation. They also provide antipyretic (fever-reducing) effects. NSAIDs are commonly used for postoperative pain control in small-animal practice. They are also used long term in certain patients with osteoarthritis. If used long term, baseline and annual blood work are ideal to use for checking kidney and liver function. Side effects of NSAID use include kidney and liver toxicity, gastrointestinal (GI) ulcers, and possible stomach bleeding. More common side effects include vomiting, diarrhea, loss of appetite, and lethargy.

Sedatives and Tranquilizers

Tranquilizers and **sedatives** are usually applied when patients are highly agitated, need assistance in easing some anxiety, or need an aid to induce sleep. Benzodiazepines and phenothiazines are examples of tranquilizers and sedatives (phenothiazines are commonly used as antipsychotics, as well). Specific examples include acepromazine, diazepam, medetomidine, midazolam, and xylazine.

It should be noted that acepromazine is not advisable for use with animals that have recently been treated for fleas using any organophosphate-based pesticide. While organophosphates are useful to kill fleas, any residual phosphate compounds coupled with acepromazine can cause negative side effects, including hypotension (low blood pressure).

Diazepam (Valium) is considered a "classical" benzodiazepine; it was the second benzodiazepine derivative developed. Others include clonazepam, lorazepam, oxazepam, alprazolam, nitrazepam, flurazepam, bromazepam, and clorazepate. Diazepam is both an anxiolytic and a sedative. An anxiolytic is a drug that relieves anxiety, while a sedative induces rest and sleep. However, diazepam can also be used as a muscle relaxant, appetite stimulant, sleep aid, and anticonvulsant. Because it can be used to address such a broad array of conditions, it has become one of the most widely used medications in the world.

Medetomidine, Midazolam, and Xylazine

Medetomidine is an alpha-2 agonist. It is manufactured under the trade name Domitor. This drug has a short elimination half-life. Medetomidine is a highly potent anxiolytic, hypnotic, anticonvulsant, muscle relaxant, sedative, and analgesic. However, medetomidine can also produce serious side effects under certain conditions, including bradycardia, hypothermia, decreased respiration, urination, occasional AV blocks, and vomiting with the accompanying potential for aspiration pneumonia. Thus, this medication should be administered cautiously, particularly to very young or very old dogs. The more significant side effects to medetomidine should be treated through pharmacological reversal of the drug.

The drug **midazolam** is manufactured under the trade names Dormicum, Flormidal, Versed, Hypnovel, and Dormonid. Midazolam can be substituted for diazepam when it is advantageous to do so.

The drug **xylazine** is manufactured under the trade names Rompun and Anased. Xylazine can be used as an analgesic. It is also useful for muscle relaxation, anesthesia, and sedation. The more serious side effects of xylazine include: bradycardia, cardiac conduction disturbances, myocardial depression, and vomiting. The reversal drug for xylazine, yohimbine, may be used when severe side effects persist.

Benzodiazepines

Benzodiazepines act as sedatives through depression of the limbic system, the thalamus, and the hypothalamus. Benzodiazepines also have muscle-relaxing effects caused by the inhibition of the neurons on the spinal cord. Benzodiazepines such as diazepam are anticonvulsants as well as anxiolytic (antianxiety) drugs (alprazolam) that are primarily metabolized through the liver and excreted through urine and should be used with caution in patients with kidney or liver disease. Benzodiazepines are absorbed quickly and completely. Some patients may experience central nervous system (CNS) depression, ataxia, weakness, disorientation, nausea, and vomiting; other patients may exhibit CNS excitation followed shortly by CNS depression.

Alpha 2 Agonists

Alpha 2 agonists, such as dexmedetomidine, xylazine, and medetomidine are sedatives that also provide analgesia and muscle relaxation. The α_2-agonists should be used with caution because they can have cardiovascular side effects such as bradycardia (slow heart rate), hypertension (high blood pressure), and a reduced cardiac output. They should not be used in patients with cardiovascular disease, liver disease, or kidney disease. The α_2-agonists such as dexmedetomidine can be used as a premedication for general anesthesia, greatly decreasing the amount of induction agent and inhalant needed to maintain the patient. Fortunately, dexmedetomidine can be reversed with atipamezole, which is the appropriate way to treat for bradycardia rather than using an anticholinergic, such as atropine, because it can cause the heart to work harder than it already is.

Anticonvulsants

Anticonvulsants are used for controlling seizures, both preventatively and when in progress. Two types of oral medications commonly given to seizure-prone animals in the home or field setting are phenobarbital and potassium bromide.

Benzodiazepines are tranquilizers that can also be used to control seizures. Phenobarbital is given to cats and dogs for long-term seizure control; it is administered orally and can be given by owners at home. Potassium bromide and sodium bromide can be used to control canine seizures when phenobarbital alone isn't effective.

Domitor

Domitor (medetomidine hydrochloride) is a sedative used to facilitate the handling of animals during clinical examinations or when undergoing difficult or uncomfortable medical procedures. For example, an animal that has come into contact with a porcupine may need to have the quills removed and can be given Domitor as a calming sedative. However, the animal must not need a drug that produces muscle relaxation such as that required for respiratory intubation. At the conclusion of the procedure, the animal can be given atipamezole to reverse the effects of the Domitor.

Atipamezole

Atipamezole is given to the patient by intramuscular injection. Atipamezole is fast-acting, so the patient should recover from the effects of the sedative within 5-10 minutes. Some animals may experience transient behavioral problems, such as a readiness to attack or extreme nervousness, so due caution should be exercised. The animal should be placed in a quiet and darkened recovery area that is not otherwise utilized while the animal is regaining consciousness and the effects of the sedative are wearing off.

In addition, the animal should be monitored for other side effects, in particular, the animal's blood pressure should be checked as the drug tends to induce hypotension. In some cases, the animal's heart and respiratory rates may rise. The patient should also be monitored for nausea and vomiting. Finally, the patient may also experience symptoms of diarrhea, hypersalivation, shivering or tremors, overstimulation, and nervousness.

Pregnant or nursing animals should not be given the drug, as the fetal and developmental effects are unknown.

Stimulants and Antidepressants

The breathing center of the brain is stimulated via neural, chemical, and hormonal signals that control the respiratory rate, tidal volume, etc. This center can also be stimulated by intravenous administration of stimulants, such as doxapram hydrochloride. Some patients may require this treatment for respiratory problems, particularly those that have been brought about by medication overdoses, lung diseases, or from the postoperative effects of general anesthesia.

Toxicity is the threshold at which a drug begins to cause untoward effects or outright physiological damage, coupled with how quickly that damage escalates with increasing levels of the drug. Virtually all stimulants can become toxic in animals as dosages are increased. Examples of stimulants that may readily cause this effect include caffeine, amphetamines, and theobromine.

Antidepressants are used to reduce symptoms of depression. Antidepressants may also be applied in the treatment of separation anxiety or canine cognitive dysfunction. Clomipramine, also known as Clomicalm, is an antidepressant often used for separation anxiety, a condition in which the patient experiences a high degree of anxiety or stress when separated from a primary caregiver or companion. Selegiline, also known as Anipryl, is an antidepressant used for canine cognitive dysfunction.

Drugs That Affect the Autonomic Nervous System

The **autonomic** (i.e., unconscious, self-regulating) **nervous system** is divided into sympathetic and parasympathetic. The **sympathetic system** (fight-or-flight) manages rapid-demand changes, while the **parasympathetic system** (rest-and-digest) modulates and complements those responses, seeking balance over time. The enteric system regulates autonomic digestive system processes.

Autonomic changes can be caused by cholinergic and adrenergic agents. In general, adrenergic agents stimulate sympathetic processes (principally by releasing epinephrine and norepinephrine), while cholinergic agents engage parasympathetic processes (principally by producing, altering, releasing, or mimicking acetylcholine). Both of these agents can be circumvented by adrenergic blockers and anticholinergics.

For example, the cholinergic drug pilocarpine reduces intraocular pressure, while metoclopramide stimulates the gastrointestinal system, and Urecholine quickens the urinary system.

Anticholinergics

Anticholinergics include aminopentamide, atropine sulfate, and glycopyrrolate. Aminopentamide has the ability to slow down gastrointestinal motility (movement). Atropine sulfate and glycopyrrolate can cause the pupils to dilate and the heart rate to increase, as well as secretions to dry up. Anticholinergics normally produce adverse effects if administered in the wrong dosage.

Anticholinergic medications may be used to block nerve impulses from reaching the vagus nerve. Examples of anticholinergics include atropine and glycopyrrolate. Pharmacologically blocking this nerve with a vagolytic medication is necessary when the veterinarian is treating bradycardia in a patient. Anticholinergics and opioids can be used in conjunction with each other.

The synergistic effects of these drugs can produce lower levels of salivary and tear secretions. Anticholinergics can also diminish bronchodilation. Contraindications associated with anticholinergics include administration to patients at high risk for tachycardia (often geriatric patients), those with a history of congestive heart failure, and patients with constipation or ileus.

Gastrointestinal Drugs

Emetics

Emetics are drugs which are used to induce vomiting. Typical applications include emptying stomach contents of contaminated foods or poisonous substances. Upon ingestion of the drug, the animal vomits up the contents of its stomach. These drugs should not be used in situations where regurgitation can cause further damage (i.e., where the substance may be better neutralized by other treatments). Generally, the contents of the stomach can be safely regurgitated when a noncorrosive toxin has been swallowed by the patient. The noncorrosive toxin must be eliminated from the patient's stomach as soon as possible. The administered emetic will produce the desired results quickly.

Emetics are also beneficial prior to anesthesia in cases where the patient has ingested food shortly before surgery, creating a risk of anesthesia-induced emesis and pulmonary aspiration. Emetics work by irritating the gastric mucosa, which then stimulates the central nervous system and causes vomiting to occur. Examples of emetic drugs are apomorphine and hydrogen peroxide.

Antiemetics

Antiemetics are beneficial in the treatment of burdensome nausea symptoms. Antiemetics are employed to stop or reduce patient vomiting. The selection of the antiemetic will be made after due consideration of the causes contributing to the vomiting. Some patients vomit as a result of motion sickness (often induced by automobile or boat travel). Patients with motion sickness have been known to respond favorably to chlorpromazine, diphenhydramine, and dimenhydrinate. Patients who suffer from gastrointestinal spasms may respond well to metoclopramide or aminopentamide. These medications may also help improve peristaltic movement in the gastrointestinal system.

Antidiarrheals

The patient with watery, diarrheal bowel movements may benefit from **antidiarrheal** drugs. However, the veterinarian should investigate the underlying cause of the diarrhea before administering an antidiarrheal drug. For example, hypersecretions (diarrhea) may be caused when bacteria emit poisons that induce fluid retention in the bowel and accelerate the excretory process. Common treatments for diarrhea include loperamide and diphenoxylate. Other diarrhea medications include aminopentamide and various antispasmodics. Some diarrhea treatments like bismuth, kaolin, pectin, and activated charcoal do not require a prescription.

Bulk Laxatives

Constipation is a condition in which the intestinal tract is blocked or obstructed with an accumulation of hardened and somewhat dehydrated fecal matter. This condition can often be alleviated with the administration of a laxative. **Laxatives** soften the stool, and thereby ease the constipating symptoms.

Bulk laxatives use insoluble, water-absorbing fiber that can often relieve constipation. Undigested fiber is transported via the GI tract where peristalsis (fecal-moving muscle contractions) pushes along the swollen, fibrous bulk that has taken on water. However, bulk-producing laxatives are unable to work without the addition of water and other liquids into the body. Thus, the patient must be encouraged to take adequate fluids to ensure the laxative works correctly and to avoid otherwise dehydrating the bowel and its contents further.

Emollient Laxatives

Emollient laxatives (stool softeners) contain a surfactant such as docusate that helps to "wet" and soften the stool. Emollient laxatives may take a week or longer to be effective. Even so, they are used frequently by postoperative patients, especially after surgical anal sac removal. They include lubricants such as mineral oil, white petrolatum, glycerin, and cod liver oil. These lubricants work to ease the friction between the stool and the intestinal tract. The involved surfaces become coated in a waterproof covering of indigestible grease or oil. This coating not only fills the entire GI tract, but covers and mixes with the feces as well. Water consumption is maintained to keep the stool soft. The lubricant and water are beneficial in producing fecal matter that is softer and more easily expelled.

Cathartics

Saline (or **osmotic**) **cathartics** osmotically induce the movement of water into the small intestines, and thereby swiftly drain the lower intestines of its contents.

Hyperosmotic cathartics such as magnesium salts and certain kinds of disaccharides are able to draw water from the surrounding tissues, thereby softening the feces. Some disaccharides are irregular sugars which cannot be digested by mammals. One example is lactulose, which remains undigested throughout the gastrointestinal tract. Inside the large intestine, lactulose attracts bacteria which produce acids and thereby bring water into the bowel. The resulting hydration can relieve the dry hardness of the feces and aid in their expulsion.

Irritant cathartics include castor oil and bisacodyl; they irritate the bowel, increasing peristalsis. Contraindications include suspected obstructed bowel and tenesmus.

Ulcers

Ulcers are sores which are found on the membranous lining of the digestive system. There are drugs, known as antiulcer drugs, which can reduce the formation of these sores. Antiulcer drugs are listed under 4 classifications: antacids, H_2-receptor blockers, proton pump inhibitors, and cytoprotective agents.

The stomach contains gastric parietal cells which produce stomach acid. Parietal cells interact with the proton pump or the ATPase pump, which is responsible for the release of histamine. Histamine is the most important positive regulator of the secretion of gastric acid in the stomach. If histamine is not released, then the proton pump cannot produce acid as readily. When stomach acid levels fall, ulcer healing can more readily take place.

Antacids

Antacids reduce acidity in the stomach; high levels of acidity may overwhelm the protective mechanisms of the stomach lining, causing discomfort (i.e., "heartburn" or pyrosis). Most antacids are designed to produce a chemical buffer which results in a rise in overall gastric pH measurements. Following treatment with a non-systemic **buffering antacid**, any stomach contents that reflux up into the esophagus will no longer cause the painful, burning symptoms characteristic of acidic fluid exposure.

Common non-systemic antacids contain calcium, magnesium, or aluminum (Tums, Rolaids, Maalox, milk of magnesia, and Amphojel).

H2 Blockers

Histamine H_2-receptor antagonist antacids reduce the amount of gastric acid produced. As histamine is the most important positive regulator of gastric acid production, blocking histamine receptors interrupts the production cycle. The H_2-receptor is a cell that can be motivated to create histamines in the stomach responsible for gastric secretions. Drugs which block the H_2-receptor thus stop some of the production of gastric acid.

Common H_2-receptor antagonists include cimetidine, ranitidine, and famotidine (with trade names of Tagamet, Zantac, and Pepcid, respectively). However, there are other receptors which can also produce acid in the stomach which are not effectively held in check by the H_2-receptor–blocking drugs. Thus, other adjunctive treatments and management approaches may be necessary.

Proton Pump Inhibitors (PPI)

Animals who don't respond to traditional antacids and acid blockers may require acid control treatment with a **proton pump inhibitor (PPI)**. The gastric hydrogen/potassium ATPase enzyme is often called the "proton pumps" (acidification) system of the stomach. PPIs denature the ATPase enzyme and allow it to be digested, stopping acid production by up to 99%.

The quantity of acid can be measured in proportion to the number of protons found in the stomach. The acid is reduced as the relative amount of proton pumps are prevented from secreting acids in the stomach. The proton pump inhibition systems, such as omeprazole, are considered to be powerful antacids.

Other Antiulcer Drugs

Another type of antiulcer drug is sucralfate or Carafate. This drug creates a protective lining along the surface where the ulcer has formed. Similarly, misoprostol (Cytotec) also forms a protective coating by increasing the production of mucus in the lining of the gastrointestinal tract.

However, the absorption of some medications may be impaired by antacids. Thus, absorption factors as related to gastric acidity should be considered when treating a patient—particularly one who has been given proton pump inhibitors—as the reason for impaired absorption may be the stomach's newly raised gastric pH levels.

Endocrine Drugs

The **endocrine system** regulates, controls, and adjusts the provision of chemical energy, enzymatic catalysts, and nutrients as needed for a healthy metabolism. Thus, endocrine disorders can be quite complex and damaging.

Hyperthyroidism

The thyroid is part of the endocrine (glandular) system. An overactive thyroid produces an overabundance of the hormones thyroxin (T4) and triiodothyronine (T3), diagnosed as **hyperthyroidism**. This condition is rarely diagnosed in canines and is more commonly found in felines.

Upon further inspection, the cat will usually be secondarily diagnosed with a thyroid tumor. The tumor is typically comprised of thyroid cells, thus accounting for the increased production of thyroid hormones. Felines diagnosed with hyperthyroidism can range from 4–22 years of age. Some cats suffering from hyperthyroidism may experience weight loss, while others may have an increased appetite. The condition can be exacerbated by a heart murmur or elevated heart rate. The cat may also exhibit marked thirst and an excessive need to urinate.

TREATING HYPERTHYROIDISM

Hyperthyroidism can be detected through a simple blood test. In most cases the veterinarian will surgically remove the diseased thyroid—often referred to as **surgical ablation** (i.e., removal or reduction) of the thyroid. However, this surgery does come with significant risks to the parathyroid gland. The parathyroid gland is responsible for producing hormones that regulate calcium and phosphorus in the body's skeletal system. The removal of the entire thyroid will precipitously cause hypothyroidism, and even partial ablation often produces a change from hyperthyroidism to hypothyroidism. In cases of hypothyroidism the animal will require thyroid supplements to regulate the body's metabolism. Periodic blood tests will be necessary to determine how much of the supplement needs to be administered to the animal. Alternatives to surgical ablation include radioactive and chemical ablation.

ANTITHYROID AGENTS AND RADIOACTIVE IODINE TREATMENT

There are alternative treatments for hyperthyroidism that are not surgical in nature, including radioactive iodine treatment and antithyroid agents such as methimazole, marketed as Tapazole.

Tapazole is beneficial in obstructing enzymatic processes in the thyroid necessary for the production of triiodothyronine (T3) and thyroxin (T4). The animal should be monitored for side effects following this treatment, as it may induce vomiting, malaise, and fatigue.

Radioactive iodine treatments make use of the thyroid's natural demand for iodine. The thyroid is the only organ in the body that requires iodine to work properly. The thyroid absorbs radioactive iodine the same way that it absorbs normal iodine. Hyperplastic tissue tends to utilize greater quantities of iodine than normal thyroid tissue. Thus, this abnormal tissue is exposed to greater levels of radiation from the radioactive iodine. The radiation works to destroy the tumor and/or reduce the numbers of hormone-producing cells. This treatment usually does not harm the majority of normal cells found in the thyroid.

HYPOTHYROIDISM

Hypothyroidism may cause a myriad of other conditions and symptoms. For example, excessive weight gain may create secondary problems. Not only can the animal's joints and cardiac and respiratory status be compromised, but when muscle and other tissues atrophy and waste away, accumulating fat may infiltrate where the tissues have become structurally diminished. Further, because normal thyroid hormone levels are necessary for healthy hair and nails, an animal's fur may thin and appear dull and lackluster, and the nails and the skin may become cracked and flaky. The animal may also exhibit marked alopecia—a condition in which its hair falls out. The animal's skin may exhibit hyperpigmentation.

The animal may also suffer from anemia and/or high blood cholesterol. Anemia is a blood disorder characterized by hemoglobin deficiency and reduced numbers of red blood cells. This may lead to fatigue. Additional symptoms include constipation, poor blood clotting, susceptibility to infections, depression, mental dullness, cold intolerance, and mild bradycardia.

The animals most commonly affected by hypothyroidism are dogs ranging in age from 4-10 years. The dogs are more typically medium or large in size. Smaller dogs do not develop hypothyroidism as often as larger-sized dogs.

TREATING HYPOTHYROIDISM

Hypothyroidism can sometimes be the result of a hypothalamus or a pituitary gland dysfunction. The hypothalamus releases a hormone called **thyrotropin releasing hormone** (TRH), which stimulates the pituitary to release a hormone called **thyroid stimulating hormone** (TSH). TSH in turn stimulates the thyroid to produce its metabolic regulatory hormones, triiodothyronine (T3) and thyroxin (T4). A breakdown at any point in this system of endocrine relays will result in hypothyroidism. Thus, the production and release of TRH and TSH is critical in the regulation of thyroid hormones required for a healthy metabolism.

In the event that the thyroid's production levels of T3 and T4 are diminished—whether due to hypothalamus or pituitary dysfunction, or due to dysfunction of the thyroid gland itself—the patient's condition will be diagnosed as hypothyroidism. Hypothyroidism can be detected through simple blood tests. The blood tests are analyzed based on measurements of T3, T4, and TSH. The veterinarian will use this data to determine the medications that the patient needs. The patient may be given supplemental thyroid hormones, as T3 and T4 can be produced synthetically.

Supplemental Medications for Hypothyroidism

Hypothyroidism causes a slowing of the animal's metabolic rate due to a decrease in thyroid hormone production. Resolution of persistent hypothyroidism requires the administration of supplemental thyroid hormones. Natural thyroid hormones are available from desiccated porcine (pig) thyroids. However, obtaining accurate standardized dosages may be problematic. Synthetic T3 and T4 are both available, but the veterinarian will normally select T4 to be administered due to the complications involving T3 supplementation. T3's dosage is often difficult to regulate, and overmedicating the patient is an ongoing challenge.

T4 supplementation alone may be sufficient, as the thyroid is able to transform some T4 into T3. However, this is not always the case with a malfunctioning thyroid, and thus combined synthetic T3/T4 supplementation may sometimes be required. The animal's hormone levels and reaction to the drugs should be monitored to ensure proper dosage and medication management over time. Periodic blood tests will be beneficial in determining how much of the drug needs to be administered at optimum intervals. Careful ongoing monitoring of the patient's blood levels should produce the data needed to successfully regulate the animal's metabolic functioning.

Reproductive Drugs

Estrogens are steroid hormones that promote female characteristics in the body.

The synthetic estrogen diethylstilbestrol (DES) is used to prevent pregnancy when breeding of the animal was not planned by causing the fertilized egg to be reabsorbed. Potential negative side effects include bone marrow suppression, aplastic anemia, pyometra, or death.

A semi-synthetically produced estrogen, estradiol cypionate (ECP) is used for hormone replacement therapy, to prevent embryo implantation within 72 hours of mating, and to treat animals that are experiencing urinary incontinence. Some horses respond favorably to this drug and become more responsive to the sexual advances of other horses. However, this drug should not be given to animals that are pregnant. To date, the drug ECP has not been reported as having serious side effects.

Oxytocin facilitates the birth process and increases milk production. Oxytocin is a drug which causes the smooth muscles to contract, helping the uterus to discharge its contents. It should be administered when the cervix is dilated. The cervix is the lower portion of the uterus with an opening, called the **os**, which connects the uterus to the vagina.

Prostaglandins

Prostaglandin is a naturally occurring hormone in female mammals. Ovulation occurs when an egg reaches the right stage to be released from the ovary, and the corpus luteum develops from an ovarian follicle following this release. Secreted by the uterus, prostaglandin controls the length of time that the corpus luteum exists. The corpus luteum is a yellow mass of tissue that manifests itself after ovulation has occurred in the mammal and is necessary to establish and maintain a pregnancy.

This process produces optimum conditions for fertilization of the egg. Gloves and other protective covering should be worn whenever administering this drug to an animal, as the drug can be absorbed through the skin.

The synthetic prostaglandin **dinoprost** accelerates the birthing process. Dinoprost can also be used to bring about a premature end to a pregnancy by inducing labor resulting in a miscarriage.

Progestins

Progestins are beneficial to animals that are having difficulty adjusting or controlling periods of sexual excitement during their estrous cycle.

Animals typically experience a stage of sexual inactivity just after a breeding period, which is known as the transitional anestrus stage. Progestins can be administered to animals in the anestrus stage to keep them from entering the proestrus period in preparation for sexual activity. The proestrus period is the stage immediately preceding estrus, which is the period of heightened sexual responsiveness and fertility.

One example of this medication is megestrol acetate. Similar to naturally occurring progesterone, megestrol acetate has anti-estrogen properties that produce the necessary effects. Gloves and other protective covering should be worn when administering progestin drugs, as the liquid form can readily be absorbed through the skin.

Diabetes Mellitus

Diabetes mellitus (DM) occurs when the body's ability to regulate blood glucose is impaired. DM causes hyperglycemia and glucosuria. Type 1 diabetes (insulin-dependent diabetes mellitus) is caused by damage to the pancreatic beta cells, resulting in decreased insulin production; it occurs most commonly in dogs. Type 2 diabetes (noninsulin-dependent diabetes mellitus) describes a decreased sensitivity to the amount of insulin produced; it occurs most commonly in cats.

Insulin is a polypeptide hormone which is secreted by beta cells found in the islet of Langerhans, in the pancreas. It is responsible for moving glucose out of the blood and into the cells, where it is used for energy or stored for later use.

Insulin and Insulin Facilitators

There are two types of medications which a veterinarian might prescribe for treatment of diabetes. These medications are synthetic insulin and insulin facilitators such as sulfonylurea-based medications.

Fast-acting insulin, such as Vetsulin, is given to patients who require their blood sugars to be decreased rapidly.

Patients who require a daily control method should be given NPH, insulin classified as an intermediate acting hormone.

Insulin can also be blended with protamine for an extended-release product, which can also be given through injections. Animal patients with diabetes will benefit from the administration of protamine zinc insulin.

Insulin facilitators can be used to treat some diabetic patients who still produce some natural insulin. One classification of these medications is the sulfonylureas. A common sulfonylurea-based antidiabetic drug is glipizide (Glucotrol), which is given to animals which still possess the ability to produce some insulin by natural means, but with a diagnosis of insulin-independent diabetes. This medication is best if given twice a day during mealtimes.

Diabetic Ketoacidosis

Diabetic ketoacidosis (DKA) occurs when fatty acid–derived ketone bodies become the primary cellular energy source when glucose cannot be moved into the cells for metabolism. The metabolism of fats produces an acidic state in the blood which often further complicates the diabetes, and rising levels of ketones may become toxic. Thus, animals with DKA may be very ill, vomiting, and depressed.

The condition may cause the patient to present with "fruity" smelling acetone breath as the ketone concentration rises. Blood or urine testing will definitively reveal the level of ketones. Treatment typically involves intravenous fluid replacement (to correct dehydration and dilute acids and ketones) and the administration of insulin until the situation becomes more stable.

INSULIN-SPECIFIC SYRINGES

Insulin is always taken by injection, as it cannot tolerate the digestive process. Insulin syringes have been specifically designed for the administration of a given solution strength of insulin. For instance, the syringe marked with U-40 is for patients in need of 40 units of insulin hormone, while the syringe marked with U-100 is for patients in need of 100 units of insulin hormone. Therefore, use of the wrong syringe can result in the wrong dosage of insulin. This can potentially result in the death of the animal.

IMMUNOLOGIC AGENTS

IMMUNOSUPPRESSANTS

Some diseases trigger the immune system to such a degree that the animal is harmed. Harmful effects arising from an overactive immune system can be relieved with the administration of immunosuppressants. These same drugs have also been used in the treatment of patients that have received organs or tissues from donors. The immune system will try to attack and destroy donated organs, as they are seen as foreign invaders. However, immunosuppressant drugs can help the body to accept the organs or tissues more gradually, while holding an aggressive immune system at bay.

Patients with autoimmune disease may also benefit from the administration of these drugs. Diseases that fall in this category include autoimmune thyroiditis, autoimmune adrenalitis, IMHA (immune-mediated hemolytic anemia), myasthenia gravis, various skin autoimmune diseases, and more.

Drugs that are classified as immunosuppressants include glucocorticoids (such as prednisone), azathioprine (Imuran), cyclosporine (Sandimmune), mycophenolate mofetil, leflunomide, and cyclophosphamide.

IMMUNOSTIMULANTS

Immunostimulants work to increase the body's immunological response against unwanted viruses and cancer cells. The animal diseases that are most commonly treated with immunostimulants include FeLV or feline leukemia virus, FIV or feline immunodeficiency virus, and canine lymphoma. Dogs that develop canine lymphoma can receive a boost to their immune system through the administration of canine lymphoma monoclonal antibodies. The abbreviated term for canine lymphoma monoclonal antibodies medication is CL/MAb 321. These antibodies are produced in a laboratory. The animal will benefit greatly when the stimulated immune system begins to inflict damage on cancer cells.

Acemannan is an immunostimulant that is beneficial in the treatment of patients with FLV, FIV, and specific cancers. Acemannan is produced by synthesizing Aloe vera and Propionibacterium acnes. The trade name for acemannan is Immunoregulin.

RESPIRATORY AGENTS

Antihistamines can keep the body's histamine response from further affecting the respiratory tract.

When inflammation in the lungs is severe, the application of **corticosteroids** is also recommended. In addition, excess fluids can be eliminated from the lungs when a patient is given **diuretics**. Finally, when a condition is present that seriously compromises breathing or airway perfusion, the recommended procedure is to give the patient supplemental oxygen.

Stimulants are sometimes given to patients to temporarily increase their respiratory function. Doxapram is a known stimulant that has the ability to transiently boost the respiratory rate in animals being treated for respiratory related problems.

Decongestants

Decongestants are normally used to reduce sinus and nasal congestion accompanying a cold. Patients will often have copious amounts of fluid or mucus built up in the nasal and sinus cavities, and decongestants can help them breathe easier. They typically work to constrict blood vessels in the nasal passages, thereby reducing nasal swelling and allowing air to pass more easily. However, decongestants can also serve other purposes. For example, the decongestant phenylpropanolamine can be used to treat urinary incontinence in animals. Urinary incontinence (where the animal is unable to adequately control the bladder) can become a significant problem for animals as they age.

Cough Medication

Antitussives such as codeine (i.e., dihydrocodeine phosphate) suppress or reduce the cough reflex. Antitussives can be administered to a patient with a dry, hacking cough. However, antitussives may be **contraindicated,** or inadvisable, for productive coughs, which may respond better to **expectorant** medication to aid in clearing congestion. A productive cough is beneficial because it decreases mucus and other organic debris that may otherwise accumulate in the airways. Antitussives can also be used to treat **tracheobronchitis**, which is commonly referred to as **kennel cough**. Three examples of antitussive medications are butorphanol, dextromethorphan, and hydrocodone.

Expectorants are used to increase the fluidity or the liquid consistency of the mucus in the airways. Mucus that has greater fluidity is easier to expel or to cough up. Human expectorants sold over the counter have not been found beneficial to animals. Instead, mucus in animals can best be thinned by moistening the air they breathe through humidification.

Mucolytic agents are beneficial in the improvement of bronchial airflow. Mucolytic agents are able to reduce the viscosity of the mucus, allowing it to be more readily broken up. Acetylcysteine is a mucolytic drug that can be given by inhalation, orally, or intravenously.

Bronchodilators

Bronchodilators stimulate Beta-2-receptors in the lung, relaxing the smooth muscle in the terminal bronchioles to improve bronchial airflow.

Some common bronchodilators include albuterol, terbutaline, aminophylline, and theophylline. The general side effects associated with the use of albuterol are related to the amount of medication that has been administered, and they are not usually long-lasting. However, caution should be used to reduce the likelihood of exhaled air entering the injection vials, as carbon dioxide can substantially accelerate the effects of aminophylline.

Topical Agents

Topical medications are drugs which are applied to the skin's surface and to the mucous membranes of the body. Mucous membranes line the surface of all moist body passages and include the eyes, inner ears, nostrils, tongue, rectum, urethra, and vagina. Mucous membranes can be very sensitive, and thus application of topical medications to these tissues requires special preparation.

Topical medications can be applied otically as ear drops; ophthalmically as eye drops or ointments; intranasally as drops, creams, or ointments; and sublingually by placing the medication under the tongue. Cream and ointment topical medications can be applied directly to rectal and vaginal areas. The veterinarian should follow the instructions packaged with a medication explicitly.

Particular caution is also required to compensate for animal biology and behaviors. For example, animals are known to pass their tongue over injured regions of the body in a cleansing and mollifying action. However, some human topical products can be poisonous to the animal. Topical treatments have a tendency to be poorly absorbed by the animal's system as a whole. Other topical drugs like nitroglycerin and certain pour-on preparations will produce a systematic effect.

Anesthetizing and Lubricating Ophthalmic Agents

There are **ophthalmic anesthetics** that can be applied to the eye to numb and reduce the sensation of feeling in exposed eye membranes. Topical anesthetics appropriate for use in the eye which can produce this result include proparacaine and tetracaine.

Individuals may have environmental or health situations arise which reduce the natural lubricants of the eye (tears). For transient relief, drops of "artificial tears" are available. Conditions which cause enduring dryness of the eyes require more aggressive intervention. The disease keratoconjunctivitis sicca causes a patient to become incapable of producing adequate tears. Patients suffering from keratoconjunctivitis sicca can be given a medication called cyclosporine. Cyclosporine seems to both reduce inflammatory cells and increase the number of mucin-secreting goblet cells, thus gaining the patient the ability to make tears in greater amounts.

Other anti-infective and anti-inflammatory agents can be applied in the treatment of the eyes. These drugs can reduce infection and irritation. However, the veterinarian should not use any medications with a steroid base for patients afflicted with a corneal ulcer.

Mydriatic and Miotic Agents

Mydriatics are medical agents which produce a dilation of the pupils in the eyes. Tropicamide is fast-acting and beneficial when the patient requires an examination of the interior of the eye (e.g., the ocular fundus).

Miotic agents constrict the pupil. A patient with glaucoma may be given a miotic agent called pilocarpine to constrict the pupil, which is necessary to transiently increase the intraocular pressure. **Glaucoma** is a disease that presents with abnormally high intraocular pressure. However, a temporary increase in pressure, such as that caused by constriction induced via a miotic agent, allows the excess aqueous humor (i.e., the transparent fluid in the eye) to drain away. This ultimately reduces the intraocular pressure that so often damages the sensitive interior structures of the eye.

Chelation and Antidotes

Chelation Therapy

Chelation therapy treats heavy metal toxicity from substances such as lead, mercury, and arsenic. Chelation therapy incorporates chelating (binding) agents that chemically bond with these metals, giving the animal a safe way to discharge the poison from its system.

Succimer (DMSA), dimercaprol, calcium EDTA, and penicillamine are all chelating agents applied in the treatment of heavy metal poisoning in animals. Succimer is a powder that has the ability to combine its white crystalline base with mercury or other heavy metals through a chemical binding process. Succimer can bind itself to the poisons in the brain by breaking through the blood-brain barrier which normally limits what can diffuse from the blood into the brain.

Dimercaprol (BAL, or British anti-Lewisite) is produced in a peanut oil base and works by joining the target heavy metals with its two nonmetallic thiol groups. Dimercaprol is transparent, thick, and has a narrow therapeutic index.

Penicillamine (Cuprimine) is a penicillin derivative, although it has no antibiotic properties. Penicillamine acts against lead, mercury, and arsenic.

Once chelated, the animal urinates to rid itself of the poisonous metal, bound with the chelating agent.

Acetylcysteine

As an antidote, **acetylcysteine** provides important protective effects against acetaminophen overdose. When metabolized in the liver, acetaminophen produces a toxic byproduct, NAPQI. This metabolite is typically removed from the body by glutathione, found in the liver. In situations of overdose, however, there are insufficient reserves of glutathione. Acetylcysteine is able to stimulate the production of glutathione and bind with NAPQI, reducing its liver-toxic effects.

Unopened vials of acetylcysteine solutions should be kept at room temperature to ensure optimal results. However, upon opening the vial, it may only be refrigerated for a period of 96 hours or less. After 96 hours, any previously opened medication should not be used. The medication is typically given intravenously due to low oral bioavailability and its very unpleasant taste and odor. The patient should be observed for possible side effects, including nausea, vomiting, and urticaria (hives).

ATROPINE

Organophosphates can be found in various insecticides and herbicides that animals may sometimes ingest. Some **common insecticides** that contain organophosphates are malathion, parathion, diazinon, chlorpyrifos, and chlorfenvinphos. **Organophosphates** are readily absorbed through the skin and can also enter through the gastrointestinal and respiratory tracts of the animal. An animal that has had contact with the poison may begin to show symptoms in just a few minutes. However, some of these poisons may only show up days later. Cats are particularly susceptible to organophosphate poisoning.

Organophosphate poisoning can cause drooling, vomiting, stress defecation, diarrhea, constricted pupils, difficulty breathing (often due to laryngospasm, bronchospasm, bronchorrhea, or seizures), tremors, muscle twitching, and death.

The anticholinergic antidote, **atropine**, lowers the secretions caused by the poison and relaxes and expands the air passageways that were constricted from the spasmodic effects of the poison. The patient should be closely monitored for possible side effects: seizures, dilated pupils, and tachycardia. Early administration of atropine should substantially reduce the toxic effects of organophosphate poisoning.

ETHYLENE GLYCOL POISONING

Animals are attracted to the sweet taste of antifreeze, which contains **ethylene glycol**. Initial signs of ethylene glycol poisoning include staggering, rapid pulse, and various abnormal behaviors. These are followed by vomiting, respiratory distress, agitation, increased unsteadiness, seizures, acute renal failure, and coma.

The antidotes chiefly used are **ethanol** (drinking alcohol) and **4-methylpyrazole**. The trade name for the antidote 4-methylpyrazole is called Antizol-Vet. The antidote should be administered within 8 hours of the animal's poisoning for the best chance for survival.

CANINE JOINT HEALTH

Glucosamine naturally occurs in the dog's body and produces glycosaminoglycan, which is used to form and repair cartilage. As the dog gets older, this natural glucosamine production decreases, so the natural formation and repairing of cartilage slows, and the dog will experience joint pain. The dog's activities will continue to wear on the joints with everyday activity, and this combined with the slowed production of glucosamine leads to arthritis. Glucosamine supplements can be given to the dog to help rebuild the cartilage and provide lubrication to the joints, improving the dog's overall activity level and joint health. To help combat the pain associated with arthritis, glucosamine also has an anti-inflammatory effect.

Chondroitin is a naturally occurring main glycosaminoglycan in the dog's body found in the cartilage that is responsible for maintaining appropriate shock absorption and joint tissue health by providing elasticity and water retention in the cartilage. Chondroitin stops the production of inflammatory mediators that destroy the joints, provides increased mobility, and improves the dog's strength. Chondroitin is normally used in conjunction with glucosamine. Whereas chondroitin blocks the enzymes that try to destroy cartilage in the joints, glucosamine works to repair them.

Antineoplastic Agents

Antineoplastic agents (cytotoxic chemotherapy drugs) are beneficial in treating patients with cancer. These drugs work by traveling throughout the body and killing off cancerous cells that can develop into tumors. A tumor (neoplasm) is an uncontrolled growth of malignant or benign cells. Left unchecked, benign tumors can encroach on normal tissues and functions, and cancerous tumors can spread and overwhelm the body.

The recommended safety gear for administering antineoplastic agents includes gloves and protective clothing. The person administering this drug is at risk because the antineoplastic agent in the drug is not end-cell selective and thus will kill off both cancer and non-cancer cells in life-forms. Thus, healthy human and healthy animal cells can be accidentally destroyed by this drug when contact precautions are not followed. The antineoplastic drug works by seeking out any cell that can multiply rapidly. Typically, the gastrointestinal cells, tumor cells, bone marrow cells, and reproductive tract cells are targeted. The drug can also result in lasting harm to the DNA, which cannot be repaired.

Classifications of Antineoplastic Drugs

There are 5 classifications of antineoplastic drugs: alkylating agents, antimetabolites, plant alkaloids, antibiotics, and hormonal agents.

The starting dosage is prepared based on body surface in square meters rather than on the animal's body weight, as this figure closely approximates total blood volume. Adjustments to avoid toxicity (e.g., based on individual metabolism or liver and kidney function) may later be needed.

The veterinarian must also consider the type of cancer and its stage of progression when selecting an antineoplastic drug and in determining a specified regimen of chemotherapy. It is not uncommon for a veterinarian to select a combination of these drugs in treating a patient with cancer. However, the veterinarian should remember to always use safety equipment when handling and administering antineoplastic drugs.

Alkylating Agents

Alkylating agents are formed out of an alkyl group and small carbon-hydrogen compounds. These agents can hinder cancerous growths in three ways, all involving cellular DNA. First, they may stop tumor cell growth by cross-linking nucleobases found in the cell's DNA strands. This action renders the DNA incapable of uncoiling and separating itself for transcription, which is necessary for replication. Second, alkylating agents can attach alkyl groups to DNA bases. Sensing alteration, DNA repair enzymes will inadvertently separate and fragment the DNA in unsuccessful efforts to replace the altered DNA bases. Third, alkylating agents can also induce the mispairing of DNA nucleotides. The double-strands of DNA must pair specific nucleotides in each strand with each other in order to form and maintain the coiled, double-helix formation necessary for proper DNA function. If the nucleotides mispair with alternate nucleotides, then DNA mutations result, preventing DNA replication and subsequent cell division.

Examples

Cisplatin, carboplatin, chlorambucil, and cyclophosphamide are drugs which work with the use of alkylating agents. All can be used in animal populations, although the drug cisplatin is contraindicated for use with felines.

Some alkylating agents (and other drugs) fall into the category of **prodrugs**, which are largely or entirely inactive in their administered form. These drugs must be changed or altered by a predetermined mechanism in the body to become active. The purposes behind prodrugs are twofold: 1) to increase bioavailability (often to improve gastrointestinal absorption), and 2) to target certain cells such as cancer cells (allowing, for example, properties unique to those cells to activate the drug).

The drug known as cyclophosphamide is considered a prodrug. This drug must first be changed by the liver in order to activate the drug's alkylating agents. The patient given these drugs should be monitored for side effects such as bone marrow suppression, gastrointestinal disturbances, and hemorrhagic cystitis (severe bleeding in the bladder due to the chemotherapy).

ANTIMETABOLITES

An **antimetabolite** is a drug which has the ability to interrupt normal metabolic processes, such as cell growth. The composition of antimetabolites inhibiting cell growth is similar to the metabolites that promote cell growth. The essential difference is that the antimetabolite uses altered cell replication nucleotides in place of the nucleotides necessary to sustain cell division. Purines and pyrimidines are organic nucleotides needed for cell DNA replication. One form of cell antimetabolite uses similar-looking purine and pyrimidine analogs, but ones that are unable to complete the replication process. The tumor cell introduces these nucleotide analogs in an effort to replicate the tumor cell's DNA. However, this similar-looking compound does not produce the same results. Further, because they are made abundantly available, the antimetabolites are largely able to prevent the true purines and pyrimidines from being introduced into the tumor cell. In this way, cancerous tumor growth is substantially inhibited by the antimetabolite.

EXAMPLES

Although originally designed for use in human hosts, veterinarians can also utilize **antimetabolite drugs** to stop or interrupt the growth of cancerous cells in animals. Hydroxyurea, cytarabine, methotrexate, and 5-fluorouracil are all cell-cycle–specific drugs (i.e., drugs that inhibit the process of cell division) and are thus classified as antimetabolites. When used, the veterinarian should carefully monitor the patient for side effects, as these drugs may cause bone marrow suppression. The drug hydroxyurea is typically given to patients with blood, bone marrow, and lymph node cancers. The drug cytarabine is given to patients with leukemia. Methotrexate is given to patients with cancer of the breast, head and neck, lung, blood, and bone, and has recently also come to be used in the treatment of certain autoimmune diseases. The drug 5-fluorouracil is given to patients with bowel, breast, stomach, and esophageal cancers. However, 5-fluorouracil is not safe for use with felines.

These drugs have all been effective in the treatment of patients previously diagnosed with cancer.

PLANT ALKALOIDS

Mitotic inhibitors (Vinca alkaloids) are derived from plant alkaloids and are able to stop the cellular process of mitosis by disrupting microtubular polymerization. This process involves the joining of protein pairs, called dimers, into protofilaments and then into microtubules. A polarization process is also involved, causing the protofilaments to join only end-to-end, thereby producing long filaments capable of creating extended microtubules. Cells use microtubules to construct the cytoskeleton, mitotic spindle, and other intracellular components. These microtubules are derived from structural proteins known as tubulin. Mitotic inhibitors work to inhibit or suppress the tubulin dimers. This stops mitosis from being carried out in the cell, and thus cell replication does not take place.

Mitotic inhibitors are not target-cell specific, and toxicity must be closely monitored. Toxicity may manifest as gastrointestinal disturbances, bone marrow suppression, and alopecia. The drug is a vesicating (blister-producing) agent and does cause skin irritation when it has been exposed. The drug vincristine is given to patients who have lymphoma. The drug vinblastine is given to patients who have mast cell tumors.

ANTINEOPLASTIC ANTIBIOTICS AND HORMONE THERAPY

Antineoplastic antibiotics include actinomycin D, mitoxantrone, doxorubicin, and bleomycin, which are all created from *Streptomyces*. Actinomycin D is given intravenously. It does not cross the blood-brain barrier, and resistance to the drug is possible. It is also cell-cycle nonspecific. Mitoxantrone can be used to treat lymphoma and some carcinomas. Doxorubicin is given IV and is considered cell-cycle nonspecific. It may cause vesication and phlebitis and has more severe side effects than mitoxantrone. Bleomycin is given SC or IV and does not cross the blood-brain barrier; it can have delayed pulmonary toxicity.

Glucocorticoids are used as antineoplastic hormonal agents. They are cell-cycle nonspecific. Resistance may develop quickly, and toxicity is possible. Signs of toxicity include PU/PD (polyuria/polydipsia), immunosuppression, glucose intolerance, peptic ulcers, pancreatitis, hypokalemia, osteopenia, muscle wasting, and cataracts.

Examples include prednisone and dexamethasone, which are used to treat leukemias and CNS lymphomas.

Drug Storage, Handling, and Inventory

Storing Prescription Medications

There are specific regulations governing the safe storage of medications in veterinary medical settings. Prescription medications must be kept in a secure, locked setting within a veterinary hospital. The hospital must adequately monitor environmental conditions like the temperature, humidity, and light exposure that could affect stored medications. The medication's expiration date must be noted, and a review system must be in place to ensure expired medications are properly discarded. The expiration date is the date that the drug is deemed no longer safe for continued use.

The reconstitution, storage, and handling instructions must also be written on the label or package insert. This literature is useful for describing the care that should be taken with each stored drug. The **Safety Data Sheet** (SDS) specific to each drug is a necessary document that presents complete safety, handling, clean-up, and disposal criteria for every drug stored in the hospital. Those drugs which are labeled as hazardous must also be handled in accordance with the guidelines published by the Occupational Safety and Health Administration or OSHA, as specific to the state in which the drugs are maintained. Drugs require a written prescription before they can be given to a patient.

Schedules of Controlled Drugs

Controlled drugs are labeled in specified **schedules** ranging from I–V. Schedule I substances, such as heroin and LSD, have the highest risk of abuse and cannot be prescribed. Schedule II drugs, such as opium, morphine, fentanyl, and hydromorphone, have a high risk of abuse and severe physical and psychological dependence. Schedule III drugs, including buprenorphine, tramadol, and ketamine, have a lower abuse potential than Schedule I and II drugs. Schedule II and III drugs require strict record keeping for tracking the use or dispensation of these drugs. Schedule IV drugs, including phenobarbital, midazolam, and diazepam, have a low potential for abuse. Schedule V substances include medications that are available without a prescription such as antitussives that may contain small quantities of a narcotic drug such as codeine. Schedule II–V drugs are all accepted for medical use in the United States.

Controlled Substances Act of 1970

The United States **Controlled Substances Act** of 1970 consists of regulations governing the manufacture, importation, possession, and distribution of certain drugs within the boundaries of the United States. Subject to this Act, the FDA, or Food and Drug Administration, is also in charge of regulating any pharmaceutical drug that has the potential for abusive use. Finally, the Drug Enforcement Administration (DEA) is responsible for enforcing these drug laws and regulations.

Under the Controlled Substances Act of 1970, Schedules III, IV, and V require strict record keeping and storage arrangements.

Controlled Substances Log

There needs to be a system in each hospital that shows the balance on hand of each **controlled substance** which must be kept for a minimum of 2 years. Frequently updated written logs or computerized logs work well. The patient's name, client's name, the date, drug name, and drug amount used must be recorded. If an injectable drug is prescribed, then the amount drawn up and the amount actually administered to the patient must be recorded. Regular inventory counts should be done to ensure that the amounts correspond to the actual log books. Having one person, whether it is a veterinarian or a veterinary technician, responsible for keeping track of the controlled drug logs is ideal. This way, the person responsible will be able to notice and keep track of trends.

Handling Shortages Within the Controlled Drugs Log

If a shortage is noticed in the controlled drug log, usually it is due to a miscalculation or record-keeping error. In these cases, the record book must be calculated through to catch any adding or subtracting errors, and drug doses and strengths must be checked for accuracy. Also, checking the computer and comparing it to the log book to determine if any controlled drug prescriptions were filled and not logged will catch errors as well. If the problem is identified, then an entry can be made to correct the balance appropriately. If theft is the cause, then a report will have to be filled out for the DEA indicating what is missing. An explanation is required, but evidence is not.

Storing Controlled Drugs

Controlled drugs should be stored in a locked cabinet with hidden hinges or in a safe that is secured to a cabinet or wall that cannot be easily moved. The attending veterinarian should be the only one with access to the controlled drug unit to ensure tight security. If using a mobile unit for controlled drug storage, there should only be drugs in the unit for that specific procedure, and the rest should be kept in a secure location in the hospital. The controlled drugs should be kept in a secure, hidden, locked unit if being transported by vehicle and unsupervised.

Storing Vaccinations

Vaccines need to be stored in the dark and at a refrigerated temperature of 35–45 °F. Vaccines should be stored in a dedicated refrigerator, meaning they should not be stored in the same refrigerator as employees' food and drinks or opened pet food that is used for patients. The vaccines should be stored in the center of the refrigerator because temperatures in the fridge can vary. The temperature of the refrigerator should be monitored daily to ensure that the vaccines are kept at a regulated temperature because being exposed to temperatures outside of the recommended range can reduce the effectiveness of the vaccines. A thermometer can be kept in the middle of the refrigerator and compared to the temperature on the refrigerator itself daily to ensure that it is at the correct temperature.

Handling Vaccines

Vaccines should always be drawn up with a fresh, sterile needle and syringe, and they should not be drawn up until just before they are going to be administered. Once reconstituted, the vaccine could be more temperature sensitive; additionally, the risk of bacterial contamination increases the longer that the vaccine is reconstituted and sitting in the syringe. Vaccines should be administered within 30 minutes of being reconstituted. Certain vaccines look similar once they are reconstituted. One way to prevent one vaccine from being mistaken for another is to peel off the sticker from the vaccine vial and place it around the syringe used to draw up that vaccine. Vaccines should be mixed thoroughly before drawing them up into the syringe.

Transporting Vaccines

The priority for transport of vaccines is to maintain a temperature of 35–45 °F. While being transported from the manufacturer to the clinic, they must be kept inside of an insulated cooler with ice packs if needed. Ice packs should be wrapped in paper or some sort of layer to prevent them from contacting the vaccines, which could make them too cold. A cooler with vaccines should not be kept in a trunk or the bed of a truck because these areas could get too cold in the winter and too hot in the summer, so vaccines need to be kept in the center of the transport vehicle where it is temperature controlled. Modified live vaccines are heat sensitive, whereas adjuvanted vaccines are more sensitive to freezing temperatures, causing the adjuvant to separate from the antigen to form a precipitate that can cause local inflammation at the administration site, so maintaining the proper temperature for vaccines is crucial.

Guidelines for Dispensing Drugs

Very specific laws govern the issuance of veterinary prescription drugs. These drugs may only be given out by a licensed veterinarian using proper documentation. In addition, the drugs must be administered through a valid **veterinarian-client-patient relationship** (VCPR), which involves the following:

- The clinical judgments regarding the patient's health are decided by the treating veterinarian.
- The veterinarian agrees to be accountable for the treatments prescribed.
- The client or animal owner agrees to abide by the veterinarian's instructions for care.

The minimum level of care should include a general or preliminary exam of the patient. The veterinarian must also stay available should the patient have need of follow-up or emergency care due to an adverse reaction. If the veterinarian is unavailable, then an alternative doctor should be available to act in the veterinarian's place.

Prescription Labels

Prescription drugs are intended for the animal that has received the prescription. No other animal should be given another's prescription medications. If the state of residence requires it, then a childproof container must also be used. It is important to follow dosage amounts as provided on a typed package label. The use of abbreviations is not allowed on this typed label. The veterinarian will have specified all requisite dosing and handling information in detail on the label of the prescription. At a minimum the label will include:

- The date prescribed
- Patient name (or herd name)
- Client's last name
- Owner's address
- Veterinarian's name, telephone number, and address
- Name of the drug
- Drug ID (DIN)
- Drug concentration
- Dosage amount, frequency, and route
- Number of available refills
- Administration directions (drug given with food, on an empty stomach, or with liquids)
- Drug storage requirements
- Drug expiration date
- Drug warnings

There may be information about the species of the animal as required by individual state law. If the medication is sensitive to light, then an amber vial is used to obstruct the ultraviolet rays.

Metric Time and Date

The proper configuration used to write the **metric date** is the year/month/day/time. The time entered is based on a 24-hour block, counted from midnight to midnight. For example, the date of April 1, 2020, 7:15 PM would be given in the following format: 2020/04/01/19:15. Notice that the time is written with 4 digits and without the use of the afternoon or morning designations of PM or AM. The first 2 digits denote the hours elapsed from midnight. The 2 digits following the colon denote the elapsed minutes in the ensuing hour.

The general population of the US does not use metric time and date, and instead uses the month/day/year configuration, most commonly as 04/01/2020 or 04-01-2020. For this reason, it may be necessary to explain its use to the client.

DRUG DISPOSAL

A veterinary clinic's SDS notebook will have information on proper handling and disposal of all materials used in the hospital. Following these guidelines will prevent environmental contamination and accidental human or animal exposure.

Controlled substances that have expired or been damaged can be disposed of through "reverse distributors" who are authorized to dispose of those drugs.

Chemotherapy spill kits should be in each facility and all staff should be trained on location and usage.

Animal urine and feces may need to be collected and disposed of safely if the animal is being treated with certain antineoplastics or parasite treatments.

CRASH CART SUPPLIES AND DRUGS

The **crash cart** should be in a central location in the hospital close to an anesthetic machine in case the patient needs to be under anesthesia or receive oxygen support. Some supplies that should be available in the crash cart are catheters, tape, syringes, needles, fluid bag, Ambu-bag, and emergency drugs. Emergency drugs that are vital to include in the crash cart include epinephrine, atropine, naloxone, lidocaine, and doxapram. Epinephrine is used to treat anaphylactic reactions, and it is also used to stimulate the heart in cardiopulmonary resuscitation (CPR). Atropine is used to treat an abnormally slow heart rate and is an important drug used in CPR. Lidocaine is used to treat cardiac arrhythmias. Doxapram is used to stimulate breathing in a patient under anesthesia or after, as well as to help initiate breathing in newborn patients after a C-section. The crash cart should also include a drug dosage chart for each emergency drug.

Calculating Dosage

DECIMALS

To **multiply decimals**, first multiply the numbers as if there were no decimals present. Then, place a decimal point at the end of the number (to the right) and move the decimal place to the left by the number of spaces equal to the total number of decimal places in the original numbers.

Example: 5.68 × 1.25

The total number of decimal places = 2 + 2 = 4

At first, multiply the numbers ignoring the decimal places: 568 × 125 = 71,000

Place a decimal place at the end of this number: 71,000.

Move the decimal place to the left a total number of spaces equal to the total number of decimal places in the original numbers (in this case, four places): 7.1

To **convert a decimal to a percent**, move the decimal two places to the *right* and add a % sign.

Example: 0.30 = 30%

To **convert a percent to a decimal**, move the decimal point two places to the *left* and remove the % sign.

Example: 65% = 0.65

Review Video: Decimals
Visit mometrix.com/academy and enter code: 837268

Review Video: How to Multiply Decimals
Visit mometrix.com/academy and enter code: 731574

Review Video: Converting Percentages to Decimals and Fractions
Visit mometrix.com/academy and enter code: 287297

Converting Between Grams, Kilograms, Milligrams, and Micrograms

A gram (g) is the basic metric unit of mass or weight. All other metric units of mass are centered around the gram. Metric units of measure can be easily converted from one form to another by moving the decimal place. A kilogram (kg) is 10^3 or 1000 times larger than a gram. Therefore, to convert grams to kilograms, the decimal place must be moved to the left three places. Milligrams (mg) and micrograms (mcg) are smaller than a gram. A milligram is 10^{-3} or 1,000 times smaller than a gram, whereas a microgram is 10^{-6} or 1,000,000 times smaller than a gram. To convert grams to milligrams, the decimal place must be moved to the right three places. To convert grams to micrograms, the decimal place must be moved to the right six places.

Unit of Measure	Kilogram	Gram	Milligram	Microgram
Conversion factor	10^3	1	10^{-3}	10^{-6}
Sample conversion	0.008	8	8,000	8,000,000

Review Video: Measurement Conversions
Visit mometrix.com/academy and enter code: 316703

Dimensional Analysis

A useful method for solving problems involving unit conversions is **dimensional analysis.** In this method conversion factors $\left(\text{example: } \frac{1\text{ g}}{1{,}000\text{ mg}}\right)$ or their reciprocals $\left(\text{example: } \frac{1{,}000\text{ mg}}{1\text{ g}}\right)$ may be used to obtain the required unit. Consider this drip rate example (note: gtt = drop):

$$\text{Drip rate} = \frac{25\text{ mL}}{1\text{ hour}} \times \frac{10\text{ gtt}}{1\text{ mL}} \times \frac{1\text{ hour}}{60\text{ min}} = \frac{250\text{ gtt}}{60\text{ min}} = 4.2\frac{\text{gtt}}{\text{min}}$$

In this example, the flow rate (25 mL/hour) was given, as was the conversion factor of 10 gtt (drops) per mL. Those values plus the conversion of 1 hour per 60 minutes can be used to solve the problem.

One way to check that the problem was set up and solved correctly is to make sure the units cancel out across the problem to give the desired dimensions. This problem asked for drip rate, which is measured in drops (gtt) per unit of time (minutes in this problem). Below, the mL and hour in the numerator cancel out the mL and hour in the denominator because 1 hour ÷ 1 hour = 1 and 1 mL ÷ 1 mL = 1, so the resulting units match the units required for the answer.

$$\text{Drip rate} = \frac{25\text{ }\cancel{\text{mL}}}{1\text{ }\cancel{\text{hour}}} \times \frac{10\text{ gtt}}{1\text{ }\cancel{\text{mL}}} \times \frac{1\text{ }\cancel{\text{hour}}}{60\text{ min}} = \frac{250\text{ gtt}}{60\text{ min}} = 4.2\frac{\text{gtt}}{\text{min}}$$

Calculating Dosage

Dosage describes how much of a medicinal substance should be administered in the treatment of a given condition, along with the recommended interval of time between administrations of the recommended amount of medication. Most medications are produced as pills, capsules, or liquids, with the relative strength measured in units known as milligrams (mg) or milliliters (mL). The **dose** indicates how much of the drug is to be given to the patient at one time.

The animal's weight must be included in calculating dosage. For instance, shorthand phrases such as 100 mg/kg, mL/kg, or tablets/kg each relate to the amount of the dosage to be delivered based on the animal's weight expressed as kg or kilograms. A kilogram is the basic metric unit of mass, with 1 pound equivalent to 0.45 kilograms. Therefore, a 10-pound animal weighs 4.5 kilograms.

Use the following formula to determine dosage:

$$\text{Weight (kg)} \times \text{Dose}\left(\frac{\text{mg}}{\text{kg}}\right) = \text{Dose (mg)}$$

To calculate the dose in milliliters, you will take the dose divided by the concentration, which is decided by the manufacturer and found on the bottle of medication in terms of mg/mL. Use the following formula:

$$\text{Dose (mg)} \div \text{Concentration}\left(\frac{\text{mg}}{\text{mL}}\right) = \text{Dose (mL)}$$

Example 1

Determine the dose of 100 mg/mL cefazolin needed for an 80 lb dog (2.2 lb = 1 kg) if the dosage is 20 mg/kg.

$$80\text{ lb} \times \frac{1\text{ kg}}{2.2\text{ lb}} \times \frac{20\text{ mg}}{1\text{ kg}} \times \frac{1\text{ mL}}{100\text{ mg}} = 7.3\text{ mL}$$

Example 2

Determine the dose of Medication A for a 30 kg animal receiving a dosage of 10 mg/kg.

$$30\text{ kg} \times \frac{10\text{ mg}}{1\text{ kg}} = 300\text{ mg}$$

Medication A is dosed 10 mg/kg. Thus, an animal that weighed 30 kg would receive 300 mg of Medication A.

Example 3

Determine the dose for Liquid Drug B (concentration 40 mg/mL) if 150 mg is to be given.

$$150\text{ mg} \times \frac{1\text{ mL}}{40\text{ mg}} = 3.75\text{ mL}$$

Liquid Drug B has a concentration of 40 mg/mL, from which a dose of 150 mg is to be given. The patient would be given a 3.75 mL dose.

Solution Terminology

Dilution occurs when the ratio of substance to **dilutant** is decreased by adding dilutant to the solution. The added dilutant can consist of one or more substances that have a compatible composition. The solute must be able to be dissolved and absorbed by the diluting substance. This other substance is called the **solvent**. The final mixture is known as the **solution**. The **concentration** of this solution reflects the amount of solute that was combined with the solvent. This concentration may reflect a strong or a weak solution.

The concentration can be measured according to its percentage: volume solute per volume solvent, written as (v/v) and expressed as a percentage—for liquids, the volume of solute in milliliters per 100 mL of total solution. The concentration can also be measured as weight per volume, written as (w/v), indicating the percent mass of the solute per 100 mL of total solution. Finally, the concentration may be reflected as percentage weight per weight, written as (w/w). This indicates the weight of the solute per 100 g of the total solution.

EXAMPLE

Determine the volume of solvent required for 50 g solute to yield a 0.25 g/mL solution.

$$50\text{ g} \times \frac{100\text{ mL}}{25\text{ g}} = 200\text{ mL}$$

STOCK AND WORKING SOLUTIONS

Pure solutions (or pure solids) that are free from contamination or foreign substances are written as a 100% solution or 100% concentration. A **stock solution** is the product of combining a pure solution or solid with the appropriate amount of solvent through the process of dilution. The solvent is mixed into the pure solution in an effort to weaken or reduce the concentration of the solute in the solution. To increase the concentration of a solution, mix a new solution that has not been diluted as much—or add more solute (i.e., the active ingredient). Alternatively, add more of the pure solution to the solvent to obtain a stronger concentration.

SOLUTION CALCULATIONS

To determine any change in concentration between an initial and final solution, use the equation:

$$M_1V_1 = M_2V_2$$

M1 is the solute concentration in the initial (stock) solution, M2 is the solute concentration in the final solution, V1 is the volume of initial (stock) solution used, and V2 is the total volume of the final solution. To create a specific dilution, determine the volume of solvent (Vs) to mix with the selected volume (i.e., aliquot) of stock solution (V1). This can easily be computed using $Vs = V2 - V1$.

SAMPLE RATIO AND PROPORTION CALCULATION PROBLEM

You are to prepare an IV for a patient that contains potassium chloride 10 mEq in 500 mL. All you have in stock is potassium chloride 40 mEq/10 mL. How much of the stock solution should be added to the 500 mL IV bag in order to prepare the 10 mEq solution?

In order to solve this type of proportion problem, it is easiest to use cross multiplication. In cross multiplication, you summarize the information into two fractions where three values are known, and one value is unknown. Then, you cross-multiply to solve for the unknown value.

We know that the stock solution we have contains 40 mEq/10 mL, so this is our first fraction or proportion. We also know that we need to end with 10 mEq, but we don't know how much volume equates to 10 mEq. Therefore, our second fraction will be 10 mEq over an unknown volume:

$$\begin{aligned}\frac{10\text{ mEq}}{?\text{ mL}} &= \frac{40\text{ mEq}}{10\text{ mL}}\\ 10\text{ mEq} \times 10\text{ mL} &= 40\text{ mEq} \times ?\text{ mL}\\ ?\text{ mL} &= \frac{(10 \times 10)}{40}\text{ mL}\\ &= 2.5\text{ mL}\end{aligned}$$

The correct answer is 2.5 mL. This means that 2.5 mL of the 40 mEq/10 mL stock solution must be added to the 500 mL IV bag in order to prepare a 10 mEq/500 mL solution (although in reality the exact concentration would become 10 mEq/502.5 mL because nothing would be removed from the 500 mL IV bag when the 2.5 mL is added).

It's always a good idea to review your answer to ensure that it is reasonable. If the stock solution is 40 mEq/10 mL and we need 10 mEq, that means that our answer will be one-fourth of 10 mL because 10 mEq is one-fourth of 40 mEq. Because 2.5 mL is one-fourth of 10 mEq, our answer is correct.

Drop Factor and Drip Rates

Medications may be administered through IV tubes over time. The number of drops per cc or mL of fluid is known as the **drop factor**, which is dependent on the diameter of the IV tubing. Three common IV tube drop factors are 15 gtt/cc, 10 gtt/cc, and 60 gtt/cc (also known as "micro drip tubing"). The drop factor is printed on the IV packaging. Facilities use 60 gtt/cc for situations needing close monitoring (e.g., very small animals, vasoactive medications).

Drip rate is the number of drops delivered during each 1-minute interval—often written gtt/min, or "guttae" (drips) per minute. A prescribed delivery rate may be given: a 0.5 L solution with 15 drops/mL for 3 hours. To determine the proper drip rate, take the time in hours and compute: 3 hours multiplied by 60 minutes equals 180 minutes total. The second step is to take the 0.5 L (500 mL) and multiply by 15 drops/mL, totaling 7,500 drops. 7,500 divided by 180 minutes equals a drip rate of 41.67 gtt/min. Note: drip rate must never be confused with flow rate—which is the rate of delivery provided by an IV infusion pump, independent of drips per minute.

Review Video: Calculating IV Drip Rates
Visit mometrix.com/academy and enter code: 396112

Determining Fluid Rate

The **fluid rate** will be determined based on the percent of dehydration, ongoing losses such as diarrhea, and the maintenance requirement. The percent of dehydration is determined by taking the animal's weight in kilograms multiplied by the percent dehydration in decimal form. Ongoing losses may be estimated or measured accurately; for example, urine can be measured if a catheter is placed and a collection system is attached. **Maintenance fluids** are the required amount of fluid needed per day, and this is calculated at 40–60 mL multiplied by weight in kilograms. In order to calculate for the patient's fluid deficit, the patient's body weight in kilograms is multiplied by the percent dehydration (in decimal form). This will result in the weight of fluid that is deficient. Because 1 kg is equal to 1 L, the result will be the amount that the patient will require to become rehydrated in liters (multiply by 1,000 to get the amount in mL) if there are no ongoing losses (e.g., urine, vomiting, diarrhea). If there are ongoing losses, they are added to the fluid deficit.

For example, a 25 kg dog presents with a 6% fluid deficit. To calculate the fluids required to replace the deficit, the following is calculated:

$$25 \text{ kg} \times 0.06 = 1.5 \text{ L}$$

$$1.5 \text{ L} \times 1000 \frac{\text{mL}}{\text{L}} = 1500 \text{ mL}$$

This dog requires a fluid infusion of 1500 mL for fluid replenishment.

Sensible and Insensible Fluid Losses

Sensible losses are losses that can be measured, such as urine. Urine can be measured if a urinary catheter is placed and a collection system is attached. The collection system can be emptied and measured throughout a hospitalization. Insensible losses cannot be measured and can only be estimated by the veterinarian. **Insensible losses** include losses due to fevers, excessive panting, respiratory loss, and fluid lost in feces. Both categories of loss must be included in the calculation for the total fluid deficit. Crystalloids are used to maintain the fluid level of the patient to keep up with the sensible and insensible losses in patients that are not eating or drinking as they should under hospitalization.

Sample IV Flow Rate/Drip Rate Problem

An IV antibiotic was prescribed for a patient to be administered at a rate of 25 mL/hour. What volume (in mL) of IV solution would be needed to last 8 hours? What is the drip rate if the IV is running through at a rate of 10 gtt/mL?

Flow rates can be expressed in mL/hour or mL/min depending upon what type of pump is being used to administer the IV:

$$\textbf{Flow rate} = \frac{\text{mL of IV solution}}{\text{hours or minutes}}$$

In this problem, the IV flow rate is given, and it is asking how many mL of solution are needed to run over an 8-hour time frame. In order to figure this out, the flow rate must be multiplied by the time period:

$$\text{Flow rate (mL/hour)} \times \text{hours} = \text{total mL administered}$$

$$25\ \text{mL/hour} \times 8\ \text{hours} = 200\ \text{mL administered over 8 hours}$$

The drip rate is the number of drops of IV solution that are administered per minute.

$$\textbf{Drip rate} = \frac{\text{gtt of IV solution}}{\text{minute}}$$

In order to calculate the drip rate from the flow rate, the mL of solution must be converted into drops (gtt). A conversion factor will be given for this. In this problem, the rate is 10 gtt/mL. If the flow rate is given in hours, then the time must be converted into minutes to calculate the drip rate.

$$\text{Drip rate} = \frac{25\ \text{mL}}{1\ \text{hour}} \times \frac{10\ \text{gtt}}{1\ \text{mL}} \times \frac{1\ \text{hour}}{60\ \text{min}} = \frac{250\ \text{gtt}}{60\ \text{min}} = 4.2\frac{\text{gtt}}{\text{min}}$$

Sample Amount of Glucose in Solution Problem

How many grams of glucose are there in a 500 mL bag of glucose 5% solution? How many grams are contained in a 500 mL bag of glucose 0.5% solution?

A concentration is the amount of substance in a volume of solution. Concentrations can be expressed as weight to volume (g/100 mL), volume to volume (mL/100 mL) or weight to weight (g/100 g).

A percentage is the quantity of substance in 100. Because concentrations are also expressed as an amount per 100, no conversion or decimal place movement is required to convert the percentage into a concentration. To solve this problem, multiply the concentration of the solution by the volume of the bag to find the total amount of glucose contained within the bag:

$$\text{Glucose 5\%} = \frac{5\ \text{g}}{100\ \text{mL}} \times \frac{500\ \text{mL}}{\text{bag}} = \frac{(5 \times 500)}{100} = 25\ \text{g}$$

$$\text{Glucose 0.5\%} = \frac{0.5\ \text{g}}{100\ \text{mL}} \times \frac{500\ \text{mL}}{\text{bag}} = \frac{(0.5 \times 500)}{100} = 2.5\ \text{g}$$

Ensure that these answers are reasonable and make sense. If there is 5% glucose in a solution (5 g/100 mL), then a 500 mL bag will have five times as much as a 100 mL bag. Because 5 × 5 = 25, our answer of 25 g makes sense. For the 0.5% solution, move the decimal place to the left one place to find the answer in comparison to the answer for a 5% solution. Therefore, 2.5 g is a reasonable answer.

Calculations for Preparing Parenteral Nutrition Orders with Stock Solutions

You are preparing a total parenteral nutrition order containing glycine 10% and dextrose 30% with a total volume of 500 mL. You have the following stock solutions: glycine 20%, dextrose 60%. What volume of the stock solutions are needed to prepare the total parenteral nutrition order?

When diluting a solution or dealing with stock solutions that contain a different concentration of substance than the solution being prepared, it is easiest to use the following equation for your calculations:

$$C_1 \times V_1 = C_2 \times V_2$$

C_1 is the concentration of the stock solution, V_1 is the volume of the stock solution needed to prepare the desired solution, C_2 is the concentration desired, and V_2 is the volume of the final/desired solution.

Because we are dealing with two different substances in this problem, we will have to use this equation twice.

$$\text{Glycine } 20\% \times (\text{mL glycine } 20\% \text{ needed}) = \text{glycine } 10\% \times 500 \text{ mL}$$

$$\text{mL glycine } 20\% \text{ needed} = (10 \times 500)/20 = 250 \text{ mL}$$

$$\text{Dextrose } 60\% \times (\text{mL dextrose } 60\% \text{ needed}) = \text{dextrose } 30\% \times 500 \text{ mL}$$

$$\text{mL dextrose } 60\% \text{ needed} = (30 \times 500)/60 = 250 \text{ mL}$$

In summary, we needed 250 mL of glycine 20% stock solution and 250 mL of dextrose 60% stock solution to prepare the 500 mL solution containing glycine 10% and dextrose 30%.

Drug Administration

Products Dosed in Drops

A prescription is written for tobramycin 0.3% eye drops; instill 1–2 drops into the left eye every four hours for 5 days. The eye drops are only available in 3 mL and 5 mL bottles. The conversion factor is 15 drops/mL. What size bottle will the patient need?

Some medications require very small amounts of liquid to be administered with each dose. Therefore, drops are used as the unit of measure for each dose. Eye drops, ear drops, and some oral liquids are dosed in drops. In order to calculate days' supply for these medications, it is necessary to know the conversion factor for drops to milliliters. Drop sizes can vary, but there are usually between 15 and 20 drops in each milliliter.

Eye drop example: A prescription is written for tobramycin 0.3% eye drops; instill 1–2 drops into the left eye every four hours for 5 days. The eye drops are only available in 3 mL and 5 mL bottles. The conversion factor is 15 drops/mL. What size bottle will the patient need?

For this problem, we need to work backward to solve for the quantity needed.

$$\text{Up to two drops} \times \text{one eye} \times \text{six times a day (every 4 hours)} \times 5 \text{ days} = 60 \text{ drops total}$$

Convert drops to mL:

$$60 \text{ drops} \div 15 \text{ drops/mL} = 4 \text{ mL needed}$$

Therefore, the patient will require a 5 mL bottle to complete the course.

Note: Don't forget to multiply by two if drops are being applied to both eyes.

ABBREVIATIONS USED IN THE PHARMACY

Abbreviation	Meaning
ACE	Angiotensin-converting enzyme
AD	Right ear
ADH	Antidiuretic hormone
ADR	Adverse drug reaction
AF, AFib	Atrial fibrillation (a type of heart arrhythmia)
AS	Left ear
AU	Both ears
BID	Twice per day
BMI	Body mass index
BP	Blood pressure
BPH	Benign prostatic hyperplasia
CNS	Central nervous system
CVS	Cardiovascular system
DEA	Drug Enforcement Administration
DMARD	Disease-modifying antirheumatic drug
DVT	Deep vein thrombosis
EKG/ECG	Electrocardiogram
ED	Erectile dysfunction
FDA	Food and Drug Administration
GFR	Glomerular filtration rate (measure of kidney function)
HBP	High blood pressure
HIV	Human immunodeficiency virus
HRT	Hormone replacement therapy
HSV	Herpes simplex virus
HTN	Hypertension
Ig	Immunoglobulin
IM	Intramuscular route of administration
INR	International normalized ratio (a test used to dose warfarin)
IR	Immediate release
LMWH	Low-molecular-weight heparin
MDI	Metered-dose inhaler
MI	Myocardial infarction (heart attack)
MR	Modified release (formulation)
MRI	Magnetic resonance imaging
MRSA	Methicillin-resistant Staphylococcus aureus
N/V/D	Nausea, vomiting, and diarrhea
NSAID	Nonsteroidal anti-inflammatory drug
NSTEMI	Non-ST elevation myocardial infarction (ST refers to the ST segment)
OD	Right eye
OS	Left eye
OTC	Over-the-counter
OU	Both eyes
PCA	Patient-controlled analgesia
PE	Pulmonary embolism
PO	By mouth
PPI	Proton pump inhibitor (acid suppressor)
PRN	As needed
Q	Every, as in "Every hour": qhr

Abbreviation	Meaning
SR	Sustained release (long acting)
SID	Once per day
SQ	Subcutaneous
SSRI	Selective serotonin reuptake inhibitor (antidepressant)
STEMI	ST elevation myocardial infarction
TID	Three times per day
TB	Tuberculosis
TCA	Tricyclic antidepressant
TIA	Transient ischemic attack (ministroke)
VTE	Venous thromboembolism
XR	Extended release (long acting)

Factors Affecting Absorption of Drugs

Drug absorption frequently occurs directly through the mucous membranes and the digestive tract, as the body seeks to equilibrate by taking in the substances found in the drug. Some drugs are less soluble and may not be absorbed and distributed as rapidly as other more soluble drugs. Further, a variety of additional factors unique to the body can impact drug absorption and distribution rates, including the drug's pKa (or ionization tendency), the pH (acidity or alkalinity) of the tissues, the perfusion of the tissues, and the overall volume of distribution (or Vd).

These factors can make the drug more unstable in the stomach and/or less able to penetrate the blood-brain barrier. Further, drugs given by mouth are absorbed into the intestines and then enter the hepatic portal circulation, which transports them directly to the liver. In the first-pass effect, the liver metabolizes many drugs using a biochemical process which prevents much of the original drug from entering the systemic circulation. Alternate routes of administration include intravenous, sublingual, and intramuscular injection methods. These methods can be used to avoid the first-pass effect.

Five Rights of Drug Administration

Medicines should be given in accordance with the **Five Rights of Drug Administration**, which are designed to produce a standard for dispensing drugs properly:

- The patient has the right to be the proper recipient (i.e., drugs must not be administered to the wrong patient).
- The patient has the right to receive the proper medication (i.e., the wrong drugs must not be given to the properly identified recipient).
- The patient has the right to receive the proper dosage.
- The patient has the right to be given the drug by the proper route (oral, injection, etc.).
- The patient has the right to receive the medication on time.

To facilitate these rights, the attending veterinarian is responsible for ensuring that the medication orders are clear and easily understood. The drug's label should be checked carefully, ideally 3 times, before being given to the patient: 1) when it is taken off the shelf, 2) when the dosage is being prepared (pills counted, injectables drawn up, etc.), and 3) when the dosage is being administered to the patient.

Drug Reference Materials

A review of the package insert or other drug reference material is required to gain specific knowledge about a drug's potential for harm, as well as its intended beneficial effects. In reading the indications for a drug, one should note the explanation concerning the expected therapeutic benefits. One should also note the appropriate use and application of the drug. Further, the literature should indicate if there are any known precautions or special considerations necessary to safely take the drug. Likewise, the literature should also note any explicit contraindications.

Contraindications are specific actions that are inadvisable to take while using a certain drug (i.e., concurrently taking certain other prescriptions, over-the-counter medications, or vitamins; eating certain foods; or engaging in certain activities). These actions could lead to adverse consequences. The literature should state any mild or significant side effects that could arise with typical usage of the drug. The literature may also provide directions to follow should accidental overdose occur, or steps to take in the event that serious but unintended effects of the drug arise.

Dosage Schedule and Tolerance

The package inserts or drug reference material includes information on when and where the drug should and should not be taken. For example, there may be a warning that the drug should be taken only on an empty stomach, or only with meals. Further, warnings may advise against certain activities or going out for prolonged periods in the sun. The literature should include information concerning appropriate dosages along with the required administration method (oral, suppository, patch, etc.) and the amount of the drug to be administered at requisite intervals.

There are times that the body can build up a tolerance for a drug, and warnings to this effect may also appear in any explanatory literature. Tolerance indicates that the response to the drug has lessened due to continued exposure over a long period of time. Tolerance may sometimes lead to higher amounts of medication usage than at prescribed intervals, to the point that the drug may become toxic to the body. In these cases, a drug overdose can occur. The literature should also explain what to do in cases of overdose. Both intentional and unintentional overdoses can be dangerous or even fatal, and thus will likely require prompt medical attention.

Extra-Label Drug Use (ELDU)

The **Federal Drug Administration (FDA)** is the agency responsible for the approval of all drugs to be used in the United States. Drugs that are approved by the FDA are approved for use under the specific conditions and diseases against which they were tested. However, not all drugs are used solely for the purposes approved by the FDA. In certain circumstances, the known pharmacological properties of a drug may suit it well for treating other diseases and conditions.

Therefore, a veterinarian may sometimes apply a drug in a manner other than for its approved purpose. In recognition that it is not possible to test every drug for every possible use, the FDA has made provisions for certain "off label" drug use or **extra-label drug use (ELDU)**. However, ELDU practices in veterinary medicine are still regulated by the **Animal Medicinal Drug Use Clarification Act (AMDUCA) of 1994**. This act specifies that ELDU medications can only be prescribed: a) by a licensed veterinarian, b) when the veterinarian has a legitimate veterinarian-client-patient relationship, and c) when no contaminants will result when the medication is provided to food-producing animals.

Animal Medicinal Drug Use Clarification Act of 1994 (AMDUCA)

Further ELDU criteria as clarified by the Animal Medicinal Drug Use Clarification Act of 1994 include the following: Medications considered for ELDU must still be listed for at least one approved purpose under FDA regulatory criteria before being administered to an animal or to a human being. The ELDU was not created to facilitate the mass production of drugs targeted for ELDU applications; instead, ELDU applications must be solely for therapeutic reasons in individually determined cases. The ELDU is applicable to those drugs that are given in the manufactured form of the drug or dispensed in a water solution.

ELDU strictly forbids the use of any drug that can become a contaminant to the human food supply or the environment. Specifically, any remaining residue that can risk or have a negative impact on the well-being of individual consumers or the community is strictly prohibited from use by the ELDU. Once the FDA has issued a ban against a specific ELDU drug application, that ELDU option is no longer permitted.

Eliminating Drugs from the Body

Elimination occurs by a metabolic process of breaking down and reconfiguring the original substance until it can be successfully excreted. The liver is the primary organ in this metabolic process, although other organs may be involved, as well. The liver uses enzymatic systems to change or break down the drug, which is then referred to as a metabolite. Some common examples of enzymes involved in these metabolic processes include cytochrome P450 oxidase and flavin-containing monooxygenase.

Some metabolites can be more potent or toxic to the animal than the original drug. Once a water-soluble metabolite is formed, the kidneys remove it from the body via the **urine**. Metabolites may also be excreted in **sweat** and **feces**. However, a patient that has poorly functioning kidneys or a damaged liver may not be able to metabolize and discharge drugs at a sufficient rate to avoid a systemic build-up and consequent toxic effects.

Drug Withdrawal Times

A drug introduced into an animal that is a future food source has the potential to be passed on to the consumer. Therefore, any drug that is administered to a food animal must be carefully monitored. The timing of the withdrawal of any medication before slaughter is particularly important to ensure that the drug is fully metabolized and excreted out of the animal, and thus is not passed on to the human consumer.

Requisite withdrawal timelines are printed on the outside label of the drug's container. There is also printed material available in other publications to give the veterinarian more information about necessary withdrawal procedures. Drugs which are extra-label, or ELDU drugs, have particularly strict guidelines for early withdrawal from animals to be used as food products. By contrast, ELDU drugs administered to companion or service animals (dogs, cats, horses, mules, etc.) do not have similarly strict withdrawal procedures.

Residual Drugs in Food Source Animals

Residual medications in food source animals may induce a number of negative consequences in human consumers. The adverse effects that the human consumer may experience include a number of severe medical conditions. One danger is a **systemic toxicological effect** (a poisonous condition) that impacts the entire body. Another danger is the likelihood of **mutagenicity**, as some residual drugs may cause the cells in the body to mutate or change. Other residual drugs may become **carcinogenic**, predisposing the consumer to develop cancer. Still other residual drugs may affect the reproductive system. These drugs can prevent pregnancy or cause harmful or even **teratogenic** (i.e., non-inherited deformative) side effects in the unborn fetus.

Further, some residual antimicrobial drugs may alter the human intestinal flora and cause digestive ailments. The overuse of antimicrobials may also cause virulent bacteria such as Salmonella and Campylobacter to become drug resistant. Where withdrawal delays occur, testing can become necessary. However, drug residue studies can be expensive, and there is little incentive to carry out these examinations. Thus, careful adherence to drug administration and withdrawal guidelines is essential.

Administering Drugs and Taking Samples in Cattle

The **jugular vein** is the ideal spot to administer large amounts of fluids and/or medications to an animal. The animal's head is held immobile through the use of a head catch device, pulled away from the side of the animal needing treatment. The syringe must be of adequate size (measured in mL or cc) for the liquid being injected. The needle used usually ranges from 16-18 gauge (the smaller the number the larger the bore) and 1-3 inches in length.

The **tail vein** is ideal for smaller quantities of fluid. Smaller cattle should be held securely in place while bending the tail straight forward from its base. The syringe must be of adequate size for the liquid being injected, with a needle that ranges in bore diameter from 18-20 gauge and about 1.0-1.5 inches in length. A smaller size syringe is applicable for the administration of more modest amounts of fluid.

The **milk vein** is another option; however, this vein does have a tendency to form hematomas. The needle used with this vein is frequently 14 gauge and 2-3 inches in length.

ADMINISTERING DRUGS AND TAKING SAMPLES IN PIGS

Swine should be given large quantities of intravenous liquid through the cranial vena cava. The mature swine requires use of an 18- to 20-gauge needle, 3-4 inches in length. This is comparable in length to a 7.5-10 cm needle. The jugular fossa closest to the manubrium sterni of the pig can be employed as a guide to ensure proper placement or alignment into the cranial vena cava. The needle must be inserted in a perpendicular direction toward the neck, facing the left shoulder.

The ear artery is known as the caudal auricular artery. This artery is ideal for giving the pig smaller quantities of liquid. The syringe should be inserted with gentle pressure. The syringe must be of adequate size for the liquid being injected. The needle used usually ranges from 18-22 gauge and 1-1.5 inches in length. This needle is comparable to a 2.5-3.75 cm needle length. Intravenous administrations given within the caudal auricular vein typically require the use of a 19- to 21-gauge butterfly needle.

Preparing Medications

COMMON PHARMACY INSTRUMENTS

A **pill cutter** is commonly used to cut pills in half or in quarters in order to get the correct strength of medication that the patient will need. A **pill counter tray** is a smooth-surfaced, plastic tray used to sort and count pills or capsules with a small plastic spatula. Using the spatula to sort and count the pills limits direct handling by the veterinary technician and allows for a more convenient and accurate count. Depending on the veterinarian's instruction, the veterinary technician must be able to calculate the appropriate amount and strength of medication to go home with the patient. For example, the veterinarian asks for 30 days' worth of cefpodoxime 100 mg tablets to be given at half a tablet twice daily. Using the pill counter tray and spatula, in increments of 5, count out 30 tablets. Then using the pill cutter, cut all of the tablets in half.

EYE MEDICATIONS

Eye medications come in suspensions, ointments, and serum drops. If the veterinarian asks to have a certain eye medication filled for the patient, the veterinary technician must create a label for the medication. You must be sure you have the patient's name, client's first and last names, and date on the label. The name of the medication as well as the strength of the medication must be on the label also. For instructions, you must include how many drops or how much ointment to apply to which eye or both eyes, how many times per day, and for how long. All instructions must be gone over with the client to ensure compliance.

EAR MEDICATIONS

In order to effectively administer ear medications to the patient, the medication must get into the ear canal where the infection is. For bacterial or yeast infections, the ears can be treated with regular ear cleanings, topical or oral antibiotics, or antifungals. Antibiotics and antifungal medications are normally administered by putting a quarter-sized amount of medication down into the ear canals and then massaging underneath the ear to move the medication further down. The ears can be cleaned with a cleansing and drying cleaner as well, which works by drying once it is inside the ear so when the pet shakes its head, the debris is expelled. Ear mites are treated by using a one-time-use medication in each ear that kills the ear mites. Veterinary staff should remind the client to come back to recheck the ears once they have finished medicating to make sure the infection has been cleared.

Oral Medications

Often, pet owners will have to administer medications orally to their pet, whether for a couple of weeks or for life. Giving a pet an oral medication in tablet or capsule form can be done for a dog by holding open its mouth wide and placing the pill as far back in the throat as possible and then closing its mouth. Hold the dog's head up and rub its neck while holding the dog's mouth shut with one hand to be sure the pill is swallowed. Sometimes it is not possible for the owner to put the medication into the dog's mouth, especially if it is trying to bite. The pill can be hidden inside a soft treat or a small ball of canned food and then fed to the dog. As for cats, the easiest way to administer a tablet or capsule is to open the cat's mouth and place the pill quickly on the back of the tongue. Because the cat's tongue is rough and the pill will stick to it, swallowing it is easy. Liquid medications are usually administered with a dropper or syringe. By placing the end of the dispenser in the corner of the pet's mouth, you can administer the medication slowly to ensure the pet swallows it all.

Chapter Quiz

Ready to see how well you retained what you just read? Scan the QR code to go directly to the chapter quiz interface for this study guide. If you're using a computer, simply visit the online resources page at **mometrix.com/resources719/vtne** and click the Chapter Quizzes link.

Surgical Nursing

Transform passive reading into active learning! After immersing yourself in this chapter, put your comprehension to the test by taking a quiz. The insights you gained will stay with you longer this way. Scan the QR code to go directly to the chapter quiz interface for this study guide. If you're using a computer, simply visit the online resources page at **mometrix.com/resources719/vtne** and click the Chapter Quizzes link.

Surgical Anatomy and Physiology

Anatomical Direction

The descriptive terms of **anatomical direction** can be grouped according to varying similarities in reference points. **Cranial** is directed toward the head. **Caudal** is directed toward the tail. **Dorsal** is directed toward the backbone. **Ventral** is directed toward the belly. On the head, **rostral** is directed toward the nose.

On limbs or appendages, **proximal** refers to a location closer to the body; **distal** refers to a location farthest from the body. **Palmar** describes the ground or bottom surface of a front foot, hoof, or paw. **Plantar** describes the ground or bottom surface of the hind foot, hoof, or paw.

Medial is directed toward the median plane; **lateral** is directed away from the median plane.

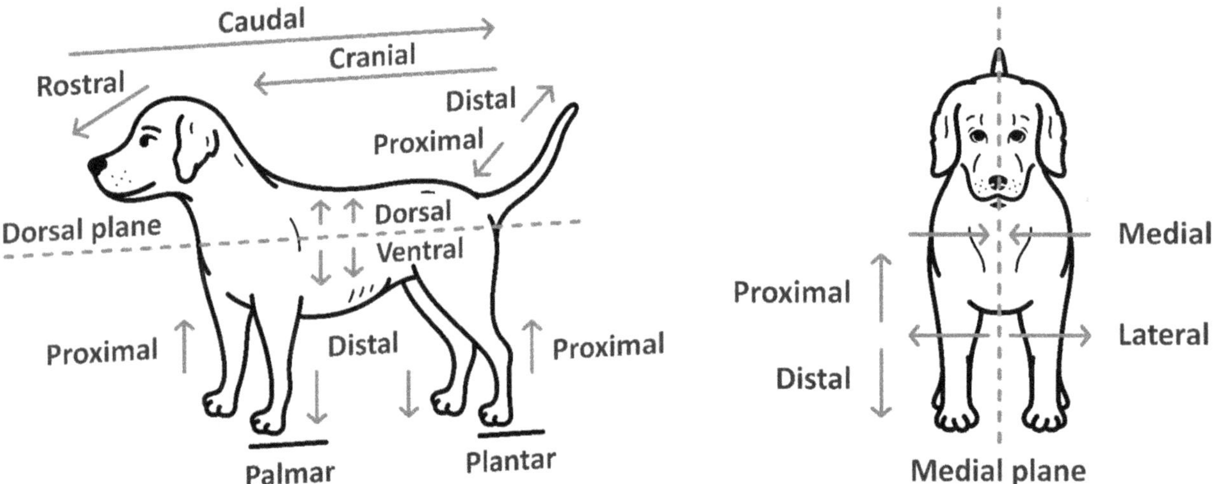

Classification and Characteristics of Bones

Bones are typically classified by shape, often using 4 categories: **long, short, flat,** and **irregular**. However, other classification systems use 6 categories: **long, short, flat, pneumatic, sesamoid**, and **irregular** (or sutural).

- **Long bones** grow primarily through a lengthening of the **diaphysis** (shaft), the midsection of the long bone. The diaphysis has two rounded ends which are called **epiphyses**. The long bone also has a marrow cavity, also called a **medullary cavity**, which is the central section of bone where the yellow bone marrow is kept. Examples include the radius and femur.
- The **short bones** share some similar structural characteristics found in the long bones. However, the short bones do not have a medullary cavity in which to house yellow bone marrow. Short bone examples include the bony digits within the hand and fingers.

- **Flat bones** are thin, level, horizontal bones that are formed from two layers of compact bone with a middle layer of cancellous bone. The skull bones, ribs, pelvis, and scapula are all classified as flat bones.
- **Pneumatic bones** have an air-filled cavity or indentation, such as those found in the sinuses.
- **Sesamoid bones** are small, short bones of an irregular spherical or sesame seed-like shape that help alleviate some of the stress caused by friction and reduce pressures otherwise applied to a tendon or joint. One example of a sesamoid bone is the patella.
- **Irregular bones** are bones with irregular shapes; they include hip bones, vertebrae, and several skull bones.

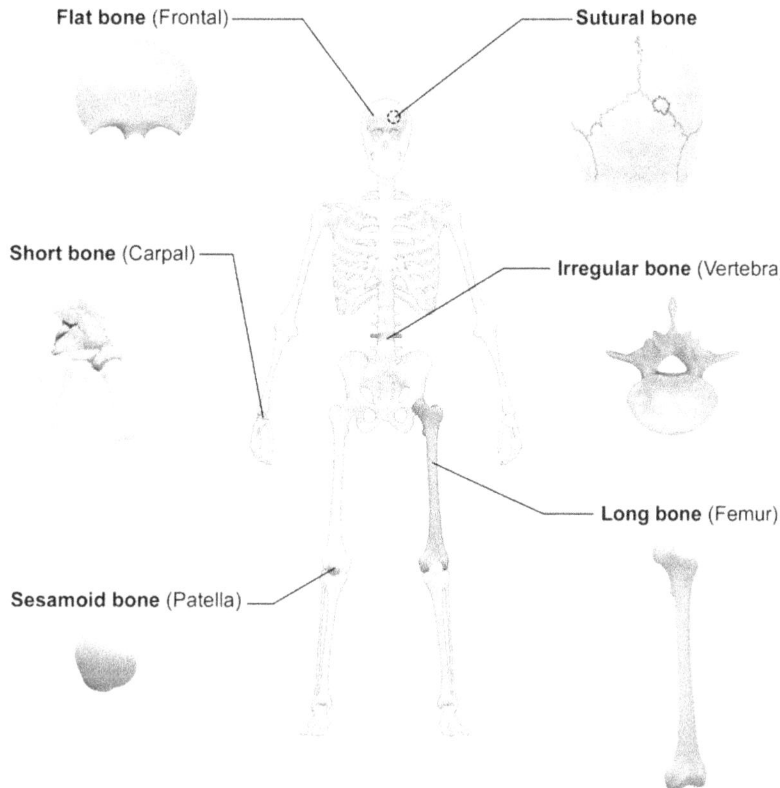

Classification of Bones by Shape

Compact Bone

There are two types of bone tissue, compact and spongy. Compact bone provides structural strength and support and allows for strenuous movement and weight-bearing activities.

Compact bone is composed of very tightly grouped **osteons** (also called *haversian systems*). Each osteon is comprised of a solid matrix of osseous lamellae (concentric rings of deposited minerals and proteins) surrounding a central canal containing blood vessels to nurture the bone. Between the lamellar rings are

osteocytes (bone cells) situated in **lacunae** (small spaces). Channels called **canaliculi** extend from the lacunae to the osteonic (or haversian) canal. Nutrition is brought in through the canaliculi, and waste is moved out.

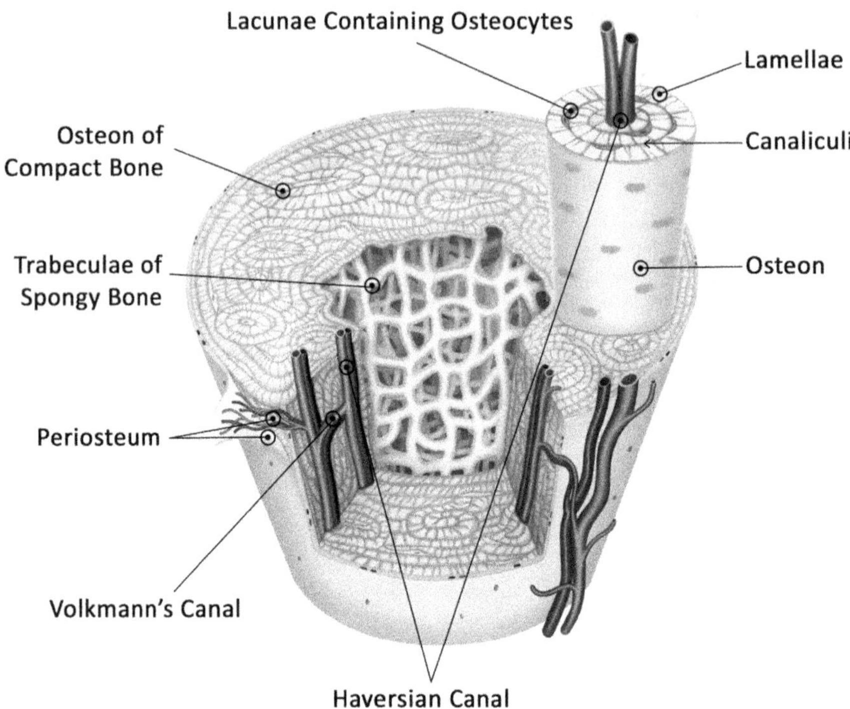

Cancellous Bone

There are two types of bone tissue: compact bone and spongy (also called *trabecular* or *cancellous*) bone. **Cancellous bone** is found inside and at the rounded ends of long bones, in the pelvic bones and breastbone. Its primary purpose is to protect bone marrow and to provide interior structural support. Cancellous bone is honeycomb-like in appearance, with cavities and spaces interspersed with bony plates and ridges known as **trabeculae**. Trabeculae are arranged to provide maximum support for stresses and loads incurred and may gradually rearrange themselves in response to new stresses or burdens.

Cancellous bone does not receive nourishment via osteonic canals (i.e., haversian systems), but rather via **canaliculi** connecting the various spaces within the trabecular structure. Osseous trabeculae may be composed of mineralized bone or collagen. **Collagen** is a connective tissue made up of fibrous proteins. The larger trabecular spaces are filled with red bone **marrow**, where the production of blood cellular components takes place.

Skeletal Articulations

A **skeletal articulation**, also called a joint, exists whenever two bones come together for purposes of movement. A **joint** is structurally created when tissue binds two or more bones together. The tissue can consist of fibrous, elastic, or cartilaginous materials. Joints can be classified by way of the type of articulation: synarthrosis, amphiarthrosis, and diarthrosis.

Synarthrosis joints are fixed in a permanent position. An example can be seen in the suture joints of the skull. **Amphiarthrosis joints** allow only limited movement, such as the pubic symphysis. Symphysis indicates that the bones merge naturally. **Diarthrosis** refers to a joint that is capable of changing position in multiple directions. An example would be the shoulder, which has the capacity for a wide range of motion.

Joint Classification

Three types of joint classifications are: fibrous, cartilaginous, and synovial. **Fibrous joints** are bony articulations joined by strong fibers. These joints are intended to move little, if at all. One example of a fibrous joint can be seen in the skull sutures. The only time these joints move is during the process of birth, to accommodate the confines of the birth canal. However, they persist in fibrous form as points of subsequent cranial growth. In late adulthood they eventually fuse.

Joints that are linked by cartilage without a joint cavity are known as **cartilaginous joints**. Cartilage is a strong, stretchy tissue. Cartilaginous joint examples include intervertebral discs and the pubic symphysis.

Synovial joints are identified by the presence of synovial fluid, a clear, viscous fluid that provides the joint with lubrication and nourishment. These joints have a joint capsule or sac which contains synovial fluid. The synovial membrane (or bursa) is a thin layer of tissue that encloses both cartilaginous and non-cartilaginous surfaces, creating a joint capsule. The synovial membrane is responsible for the secretion of the synovial fluid. The limb joints found within the body are synovial joints. Synovial joints can also be diarthrotic joints.

Muscle Tissue

Muscle tissue consists of three main subtypes known as skeletal, smooth, and cardiac muscle. **Skeletal muscle** is striated contractile tissue attached to the skeleton. It has alternating light and dark bands under microscopic view, and it is responsible for voluntary control and movement.

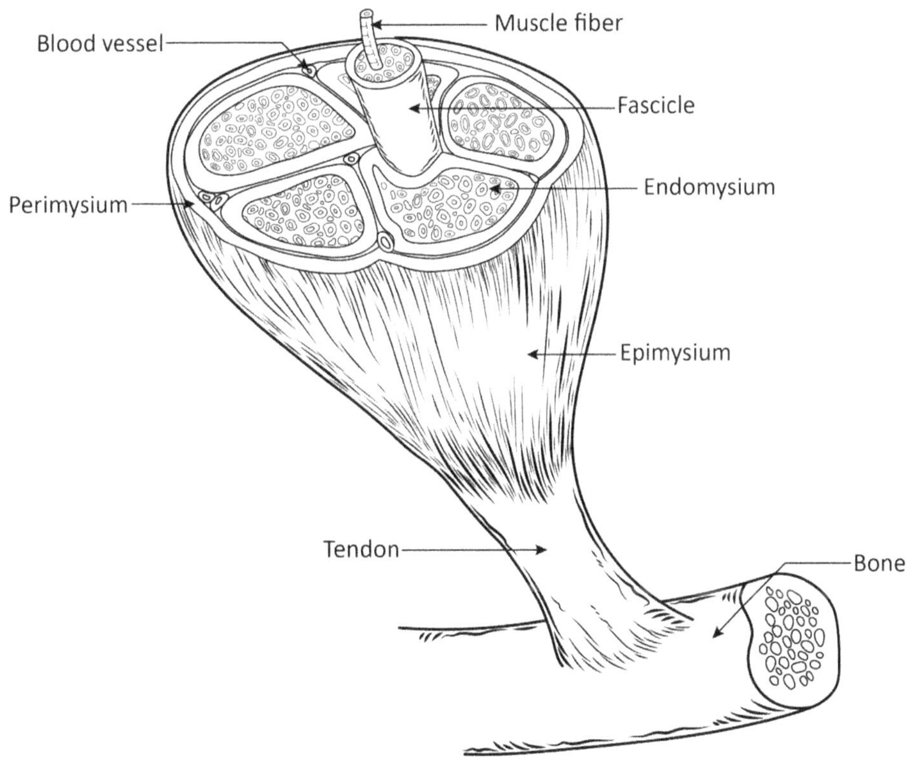

Smooth muscle is involuntarily controlled muscle and is found in the walls of the hollow organs. It moves much more slowly, has no striations, and is autonomically regulated. Hollow organs, specifically, the blood vessels, bladder, uterus, and gastrointestinal tract derive dilation, contraction, and peristaltic movement from smooth muscle.

Cardiac muscle is located in the heart. It is also striated, but unlike striated skeletal muscle, it is involuntarily controlled.

Nervous System

Neurons are nerve cells that transmit signals or impulses, to coordinate a reaction to stimuli, or to produce voluntary actions or responses. Neuroglia or **glial cells** are a network of tissues and fibers found in the brain and spinal column that provide support, protection, and nutrition to neurons, among other functions.

The **central nervous system** consists of the brain and the spinal cord. The brain itself consists of the cerebrum (the two hemispheres that collectively make up the forebrain and midbrain), the cerebellum, and the brain stem (connecting the brain and spinal cord).

The **spinal cord** is housed in the vertebral column. The spinal cord sends out nerve impulses or signals by way of efferent nerve paths and receives them by way of afferent nerve paths. Thus, afferent nerves transmit signals or sensory impulses from stimuli to the central nervous system, while efferent nerves send impulses or signals away from the brain to the organs or muscles.

The **meninges** are three layers of membranes which function to protect the central nervous system: the dura mater, the arachnoid mater, and the pia mater. The meninges are dense, fibrous connective tissues that enclose the spinal cord and the brain.

Cerebrospinal fluid (CSF) is a clear, water-like fluid found in and around the brain and the spinal cord. CSF cushions the central nervous system when jostled and is a source of nourishment for the brain. The fluid contains essential protein, glucose, and ions.

The **blood-brain barrier (BBB)** allows certain liquids or substances to pass through to the central nervous system while preventing the entrance of many others. It is yet another form of protection for the brain. Blood contains oxygen, glucose, and fat-soluble compounds that are able to pass through the blood-brain barrier. However, the blood-brain barrier keeps out waste products and many drugs.

Anatomy of the Ear

The ear is the organ responsible for hearing and balance in mammals. The ear has three main parts: the outer ear, middle ear, and the inner ear. The **outer ear** includes the pinna (the visible outside ear or auricle), the auditory canal, and the tympanic membrane or eardrum. The **middle ear** transmits sound from the outer ear to the inner ear via three articulating bones called ossicles: the malleus, the incus, and the stapes. These bones are also referred to as the hammer, the anvil, and the stirrup, respectively. The small bones vibrate to amplify and relay sound waves from the eardrum to the inner ear. The Eustachian tube links the middle ear to the nasal cavity. The liquid in the inner ear helps maintain balance. The **inner ear** consists of the cochlea and the semicircular canals. The cochlea is coiled in shape like a snail shell. The cochlea has thousands of hair cells that move in response to sound waves, generating auditory nerve impulses in response. The organ of Corti, the principal section of the cochlea, translates the neural impulses into sounds. The sound transmission is conducted by an impulse that makes its way from the brain along the auditory nerve.

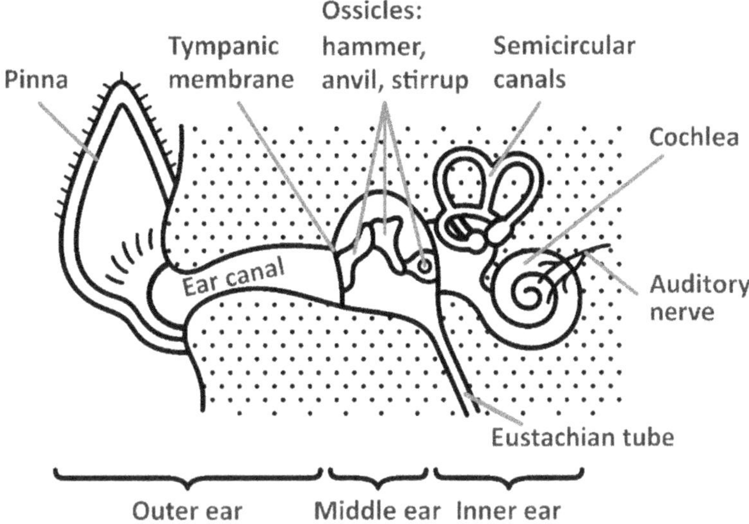

Whole Blood

Whole blood is made up of fluid and cellular substances that join to carry out specific functions within the body. **Plasma** is a very light yellowish fluid that is the primary liquid in which hematic cells are dispersed to form whole blood. Plasma is 90% water and 10% blood plasma proteins.

The hematic cells in whole blood each have a specific function within the body: Erythrocytes (red blood cells), leukocytes (white blood cells), and thrombocytes (platelets) make up the cellular components in whole blood. The substance in the plasma that is responsible for clotting is known as **fibrinogen protein**. Removal of fibrinogen protein leaves serum.

Blood transports dissolved proteins, oxygen, carbon dioxide, hormones, lipids, and metabolic end products within the body. The blood flows within the circulatory system as the heart pumps blood to the lungs before it returns to the heart and is then circulated throughout the body.

Oxygenation of Blood

The oxygenation of blood is completed by way of the cardiac cycle, through the heart's four chambers. The right atrium is the part of the heart that accepts deoxygenated blood from the superior and inferior vena cava. The vena cava is the largest vein that carries blood back to the heart. From the right atrium, deoxygenated blood is sent into the right ventricle. The right ventricle then contracts, moving the deoxygenated blood into the lungs. The lungs are responsible for the diffusion of carbon dioxide out of the blood in exchange for oxygen diffusion into the bloodstream, as gaseous molecular equilibrium is obtained. The oxygenated blood then flows out of the lungs and into the left atrium. The left atrium is the upper left chamber of the heart. Once filled with oxygenated blood, the left atrium contracts, pumping blood into the left ventricle, where its contraction pumps the blood to the aorta and to the rest of the body.

Blood Vessels

Blood is the fluid that flows within the body's vascular system, bringing oxygen and nutrients to tissues and removing carbon dioxide and other waste products. **Arterial vessels** carry oxygenated blood away from the heart, and **venous vessels** carry deoxygenated blood to the heart. The pulmonary vein is unique in that it is responsible for carrying oxygenated blood to the heart from the lungs. Oxygenated blood is blood that has been combined with oxygen, and from which carbon dioxide has been removed.

The blood is moved under pressure from the heart. Artery walls are thicker than the walls of veins, as they must sustain direct cardiac pumping pressures. However, on average, veins are larger in diameter and have many one-way valves to facilitate the passive return process. Larger arteries divide into smaller blood vessels known as arterioles. The **arterioles** distribute blood from the arteries to the capillaries.

The force of blood applied at regular intervals by way of cardiac contraction is known as **blood pressure**.

Capillary and Venous Return Systems

Capillaries have walls that are constructed from a single layer of endothelium. This allows the exchange of carbon dioxide and oxygen gases by molecular diffusion, as well as the osmotic exchange of nutrient fluids and waste molecules (such as glucose and urea) via the capillary stream. Capillaries are the smallest blood vessels in the body. They also serve as a depressurizing link between the arteries and veins in the body.

A **vein** is any blood vessel that returns blood to the heart, which usually involves the transport of deoxygenated blood; the pulmonary vein carries *oxygenated* blood back to the heart. Venous walls are much thinner than arterial walls, as they accommodate a much lower blood pressure than that of the arteries. Veins have interspersed one-way valves as an essential feature, to prevent any backflow of deoxygenated blood. Backflow could otherwise be caused by low blood pressures in the body. Venules are the venous counterpart to arterioles and carry blood back to larger venous vessels.

Pre-Gastric and Gastric Digestion

Digestion is the physical and chemical breakdown of food material so that the body can absorb and use its nutrients. **Mastication** (chewing) in the mouth is the starting point in the digestive process; the digestive process terminates in the excretion of waste.

In mammals, food enters the mouth to be ground up into smaller particles by the teeth and tongue before being swallowed. The first digestive enzymes are introduced, primarily **salivary amylase**, which breaks down carbohydrates. Once swallowed, the esophagus carries the ingesta down to the **stomach**.

Ruminant digestion varies from monogastric digestion at this point. Monogastrics have a relatively small glandular stomach. There, ingesta is physically mixed by the muscular stomach walls with both hydrochloric acid (at a pH of 1.5-3.5) and **pepsin**, an enzyme that breaks down protein. Examples of monogastrics include dogs, cats, and pigs.

Variations: Ruminants

The ruminant stomach contains four specialized compartments: the rumen, reticulum, omasum, and abomasum. Examples of ruminants include cows, goats, and sheep.

From the ruminant esophagus, ingesta is dropped past the reticulum into the rumen. The lining of the **reticulum** has a hexagonal honeycomb pattern. It acts as a garbage-catch to trap ingested non-food items such as wires or nails that might cause hardware disease. Its high surface area allows for absorption of volatile fatty acids produced in the rumen.

The **rumen** is an anaerobic fermentation vat; the rumen microbes convert carbohydrates to volatile fatty acids (VFAs) via fermentation. Protein and non-protein nitrogen are broken down to ammonia and amino acids. The rumen microbiome allows ruminants to utilize energy sources indigestible by other species.

The **omasum** absorbs water, magnesium, and bicarbonate and further grinds feed. The omasum is located between the reticulum and the abomasum. The **abomasum** is the glandular stomach compartment on a ruminant animal responsible for acid and enzymatic digestion.

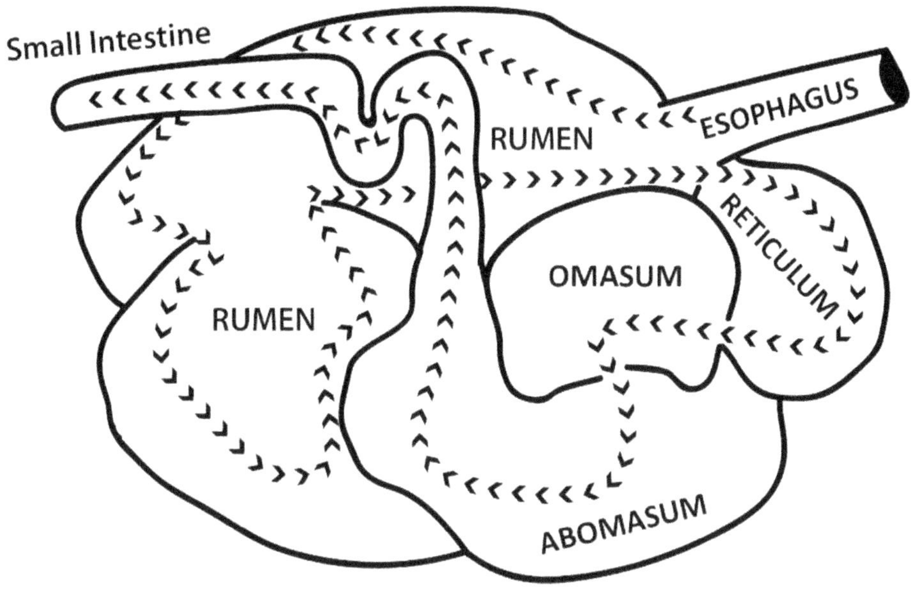

Ingesta is masticated, swallowed, regurgitated, and remasticated in a process called **rumination**, which requires as much as 150 L of saliva daily and increases the rate of digestion. The remasticated food is then re-swallowed and settles into layers of solid matter and liquid matter in the rumen.

Post-Gastric Digestion

After being acted upon by the gastric juices, ingesta becomes a softened, semi-solid mass called **chyme**, a combination of water, hydrochloric acid, and digestive enzymes. Chyme is passed from the stomach into the **duodenum**, the first section of the small intestine. The pancreas releases the enzymes **trypsin** and **pancreatic lipase** to be blended with the chyme. From there, the digesta travels to the **jejunum** and **ileum**, the second and third sections of the small intestine, and then to the large intestine, where excess water is absorbed. The ileum and the large intestine are host to considerable bacteria, many of which act to synthesize niacin (nicotinic acid), thiamin (vitamin B1), and vitamin K, which are then absorbed into the body. Finally, digesta is transported to the rectum, located between the colon and the anal canal. The body releases this undigested food as feces, which passes through the anus.

Bilirubin

Bilirubin is a brownish-yellow substance found in **bile**. It is the by-product of hemoglobin breakdown, released when aging or superfluous red blood cells are broken down by reticuloendothelial cells found in the liver, spleen, and bone marrow. Other chromoproteins may also contain heme and thus contribute to the formation of bilirubin when broken down. Bilirubin is responsible for the yellowish appearance in bruises, as well as the yellow, icteric appearance of the skin when jaundice develops, typically due to liver dysfunction. Bilirubin is formed by the metabolism of heme, which is the deep red iron-containing pigment found in the blood. As red blood cells die, they are broken down into heme and globin. Eventually the heme is changed into Fe^{2+}, carbon monoxide, and bilirubin.

Urinary System

The **excretory system** discharges metabolic waste through defecation or urination. The urinary system is made up of the kidneys, ureters, urinary bladder, and the urethra. The **kidneys** remove liquid waste from the bloodstream.

Each species of animal has a specifically shaped and sized kidney, although most are shaped in the form of a bean. The **ureters** are urinary ducts responsible for transporting urine away from the kidneys and into the bladder in mammals. The ureter is fashioned from smooth muscle. The **urinary bladder** is a hollow, stretchy sac used for urine storage. Urine is collected and stored until it is discharged. Urine ultimately passes through the urethra, which is a tube extending from the bladder to the body's exterior. The urethra is fashioned from smooth muscle, with a sphincter between itself and the bladder that operates under voluntary control for this discharge process.

Renal Structure

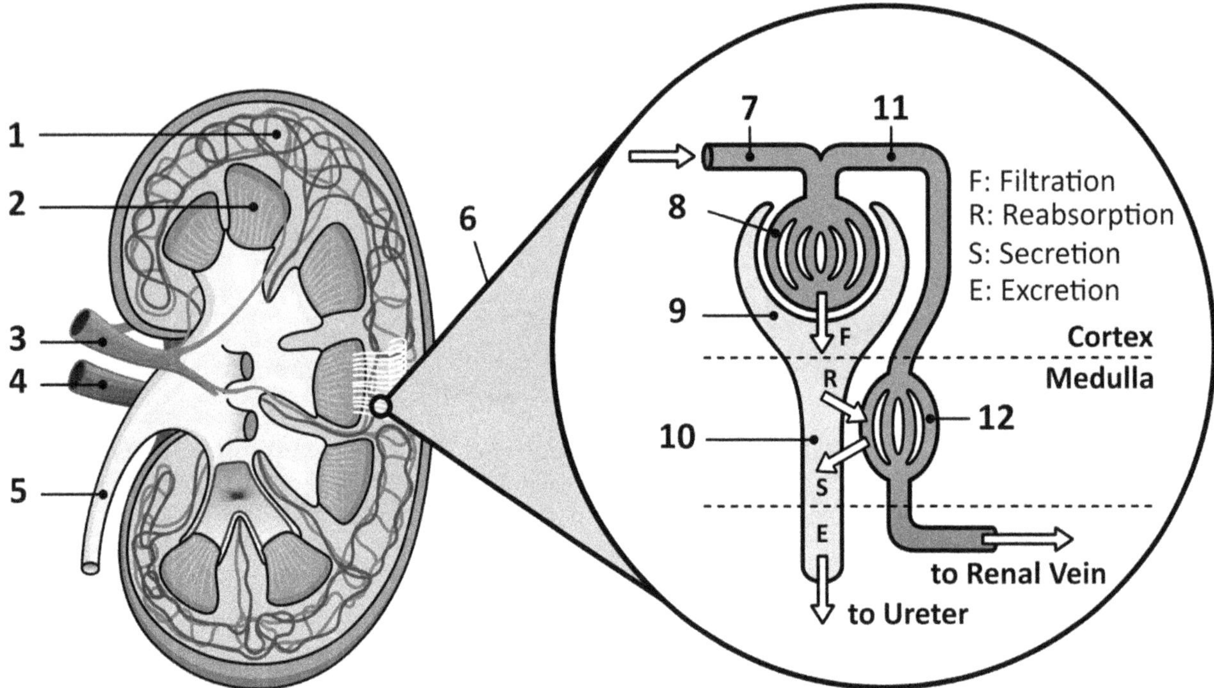

1. Renal cortex
2. Renal medulla
3. Renal artery
4. Renal vein
5. Ureter
6. Nephron
7. Afferent arteriole
8. Glomerulus
9. Bowman's capsule
10. Proximal convoluted tubule
11. Efferent arteriole
12. Peritubular capillaries

Urine Production

There are three phases of urine production: filtration, reabsorption, and secretion. **Filtration** occurs in one of the many nephrons found in the kidney. Within each nephron is a circular-shaped cluster of capillaries called the **glomerulus**. It resides under a thin, double-membraned outer covering called **Bowman's capsule**. High pressures from the renal artery force water, salt, and other small molecules out of the glomerulus. This solution of water, salt, and other molecules is known as glomerular filtrate. This solution is then filtered through Bowman's capsule. Bowman's capsule is responsible for removing waste products, inorganic salts, and excess water.

Reabsorption occurs when nutrients that are left over from this filtration process are reabsorbed into the body through renal tubules. Principally, this is carried out in the **proximal convoluted tubules** (PCTs), with reabsorbed materials entering the surrounding peritubular capillaries. The process of concentrating and absorbing salts is carried out in the nephron tubule known as the loop of Henle.

During **secretion**, blood pH is regulated in the distal convoluted tubules (DCTs) by processes of absorption and secretion, with certain substances released into the DCTs from the peritubular capillaries.

Surgical Equipment

Surgical Scissors

Scissors can be categorized based on the shape of the blade, the point of the tip, or the cutting edge, and there are a variety of scissors used in veterinary surgery. The types include:

- **Operating scissors** are very common and are used for cutting sutures and drape material.
- **Mayo scissors** are used in cutting away thick tissue or sutures in dissection.
- **Metzenbaum scissors** are used in cutting away fragile tissue in dissection because they allow delicate cuts to be made with a longer handle versus a shorter blade.
- **Iris scissors** are small, fragile, and have a very sharp, pointed tip.
- **Wire-cutting scissors** are used in cutting away wire sutures; they have a short, bulky jaw with a saw-toothed blade edge.
- **Littauer and Spencer suture removal scissors** are used for suture removal because they have blunt tips and a blade that is shaped like a finely arched hook.
- **Lister Bandage scissors** are used for bandage removal because they have flat, dense ends with dull lower-blade tips.

Thumb Forceps

Thumb forceps have a structure that incorporates the use of a spring apparatus and can be applied as either tissue or dressing forceps. They should be held as one would hold a pencil. The various thumb forceps used include:

- **Tissue forceps** are used to grasp tissue with tips that resemble teeth.
- **Adson tissue forceps** provide a strong grip. However, this strong grip does little harm to fragile tissue—largely because the structure of the Adson tissue forceps includes a solitary tooth-like tip.
- **Brown-Adson tissue forceps** are similar to the Adson forceps. However, these forceps have a wide, easy-to-hold handle and a tip with 16 thinly shaped teeth that mesh or engage with each other.

- **Russian tissue forceps** grasp hollow internal organs more easily due to their rounded tips. In the application and removal of dressing material, these dressing forceps are particularly beneficial. These forceps are structured with a smooth blade edge.
- **Dressing forceps** hold the tissue or dressings with smooth or smoothly serrated tips.

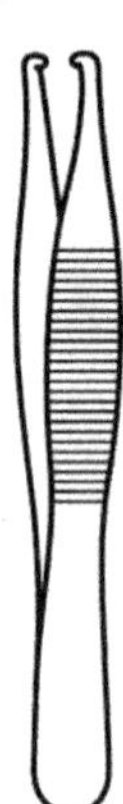

Self-Retaining Forceps

Self-retaining forceps have a ratchet-like mechanism which turns in one direction. Types include:

- **Allis tissue forceps** hold tissue in place with short, interlocking teeth.
- **Babcock tissue forceps** grasp fragile tissue without causing additional trauma because they don't have gripping teeth. The instrument has a very wide, flared tip that securely holds the tissue in place.

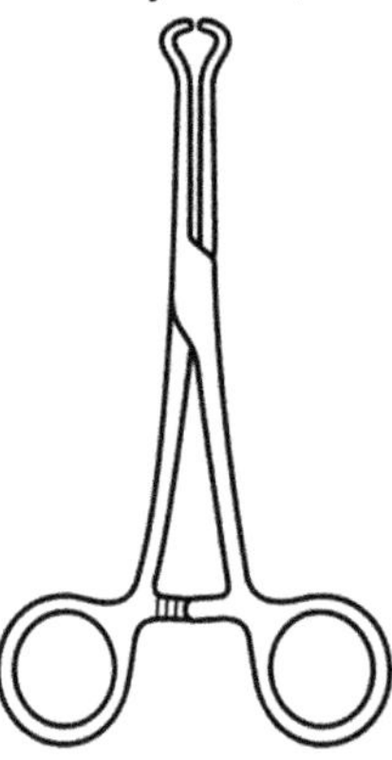

- **Doyen intestinal forceps** hold bowel in place and can close off the lumen of the bowel. However, the structure of the instrument prevents the target tissue from being crushed. It has notches like a row of teeth on a saw which extend from the top to the bottom.

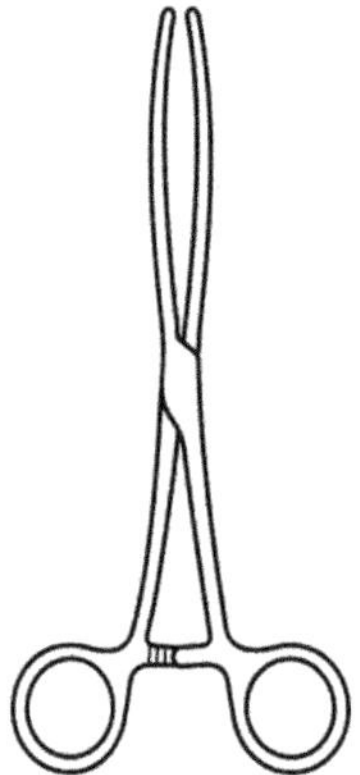

- **Ferguson angiotribe forceps** hold large bands of parallel tissues in place.
- **Sponge forceps** are used in surgical procedures or in preparation for surgery. These forceps can also provide hemostasis, which means that bleeding may be stopped. This instrument has a hole in its end which can be straight, curved, smooth, or serrated.
- **Backhaus towel clamps** firmly fix in place the drapes to folds of the patient's skin. The structure of this instrument has arched tips.

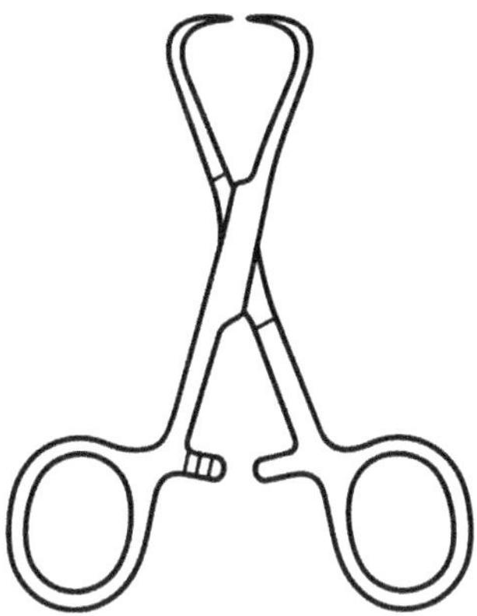

Hemostatic Forceps

Hemostatic forceps are used to stop bleeding by firmly clamping and holding blood vessels closed. They can be hinged, curved, or straight.

The Kelly and Crile forceps are applied to securely hold larger blood vessels and tissue in place. The standard length of the instrument is 12.5 cm or 4.5 inches. The **Kelly forceps** have transverse grooves which lie distally, or away from the point of attachment; Kelly forceps are applied to stump and pedicle surgical tying procedures or ligations. The **Crile forceps** have transverse grooves.

Halsted mosquito forceps are applied to capillary bleeders. They have a thin tip that may be arched or straight. The jaw has crosswise serrations. The length of this instrument is 10 cm or 4 inches.

Rochester-Pean, **Rochester-Carmalt**, and **Rochester-Ochsner** forceps have some similarities. The longest ones are the Rochester-Pean and the Rochester-Carmalt forceps: These 2 instruments are measured at 20 cm or 9 inches long. For every tooth on the Rochester-Ochsner forceps, an additional tooth has been added to the Rochester-Pean forceps. Rochester-Pean forceps have grooves which lie in a crisscross or transverse direction. Rochester-Carmalt forceps include grooves which extend from the top to the bottom of the device.

Needle Holders

Needle holders are hinged forceps that hold arched suturing needles during surgery. **Mayo-Hegar needle holders** are the heavier of the two types of needle-holding forceps used and do not have a cutting blade. The blade on the **Olsen-Hegar needle** holders cuts sutures, eliminating the need for an extra set of scissors.

Needle holders are constructed with a system of interconnected grooves on the ends. The Mayo-Hegar and Olsen-Hegar needle holders hold the needle in place during a surgical procedure. The **Mathieu needle holders** open and close at a touch of the fingers, as this instrument does not have loops for the fingers to be placed inside.

Retractors

Retractors pull back, hold, and secure tissue or organs during surgery, allowing the veterinarian unobstructed access to the operation site. Retractors can be either manually operated or self-retaining instruments. The retractors which fall into the manual operation category include: Senn, Meyerding, Hohmann, US Army, and malleable retractors.

Senn retractors are constructed with two tips consisting of either dull or sharp blade edges and are used for superficial retraction purposes on the outside of the skin. The dull blade edge is applied to regions where delicate tissue is held in place. The sharper blade edge is used to secure the fascia. Meyerding, Hohmann, and US Army retractors are applied in the securing of larger muscle mass. These instruments also serve to secure more superficial incisions that do not run as deep.

SELF-RETAINING RETRACTORS

Self-retaining retractors have a locking function and are able to retract and secure tissue. Balfour, Finochietto, Snook, and Covault retractors are all self-retaining devices. **Balfour retractors** are constructed for use in abdominal surgical procedures which are far from the surface of the skin. This instrument secures an incision's outermost layers, particularly those surrounding the abdomen. It comes in a variety of sizes. **Finochietto retractors** are applied when retraction is needed during surgical procedures in the thoracic area. Snook and Covault are instruments applied in the surgical procedures involving the ovaries. These instruments are often used in ovariohysterectomy. In veterinary medicine, they are also sometimes called spay hooks. The construction of the **Snook retractor** consists of a broad, level handle. This instrument has a smooth, curved end. **Covault retractors** are constructed with an octagonal handle, which means it has 8 flat surfaces. These retractors have a circular end that resembles a ball shape.

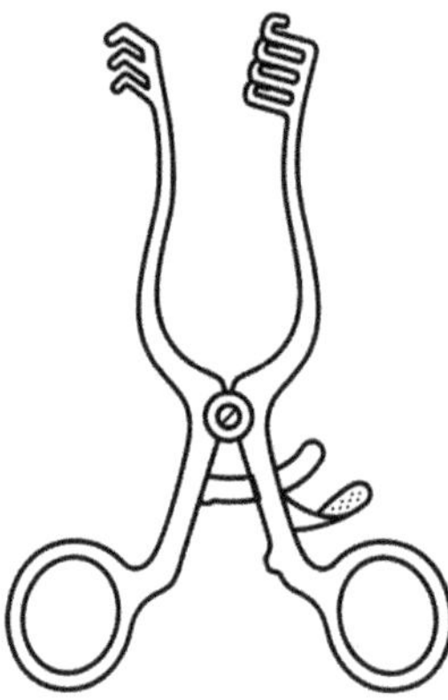

MALLEABLE RETRACTORS

Malleable (shapeable) retractors are also manually operated and are constructed to give the veterinarian the ability to bend the instrument to reach down into the deeper incisions. This malleable feature makes it easier to retract or secure areas which are normally difficult to reach. The retractors which fall into the self-retaining category include Gelpi, Weitlaners, Balfour, Finochietto, Snook, and Covault. These instruments have a locking function and are configured in such a way as to secure tissues without having to be manipulated or held in place by the surgeon or assistants. A **Gelpi retractor** is constructed with a solitary sharp end that juts outward. This instrument is applied in the retraction of incisions that are not very deep. Weitlaners are instruments which have been constructed with ends that look like the teeth on a gardening tool. These ends can be dull or sharp to the touch. Weitlaners are also applied in the retraction of incisions that are not very deep.

TYPES OF SCALPELS

The **Bard-Parker scalpel handle** is constructed with a blade that can be disconnected and removed. The reattachment of a blade is accomplished by the use of a number 3 or number 4 needle holder. The Bard-Parker scalpel handle is the most widely used in surgical procedures on small mammals. For more delicate incisions, the veterinarian will use a number 15 blade. This blade is paired with a smaller rendering of the number 10 handle. For arthroscopic procedures which delve into the inspection of the inside of the joint, the veterinarian will select a number 11 blade. The number 11 blade works well for stabbing incisions. The pointed tip construction is beneficial. The number 12 blade is constructed with a hooked end. This blade is used to take out sutures and for removal of an animal's claws.

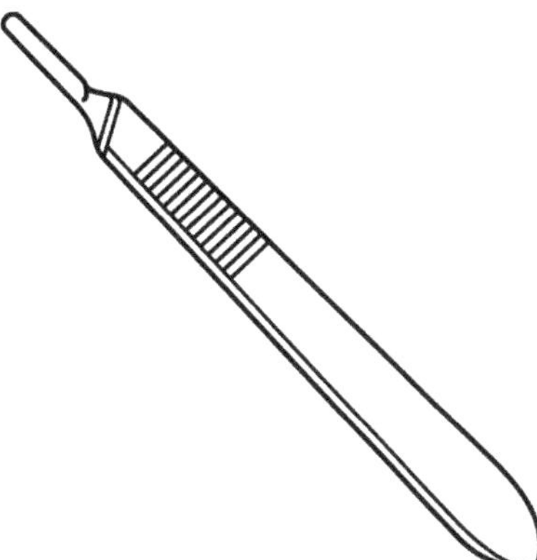

Types of Surgical Needles and Suture Material

The needle point known as the tapered point is not used for cutting. **Tapered point needles** can be constructed with or without an eye component. The eyeless needles are constructed with a swaged component. This component allows the suture end to be inserted into a hole drilled or a u-channel in the end of the needle and then crimped or bonded, avoiding the bent suture drag of an eye-insertion format. Eye-insertion, threaded needles leave the suture jutting out on either side of the needle's hole. These threaded needles can lead to some tissue trauma as the needle is passed through.

Veterinarians will select and use non-synthetic suture material known as **surgical gut.** The more widely used absorbable synthetic suture material includes polyglycolic acid, polyglactin acid, polydioxanone, and polyglyconate. Polyglycolic acid is constructed from synthetic polyester which is derived from a chemical process involving hydroxyacetic acid. Polyglactin acid is constructed from a copolymer of lactic and glycolic acids. Polydioxanone and polyglyconate are constructed from synthetic polyester.

Surgical Needle Uses

Surgical needles are found in a variety of geometric forms and sizes. The geometric shapes include arched, straight, and half an arch. The veterinarian will use the arched or curved needle most often. These arched or curved needles are gauged according to the size of the circle. The range of the circle is $\frac{1}{4}, \frac{3}{8}, \frac{1}{2}, \frac{5}{8}$ in size. The surgical needles are constructed as one-half of a circle with 2 kinds of needle points: a cutting point and a tapered point. The cutting point comes in reverse, triangular, or side cutting implementations. These needle points are best applied in the cutting of skin, cartilage, or tendons. The tapered point is not used for cutting. This is due to the rounded or oval shape of the point. The round reverse cutting points are selected for their use with torn or ragged-edged tissues.

Surgical Cleanliness

Implement Cleaning

Stainless steel instruments should not be allowed to dry without being cleaned as it may lead to staining, pitting, and corrosion of the instrument. Thus, the veterinarian should keep the implements wet until they can receive a thorough washing. The veterinarian should wash the instruments in distilled water, using approved cleaning products. The cleaning products should have a pH range of 9.2 to 11. Tap water is not recommended for use as it can cause mineral deposits to form on the instruments' surface areas.

SOAPS AND DETERGENTS

Soap can be made from potassium or sodium hydroxide mixed with natural oils. This anionic cleansing agent is a substance that is able to reduce the surface tension found in liquids such as water. However, soap is not effective in a highly mineralized liquid, such as that commonly referred to as "hard" water. Soap mixed with quaternary ammonium compounds loses its effectiveness. In addition, soap can reduce the strength of a halogen element like chlorine or iodine. Lacking true bactericidal properties, soaps should not be employed as antimicrobials or disinfectants.

Detergents are synthetically produced soaps. Detergents are classified as anionic, cationic, or nonionic. The blending of anionic and cationic detergents will counteract each other and produce an unproductive combination. Anionic and nonionic detergents function to cleanse a surface. However, the cationic detergents are the best for providing a more sterile cleanse. Detergents can be improved upon by the addition of wetting agents (surfactants), along with substances to alter the pH levels, enzymes, and non-surfactant materials. The detergent may also be supplemented with chemicals that will either eliminate or enhance the detergent's ability to produce foam or bubbles.

FURTHER CARE FOR SURGICAL INSTRUMENTS

During sterilization and storage, some metals are susceptible to **electrolytic corrosion**. This is a chemical reaction that can destroy metal surgical instruments. Following cleaning, these implements should be submerged in **surgical milk**, which coats the implements with a lubricant that inhibits rust. This is followed by a drying process which is accomplished with clean paper. Some instruments may require further treatment with lubricants.

Surgical gowns, laparotomy sheets, drapes, and skin towels should be folded accordion style. The freshly washed and dried surgical gowns should be examined for tears. If free from damage, the gown can be wrapped inside out with sleeves on top of the gown. The ties should be skillfully folded on the inside. A laundered towel should be available for drying hands after a surgical scrub. Thus, this towel should be positioned in the gown pack.

MICROBIAL CONTROL

Antibiotics kill pathogens within the body, while **antiseptics** kill pathogens on living tissues. Further, **disinfectants** kill pathogens on inanimate objects. Disinfectants may be classified in accordance with their primary functions. However, it should be noted that some pathogens may not respond to the chemical solutions specifically intended to eradicate them. Many pathogens develop resistance to certain control methods.

Some physical antimicrobial control methods include: desiccation (dehydration), filtration, freezing, moist heat (boiling, autoclaving, etc.), dry heat (incineration), ionizing radiation, and radioactive radiation. Dry heat oxidizes (burns) organic compounds with fire or a hot air oven.

The **hot oven sterilization method** requires that the oven's temperature be set at 170 °C or 340 °F for one hour. The hot oven method is most useful for substances that are in a dry or powdered form, or petroleum-based substances such as paraffin and Vaseline products. Many animal care facilities are known to use dry heat as part of their process for microbial management.

FACTORS THAT AFFECT EFFICACY

Most microbial management techniques only produce the desired results for a short time, and then only under proper conditions. The correct quantity, concentration, and contact time of the microbial product must always be utilized to produce the desired results; follow label instructions for microbial control agents. Things to note:

- Disinfectants can lose their strength when mixed with other solutions.
- The stage of development of the organism may impact efficacy of antimicrobial agents.

- Some chemicals may harm certain surfaces or cause harmful chemical reactions to occur on certain surface materials.
- Application methods may vary (spray, swabs, or immersion).
- The chemical should also be stored according to the instructions on the package.

DISINFECTANTS

Many types of chemicals can be employed to disrupt the cell growth of harmful pathogens. The chemical reactions on each involved surface and pathogen should be thoroughly understood by the person using the disinfectant. The classification of disinfectants includes low, medium, and high rankings. Chemical compounds given the highest rank are used to eradicate a wide range of organisms. High-ranking disinfectants can kill viruses that have an affinity for either lipids (fats) or fluids (water). In addition, these high-ranking disinfectants are able to eradicate bacterial spores, which can otherwise merely remain dormant on exposed surfaces.

Those disinfectants which receive a medium rank can eradicate the bacterial strain which causes tuberculosis. Disinfectants that receive a low rank can eradicate harmful vegetative bacteria.

The selection of a disinfectant should involve consideration of surface materials. The surface should not be harmed when the disinfectant is applied, nor should adverse chemical reactions occur upon contact. Finally, low-ranking disinfectants should not be overtly toxic to humans or animals. Nor should they be a fire hazard.

ALCOHOLS

Alcohols used as disinfectants include ethyl alcohol, isopropyl alcohol, and methyl alcohol. Alcohols are effective as a disinfectant against gram-positive and gram-negative bacteria and enveloped viruses.

Alcohols can be the solvent base for a variety of antiseptics and disinfectants. Alcohols are inexpensive and do not have a high risk of toxicity. Alcohol is widely used as a topical antiseptic. The recommended concentration of isopropyl alcohol is 60-70%. The recommended concentration of ethyl alcohol is 70-80%. They are generally produced in a 70% solution, as water is also needed to denature the bacterial proteins sufficient for the bacteria to die.

Alcohol will produce a burning sensation if placed on open wounds or irritated skin. Alcohol also has a tendency to dry the skin. A clotted or coagulated mass can form when alcohols are used in areas where the wound has a fluid discharge. This can also present a risk of leaving bacteria alive under the coagulum or clotted mass. Alcohol can cause a vapor-like fog to form on the outside of lenses and will cause some plastics to become hard and unyielding. Some cement will soften under the application of alcohol. Finally, the blending of some organic substances can render alcohol ineffective.

ALDEHYDES

Aldehydes consist of substantially reactive organic compounds which work against gram-positive, gram-negative, and acid-fast bacteria, as well as bacterial spores, fungi, and many viruses. Aldehydes include glutaraldehyde or Cidex, formaldehyde or Formicide, biguanide, and chlorhexidine gluconates such as Hibitane or Chlorodex.

Glutaraldehyde is not aggressively caustic but can still damage the skin and respiratory system. A more caustic form can be produced by adding sodium bicarbonate to the commercially available acidic product. It allows a cold sterilization process to take place and can be applied to surfaces like plastics, rubber, and lenses. However, glutaraldehyde can be inactivated when mixed with organic substances or hard water. Formaldehyde releases a colorless gas. However, there is a 37-40% aqueous product that is mixed with water or alcohol. The colorless gas is released from the surface that has been disinfected. Therefore, safety equipment must be worn to reduce toxic contact to the respiratory system and tissues.

Biguanide is an aldehyde-based antiseptic employed as a surgical scrub or in washing the hands. This solution has disinfectant/antiseptic properties that can be reduced when mixed with organic substances or hard water. A saline solution will render the disinfectant useless.

Halogens

Halogens are highly electronegative chemical elements. The five halogen elements are fluorine, chlorine, iodine, bromine, and astatine. Halogens are effective against gram-positive and gram-negative bacteria, as well as acid-fast bacteria, viruses, and fungi.

Iodine and chlorine are widely used to disinfect surfaces. Iodine is universally employed in blended solutions made from water or alcohol. Iodophors are disinfectant solutions. An iodophor can be dissolved in another substance to increase its wetting properties (i.e., to make the liquid spread out more readily across a surface). This not only extends the topical product's shelf-life, but also makes the product milder on the skin.

Bleach (sodium hypochlorite) is a common and inexpensive disinfectant. Bleach can be harmful when mixed with vinegar, ammonia, or rubbing alcohol. Therefore, caution must be used in its application.

Iodines and Iodophors

Tinctures are created when iodines are mixed with alcohol (ethanol). **Iodophors** are made when iodines are mixed with detergents. It is not expected that iodophors or tinctures will produce a stain or irritate the skin. However, water-based forms of iodine (certain iodophors) are known to be caustic enough to produce stains and irritate the skin. These products can also be corrosive on metallic surfaces.

Iodophors are slow to release iodine. A widely used version is known as Betadine. This is commonly used in medical facilities as a scrub prior to a surgical procedure.

Peroxygen Compounds

Peroxygen compounds are effective against gram-positive and gram-negative bacteria, acid-fast bacteria, viruses, and fungi. They cannot eradicate pinworm eggs. Peroxygen compounds are fast-acting (under 30 minutes). The humidity levels in the application area should be at 80%. The concentration levels should be at least 2%. Peroxygen compounds should not be applied to steel, iron, or rubber, as these surfaces may react to create an explosion. Peroxide can be blended safely with a low concentration of bleach. Gloves should be worn to protect the skin.

Two types of peroxygen compounds are peracetic acid and peroxide. Peroxide is widely sold in stores as hydrogen peroxide in concentrations of 3% and 6%. The manufacturer uses a brown container to reduce the rate at which the product breaks down or decomposes due to light exposure. Peracetic acid is also available for purchase in many stores. This product is sold in its liquid form.

Phenols

Phenol is perhaps the earliest disinfectant/antiseptic known, used by Joseph Lister when it was called carbolic acid. Phenols include carbolic acid, coal tar phenols, and cresol. Phenols have an active ingredient which is able to disrupt gram-positive bacteria and enveloped viruses. Synthetic phenols are blended with soaps that are not poisonous.

Quaternary ammonium compounds can reduce the active ingredient found in the phenols. However, phenols will not be deactivated by organic compounds like soap or hard water. The person applying phenol should wear gloves and protective clothing to avoid prolonged contact. Phenols have been known to produce skin lesions. The mucous membranes are susceptible to burns from exposure to phenols. Severe ulcerations can result from accidental contact with the eyes. In addition, swallowing this chemical can result in respiratory distress, including hyperventilation. This is due to the toxic effect on the brain that occurs from consumption.

Cats, rabbits, and rodents can suffer harmful effects from this toxin. Toxicity can result from dosages as low as 0.22 g/lb in dogs.

Quaternary Ammonium Compounds

Quaternary ammonium compounds (**quats**) disinfect surfaces and objects contaminated with gram-positive and gram-negative bacteria and enveloped viruses. Quats include Cetrimide, benzalkonium chloride, Zephiran, Quatsyl-D, and Germiphene.

Individuals applying these disinfectants should wear gloves and avoid contact with the skin, as these compounds can produce ill effects. They can also harm the lining of internal organs within the body. However, quats can be used safely. They do not usually cause irritation when safety measures are used, and they rank low on the toxic scales. It should be noted that some organic compounds and hard water salts can deactivate or reduce the effectiveness of quats. Conversely, quats can be strengthened by increasing the pH level. Surface areas should be rinsed thoroughly before the application of a quat solution. This should allow the quats to work on the surface without the interference of other compounds.

Sterilization

The **sterilization** process involves a complete and thorough disinfection method that employs microbicidal chemicals to eradicate the microbes. The absence of any infectious organism and its contaminants represents a state known as **asepsis**. In addition, **bacteriostatic** chemicals are often used to prevent further microbes from developing.

Radiation

Radiation is a sterilization method that employs an energy wave that disrupts cell enzyme systems and DNA. There are 2 types of radiation applied in the sterilization process.

Gamma radiation is used in the manufacturing of products sold by pharmacies, such as disposable plastics and some biological goods. It produces ionization that disrupts the stability of pathogens on the molecular level, altering the tissue and the DNA during the sterilization process. The result is the death of any exposed organism. Gamma radiation is a very effective sterilizing method, as it can pass through multiple layers of solid or fluid matter. This penetrating effect should be centralized to prevent any contact with tissues that are not meant to be disrupted by the discharge.

Ultraviolet (UV) rays are used to sterilize objects that are in close proximity and fully exposed to the UV rays. UV rays should be used on surfaces that do not have multiple layers needing to be made germ free. Although the UV ray has a low energy capacity, some (not all) transparent surfaces can be treated with UV radiation. Eye protection is necessary.

Ethylene Oxide

Ethylene oxide (EO) kills gram-positive and gram-negative bacteria, lipophilic and hydrophilic viruses, fungi, and bacterial spores. EO can be applied to surfaces that cannot be heated. EO has no color and very little odor is given off during its application. However, this substance can be dispersed quickly and is also a fire hazard that can become an explosion risk under certain conditions. EO is kept at a temperature of 70–140 °F and the application humidity levels should range from 30–40% with higher levels of humidity producing the best result. This product can be applied in a vacuum type compartment. Ethylene oxide should be blended with CO_2, ether, or Freon and produces optimum results within 1–18 hours of its use. Always dry the sterilized objects, and circulate the surrounding air for a period of 24–48 hours to dissipate any EO residue. This reduces the likelihood of contamination, as there are carcinogenic and other toxins present in EO residues. Finally, the sterilized objects should be covered in a muslin, polyethylene, polypropylene, or polyvinyl wrapper.

Air Filtration

Antimicrobial air filters allow air to pass through but remove harmful microorganisms. Animal care facilities employ this form of sterilization in many ways, including through the use of surgical masks, laboratory animal cage tops, and air duct filters. The most effective filtration screens incorporate a very dense filter that has been manufactured from a variety of products and fibers.

The three components that impact the effectiveness of an air filter are air velocity, relative humidity, and electrostatic charge. Any fragment that is larger than 0.3 micrometers will be trapped in a **high efficiency particle absorption (HEPA) filter**, which functions at an efficiency rate of 99.97–99.997%. The masks used in surgical procedures prevent the patient from becoming contaminated by the person wearing the mask. If it is necessary to prevent an infection from being transmitted to the person wearing a mask, then a mask specifically designed for that purpose should be worn. These masks are not interchangeable and should not be expected to function in the same way. Both types of masks should be replaced after a few hours' use with a clean, dry, well-fitting mask.

Fluid Filtration

Fluid filtration employs a filter which works to prevent the passage of organisms. The organisms are thus trapped inside the filtering material. The filter can apply a positive or negative pressure to allow the fluids to gain access. Bacteria can be trapped inside a filter with a pore size of 0.45 micrometers. Mycoplasmas and viruses can be trapped inside a filter with a pore size of 0.01-0.1 micrometers. Larger pathogens will need a filter with pore filters that are smaller in size. A prefilter can be employed to improve the effects of the sterilization process.

Ultrasonic Cleaner

An **ultrasonic cleaner** is recommended for use in the sterilization process. Ultrasonic cleaners have been studied and found to be 16 times more efficient than manual cleaners. All box locks and ratchets should be opened and exposed upon placement into the ultrasonic cleaner. This allows the cleanser access to hard-to-reach locations on the instrument. The ultrasonic cleaner should not be overloaded with instruments. The implements that are to be used first should go on the top of the tray. The heavier implements should be packed on the bottom of the tray. In general, it is not good practice to vary the kinds of metals placed within the same cleaning cycle.

Boiling and Steam

Boiling requires a 3-hour period to fully destroy microorganisms. The first 10 minutes of the boiling method should eradicate the vegetative bacteria and viruses. However, additional time is needed to eradicate the more resistant bacterial spores. A 2% calcium carbonate or sodium solution can improve the sterilization efficacy. This supplement will also reduce rust.

Another method that destroys pathogenic microorganisms is **steam**. Steam is reached at the same temperatures that are needed to bring a liquid to a boil. Therefore, steam can be used for sterilization. However, a longer period of time is required to achieve the same effect. Steam requires a 90-minute period to fully eradicate vegetative bacteria. However, steam alone is not an effective measure for eradicating bacterial spores from the surface of an object being sanitized. The best and most reliable method of moist heat sterilization is accomplished with vaporized water that is applied under pressure or force. The **autoclave** is a steel vessel that applies steam and pressure to sterilize the equipment used in most veterinary facilities.

Autoclave Sterilization

Surgical implements and other reusable items will need to be sterilized prior to being used again. Typically, this is done using an **autoclave**, a pressurized container that superheats water to steam clean instruments.

All autoclaves utilize a pressurized steam system to eradicate harmful organisms from the surfaces of objects. Gravity displacement autoclaves (type "N") allow gravity to exchange the air in the sterilization chamber for steam (air is heavier than water vapor and is displaced through a port in the bottom as steam enters the top). Some autoclaves use positive pressure, venting steam into the chamber only after it has been sufficiently pressurized in a separate chamber to blow all existing air out. Some use negative pressure (type "S"), provided by a vacuum pump that removes the air, achieving among the highest **sterility assurance levels (SAL)**.

The steam is able to penetrate multiple layers of material placed within the confines of the steel vessel. The increased pressure inside the vessels keeps the heated water at the boiling point. The usual time required for sterilization is 9-15 minutes. The temperatures should be at 121 °C or 250 °F to properly accomplish full sterilization. The pressure can be decreased to that at sea level to bring the temperature of the steam down to 100 °C or 212 °F. Additional pressure of 15 pounds per square inch (psi) will produce steam at 121 °C or 250 °F. Some autoclaves can be set at 35 psi to reach a steam temperature of 135 °C or 275 °F. The objects should be placed in the autoclave for the recommended amount of time to allow the steam to penetrate all surfaces.

Gravity Displacement Autoclaves

Gravity displacement autoclaves gradually replace the air inside the sterilization vessel using gravity. In these devices, the water is brought to a boil with electricity. This produces steam and pressure inside the vessel. The gravitationally lighter water vapor will begin to displace the air inside the autoclave by way of an underside vent. The vent closes when the exiting air is at the proper sterilization temperature. The interior temperature will reach 121 °C or 250 °F, at which point the sterilization will begin to be timed for the requisite exposure period.

Following the recommended time for sterilization of the contents, the heated water vapor will be released through a small narrow opening into a reservoir. The steam inside the vessel's interior will then be displaced with air that has been sanitized and filtered of impurities. Correct loading of the chamber will prevent any materials from obstructing the proper movement of steam, heat, and air. This is important, as pockets of air can limit the penetration of heated steam, keeping it from reaching all layers and surfaces inside the autoclave. Object surfaces should not be wet when taken from the autoclave if done properly.

Pre-Vacuum Autoclaves

A **pre-vacuum (negative pressure) autoclave** can be more expensive to purchase than a gravity displacement autoclave. However, the pre-vacuum autoclave can hold more objects due to its larger size and greater effectiveness. The pre-vacuum autoclave works to produce steam from a boiler or water heating tank. Then a vacuum pump works to remove the air from the loaded sterilization chamber, allowing steam (121 °C or 250 °F) to fill the empty chamber. The exposure period is timed from this point. When the exposure period is ended, the steam is vacuumed from the chamber. This allows heated, dry, sterilized air to enter the chamber to begin the drying process that takes place inside the autoclave. The vacuum action prevents air pockets from forming during the air-steam exchange process, and it also reduces the time that is required for the drying process. It is not uncommon for a pre-vacuum autoclave to come equipped with a digital display screen. Most pre-vacuum autoclaves can also print out the interior temperatures and pressures that are reached in the sterilization cycle.

Autoclave Maintenance

The autoclave reservoir must always be filled with distilled water because it will generate pure steam for sterilization unlike tap water, which can leave mineral deposits that can stain instruments and promote buildup in the autoclave itself. The chamber will be cleaned with a specific autoclave cleaner and scrubbed with a bristle brush to prevent buildup at least once a week. The gasket inside of the autoclave door will need to be wiped down weekly. The steam-line filter will need to be cleaned monthly (or according to the manufacturer's guidelines), by draining the water out, filling it with new distilled water, and running a couple of short cycles with a specialized cleaning solution.

AUTOCLAVE SETTINGS

The **wrapped goods setting** begins with steam flowing through the chamber. The setting allows for a predetermined temperature to be sustained over a measured time period. The cycle completes when the steam is withdrawn from the chamber, which returns to normal atmospheric pressure. A drying period is optional.

Hard goods are utensils made from stainless steel or other sturdy materials, including syringes, which should be separated before sterilization. They should be washed thoroughly and rinsed with deionized water before autoclaving. The **hard goods** (or **flash autoclave**) **setting** is utilized when trays, bowls, and cages are placed in the autoclave. The setting is also employed to rapidly sterilize utensils for immediate use in urgent care situations. It is not necessary to wrap hard goods for sterilization.

Liquids can be autoclaved in a flat Pyrex container with a capacity at least three times the volume of the liquid inside. The container requires a loose-fitting lid or a paraffin cover with a needle inserted in the cover to allow air to flow. There are some concerns that infective organisms may remain in autoclaved liquid. Staff should use caution in removing these liquids to prevent injury.

MATERIALS USED TO WRAP INSTRUMENTS

Sterilization drapes stop microorganisms while allowing sterilant to pass through to the instruments. Paper and linen wraps should be one-time use because they function as a mesh-type filter and after washing and being used, the spaces between the threads get larger, allowing microorganisms to get through. SMS polypropylene wraps are made of dense microfibers and are more reliable for not allowing dust and microorganisms through.

Pouch packs or **peel pouches** serve the purpose of securing single instruments, sponges, and a variety of other objects. The packs are arranged so that steam can penetrate the layers inside. The loose ends of the pack are fastened with a heat seal or taped down. The ends should be folded over so that the autoclave tape shows the date, contents, and operator.

Peel pouches are easy to open and close without tearing and dropping the sterile instrument. When packing an instrument in a peel pouch, make sure it is the right size for the instrument because if it is too small the instrument could pierce the pouch. Allow one inch of space between the instrument and all of the sealed edges of the pouch, and place the instrument so that when the pouch is opened the surgeon can grab the handle first.

PREPARING LINEN PACKS

Instruments and linens should be packed using a standardized procedure. Perforations in pans or trays should not be blocked to ensure steam flow. The instruments should be washed, rinsed in deionized water, and broken down into constituent pieces. Ratchets should be opened and unlocked for thorough cleaning.

At least two layers of material are applied in wrapping each pack. The pack is sealed with autoclave tape that has been marked with the date, contents, and operator. Each pack is marked with its own temperature-sensitive seal to indicate if the proper temperatures were reached during the sterilization process. The pack must measure no more than 30 x 30 x 50 cm. It should weigh no more than 5.5 kg. The pack density should not exceed 115.3 kg/m^3.

Two pieces of wrapping material should be folded like a diamond. The placement of the pack will go in the middle of the uppermost wrap. The corner closest to the packer will be folded over the uppermost region of the pack. A flap will be created by folding a small portion of that corner. Repeat this procedure for each corner. The final corner will be tucked under the two side corners with a small flap left to pull it open. Continue this procedure until all the layers have been folded in like manner.

Loading the Autoclave

The autoclave provides the best performance when it is loaded in such a way as to allow steam to flow freely inside its chamber. Wire mesh or perforated shelves are recommended to promote good circulation. Arrange packs with 2.5–7.4 cm (1–3 in) of space between packs. Multiple packs should be positioned on their sides in a vertical position. Specialized containers hold the pouches in place so the plastic side of one pouch is facing the paper side of the adjacent pouch. Solid pans are laid upside down or on their side. Wrapped goods are arranged on the top layer with other hard and wrapped goods. It is best to operate the autoclave with only one type of metal on the inside to prevent electrolysis.

Sterilization Monitors: Indicator Tape and Strips

Sterilization monitors are classified as follows: indicator tape, chemical indicator strips, Bowie Dick tests, and biological indicators. The veterinarian should utilize more than one sterilization monitor to maintain quality control.

The lines on **indicator tape** will change color upon contact with steam or ethylene oxide. However, this tape cannot be used to determine that a certain temperature has been reached in the sterilization process or the period of time that the sterilization process lasted.

Chemical indicator strips which have been placed under the folds of a gown will indicate if steam has reached the inside of the gown by changing color. Post-autoclave analysis of these strips can confirm that sterilization temperatures were achieved. They can also be utilized when the toxic gas ethylene oxide is used in the sterilization process instead of steam or dry heat. The paper strips are arranged outside and within a test pack in such a way as to confirm that sufficient heat, steam, or gas was able to reach and penetrate into the most interior region of the pack.

Sterilization Monitors: Bowie Dick Test and Biological Indicators

The **Bowie Dick test** employs test sheets that have been designed to indicate a consistent color change whenever air has been effectively evacuated from the sterilization chamber. It also measures when full steam penetration has been attained. This test shows immediate results via indicator tape and test sheets. However, it does not prove that complete sterilization (time duration) has been achieved.

A **biological indicator** will also ensure that heat-resistant bacteria have been adequately exposed to the sanitation process. Biological testing strips contain embedded bacterial spores, likely *Bacillus stearothermophilus*. The strips will be placed in various locations inside a fully loaded autoclave. The usual operation of the autoclave will be carried out as a full cycle, but under its minimum setting. The strips are next removed from the autoclave when the steam has been evacuated. The bacteria strips should then be incubated and analyzed as directed by the manufacturer.

Sterilization Monitors: Surface Sampling and Temperature Recording

Surface sampling evaluates whether the appropriate disinfectant procedures are applied to surfaces of surgical zones. The surface may be swiped with a sterile applicator and cultured on a suitable growth media. The surface or object being tested can also be rinsed down with a sterile solution. The solution can then be collected and examined for any contaminants that may be present.

Finally, the sterilization time, temperature, and pressure should be recorded. The **recording thermometer** keeps track of the autoclave's temperature during each cycle. Some types of autoclaves make a printout of the recorded temperatures and pressures attained during a cycle. A **thermocouple** is a device which can measure the temperature in moist or dry heat or chemical sterilization applications in the most remote region of the test pack.

Surgical Preparation

Surgical Suite Cleaning

An effective aseptic technique involves removing any debris from the area such as blood, feces, or vomit and then cleaning the surfaces with a general cleaner and wiping dry. Next, apply a disinfectant and allow it to sit for the amount of time required on the label, rinse, and then dry again. To obtain asepsis, the surgical suite must be cleaned from top to bottom daily. Start with the walls, which must be wiped down with a disinfectant, as well as all monitoring equipment, lamps, and operating tables. The floors must be swept and mopped using a mop separate from that used for the rest of the hospital.

Surgery Room Preparation

To prepare the surgical suite for a patient, a checklist is helpful. First, the surgical suite needs to be inspected to be sure it is clean of all hair and debris. Next, check the anesthetic machine to be sure that the sevoflurane or isoflurane is full and that the oxygen tank is full. Perform a leak test on the anesthetic machine with the correct-sized rebreathing bag and breathing tube for the patient's weight. Gather the supplies needed for the specific procedure to be performed such as a sterile spay pack containing the instruments and gauze, a sterile drape, a sterile scalpel blade of the appropriate size, and the appropriate size suture. Place all sterile items on the Mayo stand until they need to be opened. Any patient-warming devices should be warmed up prior to surgery, and all monitoring equipment needs to be turned on to ensure that it is working correctly. An IV fluid stand, pump, appropriate fluids, fluid line, and extension set need to be set up with the fluids run through the line to ensure that there is no air in the line. Overhead lights should be turned on and adjusted accordingly.

Preparing a Patient for Surgery

An animal should void its **bladder** before surgery, usually by walking the animal until it urinates. If necessary, the bladder can be manually expressed. Once anesthetized, the animal's hair should be removed from the incision site with electric clippers. The surgery site should then be cleared of loose hair and scrubbed thoroughly, then cleansed with a surgical disinfectant. The patient's scrubbed incision site should not be contaminated during the transfer of the patient to the operating table. Finally, the monitoring equipment should be positioned, with the patient given a reapplication of antiseptic on the incision site.

Pre-Surgery Hair Removal

The staff member who clips the hair on the animal as preparation for surgery should wear a smock over the scrubs.

For abdominal surgeries, removal of the fur is extensive. If the veterinarian is to perform surgery on a cat, then the cat's hair should be removed one clipper blade past the nipple for cats. The distance extends to at least 4 inches on each side of the midline for large sized dogs. In the case of a canine castration, the hair is removed from the scrotum, prepuce, and inguinal (groin) area. In the case of feline castrations, there is not a need to remove as much hair.

If necessary, additional hair can be removed by plucking. The hair can be pulled out by the roots in the testes and the region surrounding the scrotum. In the case of removal of claws in cats and puppies, and for tail docking, hair removal is not recommended.

After the surgical area is shaved, use a small vacuum to get the excess hair off of the surgical site.

Surgical Scrub of a Patient

There are two widely used scrub products used by veterinary clinics: chlorhexidine and povidone-iodine (an iodophor).

The patient requires scrubbing around the incision site before surgery can be carried out. This is done in a circular motion, gradually moving outward away from the incision site to get rid of any dirt and debris on the skin. Do not go back and forth over the incision with the solution, rather, make one swipe around and down, then toss. The scrub should consist of an ample lather for a thorough cleansing. The surgical site should be cleansed with the scrubbing product a total of three times. The second application should be accomplished with brand new gauze. The third application must also be done with a new gauze square. Upon the third scrub, this gauze should have no dirty residue. The procedure should be done again if the gauze is dirty, and should be repeated until the gauze comes away clean. End with the chlorhexidine solution, then spray Betadine over the surgical site, which is an antiseptic microbicide.

Surgical Scrub of Surgery Staff

Surgery staff should dress in surgical scrubs, cap, gown, and mask before scrubbing. Remove all jewelry and inspect the fingernails, which should be short and without polish. The hands are scrubbed with a sterile scrub brush and antiseptic soap, starting at the edges of the fingertips of one hand using 12 strokes for each finger, working from the pinky finger to the thumb. From there, scrub the palm, the back of the hand, and then the side of the hand.

Next, scrub the four surfaces of the wrist. The scrub continues up the arm and ends two inches below the elbow. The brush should be rinsed completely before repeating the scrub on the other hand. At the end of the scrub, rinse both hands with antiseptic soap. The hands should be held in an upward position. The drying procedure is accomplished with a sterile towel. The staff should use one side of the towel for the right hand and right arm. The other side of the towel should be applied to the left hand and left arm. These specific procedures should be followed for every surgical procedure.

Positioning Animals for Surgery

Standard **laparotomies** or surgical cuts through the abdominal wall require the animal to be in dorsal recumbency. This position is necessary for the veterinarian to perform an ovariohysterectomy or a splenectomy.

The animal having perineal urethrostomies, rectal fistulas, and anal sac surgeries should be positioned so that the veterinarian can access the lower body in the front of the animal in a ventral recumbent position. The animal's tail should be securely fastened to the top or side of the table. The animal's hind legs should be allowed to hang down over the edge of the table. It should be noted that in the case of orthopedic surgeries, it is necessary to prepare a larger surgical site so that the surgeon has a greater range of motion for the limb.

Draping the Patient

The patient must be securely positioned on the operating table, where they are given one last surgical site sterilization. The surgical team member should be fully masked and gowned in sterile garments. The team member places a drape over the patient at this time. The sterilized drape protects the patient from any contamination along the surgical site. Field drapes are positioned over unsterilized regions of the animal. These drapes are placed one at a time on the perimeters of the sterilized surgical site. The surgical team member should not try to move the drapes once they have been positioned, as this could lead to contaminants entering the sterilized surgical site. The surgical team member will use towel clamps to fasten the four corners of the drapes to the skin. The last step is to lay a large drape or laparotomy sheet over the entire region. There should be a gap left for easy access to the surgical site. This gap still covers the site, but it can be folded back to reveal the area underneath, with the final drape covering the uninterrupted sterile area.

Proper Surgical Attire

The proper surgical garments are surgical scrubs, a hooded cap called a bouffant, surgical mask, a sterile gown, and foot covers or surgery shoes. In addition, hooded caps may be needed to cover facial and neck hair.

The front side of the surgical gown, from the waist to the shoulder and down the arms, is the person's **sterile field**. This can become contaminated if proper infection control procedures are not followed. The hands should be held close to and in front of the body when not needed for the surgical procedure. The hands should also be kept above the waist and surgery table. The staff should move by passing one another with their backs toward each other, never with their backs facing the patient.

There are two types of surgical masks that can be worn by the staff. **Molded masks** are best when there is little need to cover facial hair as it permits air to escape from beneath. The **flat-style mask** has pressed folds with a metal nose band, which gives a more customized fit which does not allow air to escape as readily as the molded mask.

Operating Room Rules

The staff should obey proper procedures when opening sterile equipment packs and when handing sterile equipment to other staff members. The surgical assistant is responsible for handing off sterile equipment to the surgeon; the assistant will be diligent about using implements that are sterile beyond a doubt. Contact with a non-sterilized item will result in the contamination of both the item and the patient's incision.

Surgical assistants should be positioned to receive sterile equipment without intruding upon the sterile field or the patient. The surgical table should be kept orderly and sterile. The assistant will be responsible for handing over all instruments in response to the surgeon's need. The assistant will tap the surgeon's hand with the instrument to ensure that the proper contact has been made between the instrument and the surgeon.

Assisting in Surgery

The staff should not engage in unnecessary communication or movement. The assistant is responsible for maintaining the patient's hemostasis. This is accomplished by positioning the suction near tissue to accommodate any blood flow. The tissue should not have suction applied directly to it. The assistant will also dab the tissue region with gauze. The assistant keeps track of the quantity of gauze squares used. The assistant will dispose of the used gauze properly. The skilled assistant is responsible for drawing back the muscles and tissues with the retractor. The assistant's skill is most evident when the patient has the least amount of trauma or distress. The surgical assistant is responsible for cutting the sutures during and after the surgical procedure.

The surgical assistant plays a major role in the success or failure of the surgical procedure.

Choosing the Correct Size Endotracheal Tube (ET) for a Patient

The **endotracheal tube** (ET) allows oxygen/gas anesthetic or just oxygen to pass to and from the lungs via the trachea of the patient. The technician can palpate (feel) the patient's trachea to determine which size may fit best, or another method would be to measure the distance between the patient's nares and compare it to the beveled end of the ET tube. If it fits between the nares, then that is a good indication it will fit in the trachea. For each patient going under anesthesia, three ET tubes should be picked out: the one that the veterinary technician believes will fit the best, one a size smaller, and one a size bigger. This way, if the ET tube thought to be the best fit doesn't fit, another one is close by. Brachycephalic breeds can have deceiving tracheas compared to their face size and shape, and usually their tracheas are smaller. Intubating with the correct size ET tube is crucial because if it is too small, the patient may breathe around the tube and not stay adequately anesthetized. The largest ET tube that can be placed without causing trauma to the tissues is ideal.

Surgical Procedures

Ovariohysterectomy

A **spay (ovariohysterectomy)** is a surgery that removes the ovaries and uterus from females. The procedure is usually performed between 5 and 7 months of age; however, in large or giant-breed dogs it may be performed as late as 12–18 months. Early spaying of large and giant-breed dogs can cause delayed closure of the growth plates leading to longer and thinner bones, which increases the risk of musculoskeletal injuries such as cruciate ligament tears. Although these are the recommended ages to spay a female pet, it can be done at any time in the pet's life and should always be recommended. Female dogs that are spayed prior to their first heat cycle have a greatly reduced risk of developing mammary cancer.

Pyometra

Pyometra is defined as a life-threatening secondary infection of the uterus that must be treated as soon as possible. During the heat cycle, white blood cells (WBCs) that normally protect the uterus from infection are kept from entering the uterus, allowing sperm to enter and not be destroyed. Following the heat cycle, the progesterone hormone levels are still high for up to two months, and this causes the uterus lining to thicken to prepare for pregnancy. The lining will continue to thicken if pregnancy does not occur for several estrus cycles, which will lead to cyst formation in the tissues. Fluid secretions from the thickened, cystic uterine lining allow for an ideal environment for bacteria to grow. High progesterone levels will prevent the uterine muscles from contracting in order to expel any obtained fluid and bacteria. Bacteria from the vagina can enter through an open cervix, and an unhealthy uterus with a thickened and cystic lining will not be able to appropriately expel any invaders.

Symptoms of Pyometra

Signs of pyometra include loss of appetite and lethargy, as well as pus discharge from the vagina. Pus will only be seen from the vagina if the cervix is open. If the cervix is closed, then the pus will build up inside of the uterus (called a closed pyometra), and the patient will likely present with a distended abdomen. Dogs that present with a closed pyometra will appear to be very ill very quickly, due to the toxins released into the bloodstream that the bacteria release. More severe clinical signs in a patient with closed pyometra include vomiting, diarrhea, and polyuria (increased urination), due to the toxins from the bacteria affecting the kidneys' function to retain fluids. Polydipsia also occurs (increased drinking) to compensate for polyuria. Diagnostics to confirm pyometra include a high WBC count and globulin levels, which are proteins of the immune system. Urine specific gravity is normally low due to the effects that the bacteria have had on the kidneys. Ultimately, radiographs will confirm an enlarged uterus.

Pyometra Treatment

To treat pyometra, it is recommended to remove the infected uterus and ovaries (ovariohysterectomy). Most patients that are diagnosed with pyometra are unhealthy, which makes them high-risk surgical candidates. They will require IV fluids pre-, peri-, and post-surgery and will need a longer hospitalization stay to closely monitor their recovery.

There is a medical treatment that is not highly recommended: to give prostaglandins, hormones that lower the progesterone level, thus allowing the uterus to contract and get rid of the bacteria and pus accumulation. The use of prostaglandins does not have a high success rate, and they have multiple side effects such as vomiting, abdominal pain, and panting. If left untreated, the outcome is most likely death due to the toxic effects of the bacteria or a ruptured uterus.

Cesarean Section

There are three surgical options for a Cesarean section (C-section), including C-section only, C-section plus ovariohysterectomy, or an "en-bloc" spay and C-section. A **C-section** is done by isolating the uterus in the abdomen so the fetuses and their placentas can be identified, and an incision is made on the great curve of the uterine horns to remove the puppies. Once the puppy is removed, the fetal envelope is opened and the nasal passages are wiped. The umbilical cord is still oxygenating the puppy via the placenta, and the cord will be clamped with two mosquito hemostats and then cut between the two.

Some owners may want their dog to be spayed at the time of the C-section; therefore, an ovariohysterectomy is done after the C-section is performed. An **en-bloc spay and C-section** may also be done, which is a procedure during which the ovarian and uterine pedicles are clamped two or three times and no ligatures are done until after the entire uterus is taken out and handed to the technicians aseptically. The technicians open the uterus, remove the puppies, and resuscitate while the surgeon ligates and closes the incision.

Prepare a Patient for a C-Section

A **C-section** is a surgical procedure done to remove puppies from the mother's uterus. A hysterotomy is often done in the event of an emergency such as the dog having previous dystocia or being likely to have dystocia. Pre-medications for the mother will lower her stress, and pre-medications that can be reversed are preferred. Often, the patient having a C-section will be dehydrated, so any animal going under anesthesia for this procedure should be administered IV fluids. Dogs presenting in late pregnancy are prone to hypoxemia, so preoxygenation is required five minutes prior to induction and during induction because induction agents commonly cause apnea. The patient is dorsal, and the abdomen is surgically shaved, cleaned of any hair, and surgically scrubbed. The veterinarian removes the puppies from the uterus, clamps and cuts the umbilical cords, and hands the puppies to the technician to resuscitate.

Resuscitating Puppies After a C-Section

Three things need to be prevented when resuscitating the puppies: hypothermia, hypotension, and hypoxia. To prevent hypoxia, the nasal passages and mouth must be cleared of any secretions. This is normally done by gently using a bulb syringe because too much suction can damage the tissues of the pharynx and larynx. Rubbing the puppy's thorax will stimulate it to breathe and help to clear the lungs of fluid, which will result in less heat loss. Once the puppies are moving and breathing on their own, they can be placed in a box with warm towels or towels over a warm water blanket to keep them warm. Administering IV fluids as soon as the mother arrives for surgery will help maintain adequate blood pressure for the mother and the puppies. The puppies should continue to be resuscitated until they have 10 breaths per minute and are making noise and moving around. Swinging the puppies is no longer a recommended technique for resuscitation.

Castration

Castration is the surgical removal of the testicles in male animals. In dogs, an incision is made in front of the scrotum where the testicles are removed, and in cats, the testicles are removed through two incisions into the scrotal sac. Neutered dogs are less likely to display dominant behavior and aggression and are less likely to roam. Male cats that are neutered are less likely to mark their territory by urinating and are less likely to be aggressive. There is a decreased chance of testicular cancer, perianal tumors, and prostate cancer.

Ruminant Castration

In ruminant castration, the scrotum is incised, the testicles removed, and the spermatic cord and testicle-supplying blood vessels are crushed and thereby closed. Bull calves are normally castrated when they reach one to four weeks of age. It is recommended that the calf be fully vaccinated before scheduling the castration to prevent clostridial infections like botulism, tetanus, or gas gangrene. Typically, the calf does not receive any pain-numbing medications as this is considered to be expensive and unnecessary. The same reasoning is applied to the absence of a sterile field before the surgical procedure. Lambs raised for meat are not often castrated before going to market; wool-producing lambs are castrated at 1-2 weeks old. Kids, young goats, are typically castrated at 1-3 weeks old. It is recommended that lambs and kids be given vaccinations before scheduling the castration. The vaccinations will be beneficial in preventing clostridial infections like botulism, tetanus, or gas gangrene. Small ruminant animals will also receive an injection of Vitamin E and selenium at this juncture.

Open Castration

Open castration involves a surgical incision through the scrotum. An emasculator device is then applied to cut away and crush the spermatic cord (which includes the vas deferens that carries the animal's semen). The surgical site is left open to drain without any suturing. Open castrations are quicker and less expensive, and can usually be done on the farm. The Burdizzo emasculatome is applied in such a way as to only crush the cord carrying the semen, causing the testicles to atrophy and wither away without surgical intervention or loss of blood. This is similar to the emasculatome procedure performed on a calf during closed castration.

In some situations, "open" castration refers to incising (i.e., opening) the tunica vaginalis covering the testicle when removing it.

Closed Castration

A closed castration involves the suturing of the incision after castration. This is performed under sterile conditions and general anesthesia. Alternatively, it may refer to the testicles being removed with the tunica vaginalis still intact, followed by suture closure. It may also refer to an emasculatome device crushing the spermatic cord in a bloodless procedure that causes the testicles to atrophy and wither away. Other non-surgical methods can be applied. For example, an elastrator is a device that places a strong rubber band around the testicles, depriving the area of blood. This method is efficient in removing the testicles, but is not recommended for older animals. Small ruminants can be castrated using the elastrator.

Cryptorchidism

Cryptorchidism (undescended testicles) may occur when one or both testicles do not drop into the scrotum. Both testicles should have migrated to the scrotum by two months of age; if one or both have not descended, they could be hung up in the belly (abdominal cryptorchid) or in the inguinal area (inguinal cryptorchid). If a dog that is cryptorchid is not neutered, it can cause major health issues including testicular torsion and a much higher risk of testicular cancer.

A cryptorchid neuter is more involved because there may be an abdominal incision and longer surgery and recovery time. The veterinarian will palpate the subcutaneous (SQ) tissue to locate the retained testicle, and if nothing is palpated, then it is an abdominal cryptorchid. If the testicle is felt in the SQ tissue, then an incision is made right above it, and the testicle is removed rather easily. If it is an abdominal cryptorchid, an incision is made into the abdominal cavity, and once the ductus deferens is located, it is followed until the testicle is retrieved.

Common Procedures with Piglets

Pigs have a propensity to cannibalize. Thus, the pig's milk or needle teeth are cut back, as these teeth can hurt the sow or other litter-mates if left unchecked. The pig's tail is also often docked at this stage.

Male piglets should be checked for an inguinal hernia during the castration process. This appears as a bulge that abnormally sticks out through the wall of the scrotum. Pigs require an injection of iron dextran prior to the castration for a number of reasons; primarily, it will keep the animal from becoming anemic. The immature pig can be hung up by its forelegs and shaken lightly during the detection process as even the smallest of hernias will expand outwardly with a significant-sized bulge. The inguinal hernia can be repaired following a cleansing with antiseptic. The recovering animal should be housed in a small enclosure that is well maintained and kept clean.

Cystotomy

A **cystotomy** is the surgical creation of an opening in the urinary bladder wall. The most common reason to perform a cystotomy is to remove **uroliths** (bladder stones). Prior to performing a cystotomy to remove bladder stones, an abdominal radiograph should be taken to visualize the stones. The surgical procedure starts with a caudal abdominal midline incision; then the bladder should be isolated from the rest of the abdominal contents and surrounded by laparotomy sponges. Once an incision is made ventrally, the stones and calculi are removed with sterile forceps. Often, a small, sterile spoon will be used to remove the smaller particles. A urethral catheter is flushed multiple times to make sure that all of the stones have been removed, and the stones obtained are sent out to a reference lab for analysis. The bladder can be sutured with 4-0 monofilament, absorbable sutures. Multifilament suture has been known to promote urolith formation, and nonabsorbable sutures are associated with urinary calculi formation. Within 14 days, the urinary bladder regains almost 100% of its tensile strength.

Digit Amputation for Cattle

Digit amputation is a procedure used to remove an infected claw from a cow's hoof. The veterinarian will require that the cow be placed in a lateral recumbent position for this surgical procedure. The cow will be laid on its side with the infected claw facing in and right side up. The claw and the mid-metacarpus to the hoof will need to be thoroughly shaved and sterilized. This is crucial, as this claw comes into contact with manure and other substances which can lead to infection. The animal will receive anesthesia to reduce pain. This is given to the animal by way of a ring block or intravenous local. The cow will require a tourniquet—typically rubber tubing used to limit or block blood flow—applied distal to the carpus or hock to stop excessive bleeding. The tourniquet consists of a rubber tube. The veterinarian will use obstetrical or Gigli wire to sever the claw from the animal. The cow will need to have its bandage changed on a regular basis to prevent infection. The cow that is healing properly will not need the bandage if a 2- to 3-week period has passed without complications.

Dehorning

Ruminants may have their horns removed to keep them from harming themselves and others. When fully, surgically removing horns, the animal should be given a cranial nerve block or ring block for local analgesia. Goats have a low threshold for pain. Therefore, analgesic pain management is critical to the success of this procedure.

The process of removing a one- to two-week-old calf's horn-producing cells is known as **disbudding**. Goats can be disbudded as soon as the horn bud makes itself visible. The process is accomplished using an appliance known as an electric dehorner. The horn removal appliance should not be allowed to reach an excessive degree of heat, as this can lead to cerebral burns.

It is not recommended to use caustic pastes, as this could burn the animal.

A gouge-type dehorner can be employed when the horn buds are 1-2 cm long. The Barnes instrument is classified as a gouge-type dehorner.

Trimming longer horns non-surgically can be done with a Keystone or guillotine dehorner or a hardback or wire saw.

Canine Blood Donor Requirements

There are 2 kinds of dog blood types: Type A- and type A+. The A- blood type is regarded as the universal blood donor type for dogs; ideal donors can be any breed of dog and can be male or female. However, the animal should have been neutered or spayed, to reduce blood hormone levels. In addition, the animal should:

- Be larger than 25 kg or 55 lb
- Be between 1 and 7 years old
- Have received all of its vaccinations
- Have been blood typed
- Have normal results from the following tests on a yearly basis: blood chemistry, CBC, and urinalysis
- Have regular checkups scheduled at 6-month intervals
- Be free of heartworms, intestinal parasites, and infectious diseases
- Be fasted before giving blood to reduce the likelihood of producing a lipemic (fat- or lipid-laden) blood specimen

Feline Blood Donor Requirements

There are 3 kinds of feline blood types: Type A, Type B, and Type AB. Type A is the most common type found in domesticated cats. This is true of both longhair and shorthair species. However, purebreds most often have the blood type known as Type B. It is not necessary to determine the type of blood in the feline before the blood withdrawal procedure. The ideal feline blood donor will be under 8 years of age, will be neutered or spayed, and will have received all of its vaccinations. In addition, the cat will not be overweight or underweight. The ideal weight for the cat is a lean body mass of not lower than 4.5 kg or 10 lb. A cat with a good disposition and accustomed to living indoors will usually find the procedure less traumatic.

Teat Laceration Repair in Cattle and Goats

Female cattle and goats can experience trauma to a teat caused by another animal accidentally stepping on the animal's teat, leaving it unable to fully release milk from the udder. Surgical intervention is required for teat laceration repair. The cow or goat can be operated on in a variety of positions, most commonly on its side or standing, depending on the animal's size, health, temperament, and the extent of the injury.

The cow or goat undergoing surgical repair will need to be sedated, typically with the application of a ring block. The animal will need to be washed and sterilized to prepare the surgical site. The animal can have a tourniquet applied to the region to stop any unnecessary bleeding or milk seepage. The teat of the animal may also need to be fitted with a prosthetic drain to allow the injured teat to release its contents without any milking action taken. Hand-milking the animal postoperatively is not recommended, as it can disrupt the sutures. The animal can return to its milking schedule in about 2 weeks, shortly after removal of the sutures.

GI Foreign Bodies

If a dog or cat ingests foreign objects such as toys, string, bones, or any item that will not be able to pass through the GI tract, this may cause an obstruction that requires surgery to remove the object. Foreign bodies stuck in the GI tract can perforate the intestinal tract, and there is the risk of the contents of the intestine leaking into the abdomen, which can cause **peritonitis** (abdominal inflammation) and sepsis, which are life-threatening. Most GI foreign bodies require abdominal exploratory surgery under general anesthesia to remove the object. Most foreign bodies will get stuck in the stomach, requiring that a gastrotomy be performed, or in the intestines, requiring that an enterotomy be performed. Some foreign bodies may cause enough damage to the intestines such that more than one enterotomy is required. If a part of the bowel cannot be saved, then an intestinal resection and anastomosis will be performed, meaning a segment of the intestine is removed surgically and reattached to the healthy ends.

Gastropexy Surgery

A **gastropexy** is a surgery that permanently attaches the stomach to the abdominal wall. It is done to prevent **gastric dilatation and volvulus** (GDV) or "bloat," which occurs when the stomach fills with air and twists and is life-threatening. Treatment for GDV requires surgery to decompress the stomach and repair any internal damage done, as well as performing a gastropexy to prevent it from happening again. A gastropexy is done by attaching the pyloric antrum to the right side of the abdominal wall to prevent further stomach rotation. A gastropexy can be done a few different ways including belt-looped, circumcostal, incorporating, laparoscopic-assisted, or incisional. The incisional gastropexy is done by attaching the muscular layer of the gastric wall's opposite side to the right abdominal wall. Belt-looped gastropexy is done by tunneling a seromuscular flap through the abdominal wall, and circumcostal gastropexy is done by taking a seromuscular stomach flap and wrapping it around the last rib and then attaching it to the stomach wall. Laparoscopic-assisted gastropexy allows for suturing or stapling the stomach securely.

Enucleation

Enucleation is the complete removal of the eyeball due to ophthalmic neoplasms, severe corneal or scleral laceration, painful dry eye with corneal scarring, proptosis, tumors, and end-stage glaucoma.

There are two surgical options for enucleation. The **transconjunctival approach** is performed with an incision around the conjunctiva, which results in less orbital tissue loss, less bleeding during the surgery, and a faster procedure, but it should not be done on an eye that has an intraocular infection. The **transpalpebral procedure** is done with an elliptical incision around the eyelids and the globe, along with all of the secretory tissue including the conjunctiva, eyelids, and nictitating membrane being removed.

Cattle commonly develop malignant tumors arising from ocular squamous cells. The animal in need of enucleation surgery should be placed in its halter in such a way as to firmly fix the head to the side of the chute or stall. The animal's eyes should be closed fast with needle and thread. The animal's hair must be shaved and the animal should be prepared for surgery using proper sterilization procedures. The cow or goat should be given a Peterson eye block or a four-point retrobulbar block prior to the operation.

Total Ear Canal Ablation

There are three parts of the ear: the inner, middle, and outer portions. The inner ear controls balance, the middle portion holds the tympanic bulla and the eardrum, and the outer portion contains the ear canal and the pinna. A **total ear canal ablation** is the surgical removal of the whole ear canal and the pinna. This is followed by a bulla osteotomy, which is the opening and cleaning of the infected debris in the bulla. A total ear canal ablation is normally performed once medical treatment for chronic ear infections is not helping, and the patient is in constant pain. Total ear canal ablation is also recommended if there is cancer in the external ear canal. It could be a cure for the cancer depending on the size of the tumor and if it can be completely removed with this procedure.

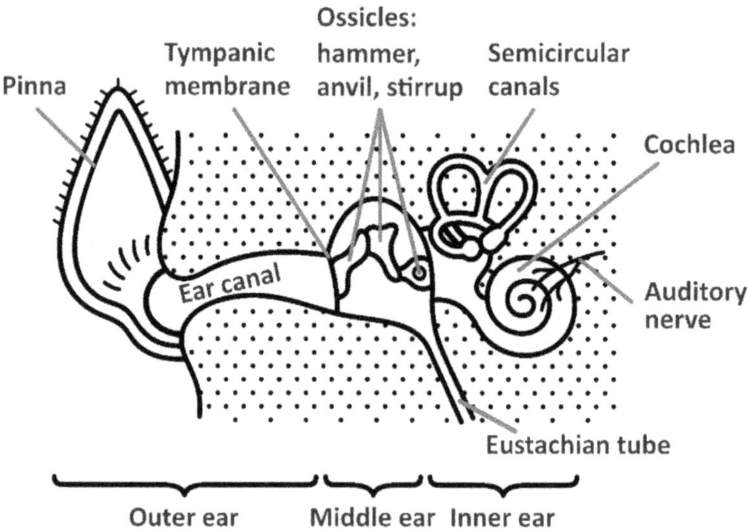

Onychectomy

Onychectomy, normally only performed on the front paws, is the removal of the claw, including the last bone in the digit. There are a couple of different surgical procedures used to perform an onychectomy. One method is to use a size 12 scalpel blade to cut out the claw. Some veterinarians use a more traditional method using a Resco nail trimmer to clip out the nail. The surgical sites are closed normally with surgical glue, and a pressure wrap is placed over the foot for 24 hours. Some veterinarians use a surgical laser to remove the claw. Using the laser results in little to no bleeding because it cauterizes the blood vessels as it cuts, and there is less swelling because it does not tear or crush the tissue. The laser will seal off the nerve endings as it cuts through the tissue, and this could reduce pain. A **tendonectomy** can also be done in which the claw is not removed, but the tendons under the paw are cut so the claws are always retracted into the paw.

Tibial Plateau Leveling Osteotomy (TPLO)

A **tibial plateau leveling osteotomy** (TPLO) surgery is performed on dogs with a torn **cranial cruciate ligament** (CCL), also commonly described as the anterior cruciate ligament (ACL). Approximately 90% of all orthopedic injuries in canines are from a torn ACL, and the TPLO surgery has been proven to be an extremely effective solution. A dog's knee is at a constant 110-degree bend; therefore, there is a constant stress put on the ACL, which is inside of the knee joint. Occasionally, this constant stress will cause injury or tearing of the ACL, which then results in the femur rubbing along the back of the tibia causing pain and inflammation. A TPLO surgery will be performed to rotate the tibial plateau where it is rubbing with the femur so that the femur will no longer be able to slide back on it, which creates stabilization for that knee. The first 12 weeks post-surgery are critical, but a full recovery usually takes 6 months. Each dog will recover at its own pace, but home rehabilitation is crucial. The owner should be made aware to avoid infection of the surgical site, and the dog must be kept from licking at the wound by wearing an Elizabethan collar. The owner must keep the dog quiet and avoid overactivity for a minimum of 8 weeks because the joint will need to heal.

TPLO PROCEDURE

A **tibial plateau leveling osteotomy** (TPLO) surgery is done to treat a cranial cruciate ligament tear by reducing the tibial plateau angle and eliminating the instability of the joint. Before the TPLO procedure, an x-ray of the stifle is taken for a measurement of the tibial plateau angle. During surgery, the joint is examined and any damaged cartilage is removed in order for the patient to regain normal function. A curved saw is then used to cut a semicircle into the inside top portion of the tibia. This cut portion is rotated to get the desired tibial plateau angle, and then a bone plate is placed on the bone holding the two pieces in the new alignment. After the surgery is complete, postoperative radiographs of the stifle are taken to ensure that the angle is correct and the bone plate placement is correct.

Suture Techniques

For surgical incisions, absorbable suture is commonly used for **closure**. The sizes of the suture material range from the largest being (0) and in numeric order—as the number rises, the suture gets smaller. Therefore, 2-0 is bigger than 4-0. The tensile strength of the suture compared to the tissue needing to be sutured will determine the suture size needed. **Subcuticular suture patterns** can be done with either continuous or interrupted sutures. Interrupted sutures are performed by each suture strand being tied and cut after the bite, giving a more secure closure. Microorganisms are not likely to migrate along this type of suture pattern, which is why it is used for wounds that are infected. **Mattress sutures** are used when there is more of a distance from one side of the wound to the other and tension is needed to bring the edges together. **Surgical adhesive** glue is a liquid wound adhesive that can be used for minor cuts or abrasions, and it is also used in feline declaws. Skin staples are commonly used to reinforce a sutured wound closure to further prevent dehiscence.

SUTURE MATERIALS

The veterinarian will apply a non-absorbable suture material in surgery. These materials are constructed from man-made and natural materials. Natural sources include silk, cotton, linen, and stainless steel. Silk does lose its ability to stretch after a 6-month period. However, silk is still beneficial as a material that will not soak up liquid. Cotton is derived from a spun cotton fiber that originates from a cotton plant.

Stainless steel has limited flexibility and can be difficult to manipulate. However, stainless steel is often used in veterinary medicine.

Non-absorbable synthetic materials include polypropylene, polyamide/nylon, and polymerized caprolactam. Polypropylene is derived from a synthetic plastic. Polyamide/nylon is derived from a polymerized plastic. Polymerized caprolactam has an outer layer that has been coated with a synthetic fibrous material. This synthetic fibrous material is applied by veterinarians in the surgical procedure to close the skin flaps after an operation.

SIZING SUTURE MATERIAL

Suture material sizes are represented by identifying numbers written as 4-0, 3-0, 0, 1, and 2. The suture material 4-0 is referred to aloud as "4 ought," with the word "ought" used in reference to the number zero.

The diameter or the width of the suture material can be determined by looking at the number with reference to zero. The larger the number, the thicker and larger the size. Therefore, a size 2 suture is larger than a size 1 suture. Contrarily, the diameter or width of the suture gets thinner as any number paired to the left of a zero enlarges. This indicates a smaller size. Thus, the size 3-0 is larger in size than 4-0. Wire suture sizes are indicated by the wire's gauge, ranging in size from 18-40 gauge. The higher gauge numbers indicate a thicker wire and vice versa. The veterinarian performing a surgery should select the best suture material and needle size based upon the surgical site, the recovery needs, and past experience.

General Knot Tying Principles

The **one-hand knot tying method** is applied in procedures where a deep hollow in the body must be reached. The solitary hand is easier to manipulate in the limited space than 2 hands or an instrument. The one-hand method uses the square knot. The two-hand method produces a uniform square knot. However, this method is time-consuming and considered to be quite tiresome.

The relationship between suture security and tying technique has been discussed as 2 variables where one increases as the other decreases, and vice versa. To complete the knot, the veterinarian must apply enough force to each strand to construct a secure square knot. For adequate interrupted sutures, the veterinarian selects a synthetic material with 3-mm tags. However, surgical gut tends to become larger and loosen. Thus, surgical gut tags are about 6 mm long. The veterinarian will eliminate any frayed or damaged suture material in the construction of the knot. The veterinarian will only apply instruments on the boundaries of the material. The recommended number of throws (suture strands) designated for the specific suture material will be used to create the knot. This will limit the mass of the knot and reduce ill effects on the tissue.

Square Knot

The **square knot** is applied at the beginning and end of both the interrupted suture pattern and the continuous suture pattern. The square knot is the knot most preferred by surgeons in tying off a suture securely. The square knot is created by making 2 casts with the suturing material. The casts are directed in a reverse route between each cast. The cast is completed by manipulating the tags to exit on the matching side of the loop. The surgeon will apply constant pressure when the knot is tightened securely. Most suturing material requires that the square knot have at least 3 casts. Some have more than 3, depending upon the material that is used in making the square knot. The surgeon will use as many casts as necessary in tying off a square knot securely. However, the bulkiness of the knot will increase as more casts are used.

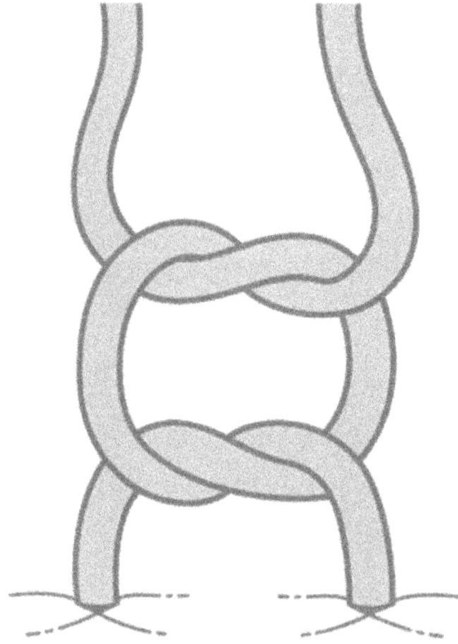

Knots tied off without this reversal are considered to be **granny knots** that have the tags on the opposite sides of the loop. The granny knot is not used by most surgeons due to the fact that this knot may slip and lose its hold.

Surgeon's Knot

The **surgeon's knot** begins the same way as the square knot, but the strand is passed through the loop twice on the first cast. This knot is also tied off similarly to the square knot, with an additional cast that creates more friction on the first pass. The surgeon's knot is to be applied in instances where the tension on the tissue presents a problem in using a square knot. However, this knot can be problematic because of its knot mass and its asymmetrical form, which is not usually beneficial in surgical procedures.

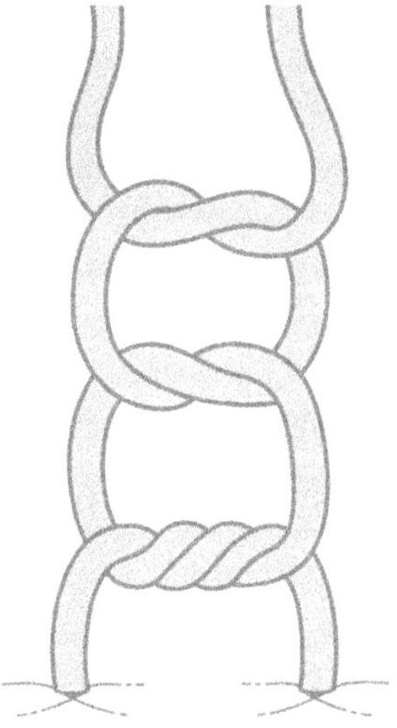

Buried Knot

The **buried knot** is used when a subcuticular or intradermal pattern is required. The buried knot incorporates a square knot in its tying-off pattern. The suture is passed on the nearby side from close to the surface to deeper into the incision and then crossed to the farthest side and passed from deep in the incision to close to the surface. This technique allows the knot to be hidden deep within the skin's tissue. This pattern can be described as an interrupted suture pattern that has been turned upside down.

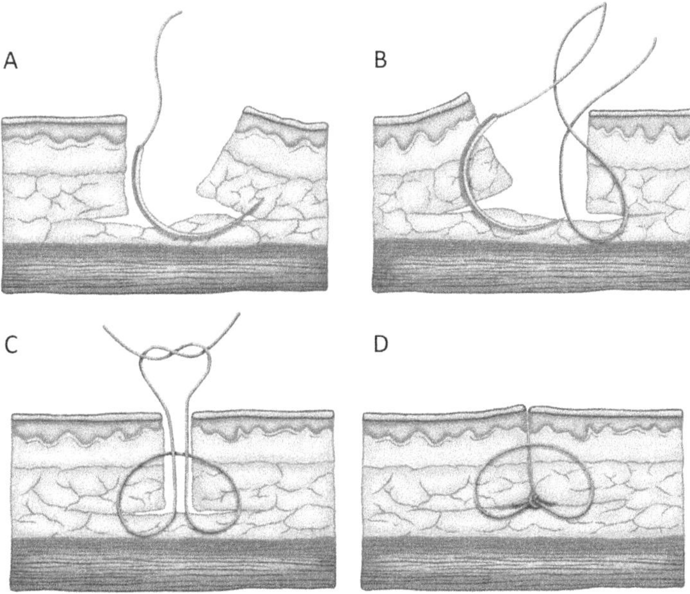

Buried Knot

Suture Patterns

Sutures can be applied in an interrupted or continuous pattern. Sutures which are considered to be **interrupted** are those that are cut and tied off at the end of every stitch. Uninterrupted and **continuous** sutures are those cut at the end of the entire suture procedure only; a **closing stitch** is applied at the end of the wound or incision site.

The advantages of interrupted suture patterns include that precision can be applied to the entire suture line so that the failure of one knot does not result in a significant failure along the entire suture line. However, it is time-consuming, requires more suturing material than is used in a continuous suturing method, and may more easily introduce foreign substances and debris along the incision site line.

A disadvantage of continuous sutures is gauging wound approximation and tension. The continuous suture procedure cannot be regulated and adjusted with precision during the suture procedure. By contrast, interrupted sutures allow for readjustments in tissue margin matching and tension with each new suture.

Appositional sutures bring tissues together. **Inverting** patterns turn the incision edges towards the patient.

SIMPLE RUNNING TECHNIQUE

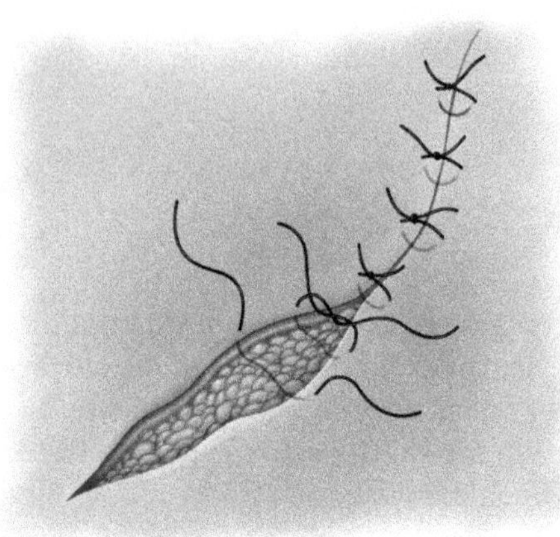

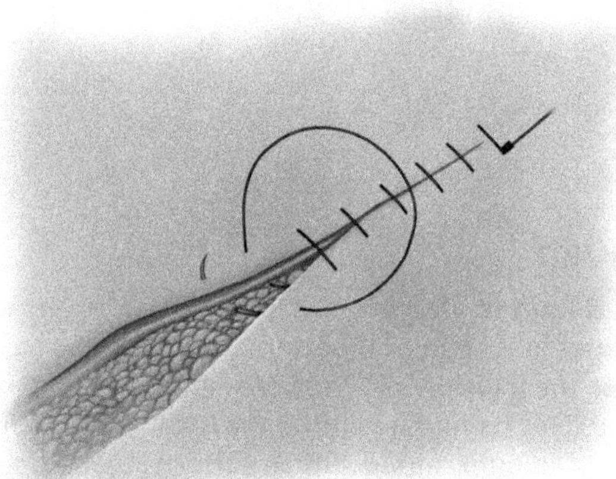

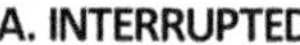

A. INTERRUPTED

B.CONTINUOUS

Simple Continuous Pattern

The appositional **simple continuous pattern** is initiated with two square knots and begun with four casts of the suture material. A simple continuous suture pattern can be cast in two different ways. The first method involves casting the suture just beneath the skin, where the sutures can be placed in a parallel position towards the tissue edges. The suture can also be placed towards the front, on the surface of the skin, leaving the visible sutures at an angle near the edge. However, this suture pattern often gathers into creases, and the skin's edges may constrict to prevent the proper air and blood flow.

Even so, the simple continuous pattern is sturdy and easily produced. This pattern is particularly valuable in the applications concerning the skin, subcutaneous tissue, fascia, the gastrointestinal tract, and the urinary tract. However, if there is a noticeable break along the suture line, the knot may fail to hold.

Ford Interlocking Pattern

The appositional **Ford interlocking suture** can be called the blanket stitch or the continuous interlocking suture. The interlocking loop is created by moving the needle above the trailing suture material after every stitch. The suture is initiated with 4 casts, and requires 4 casts on the end with a final loop to the loose end. The end is tied with a knot. This suture pattern is not economical because of the excessive suture material that is used. However, the suture does provide an airtight and watertight seal similar to the simple continuous pattern. There is a similar disadvantage in the strength and integrity of the suture line. A failure of the beginning or ending knot can cause the suture line to fail in its entirety. However, the failed knot of the Ford interlocking suture will not be as risky as that of the simple continuous suture because the knot found on the Ford interlocking suture is harder to remove. Other risks include poor wound margin approximation and potentially marked tension. The precision of the tension given to the sutures cannot be regulated or controlled with certainty using this method.

This suture is found on the top side of the skin.

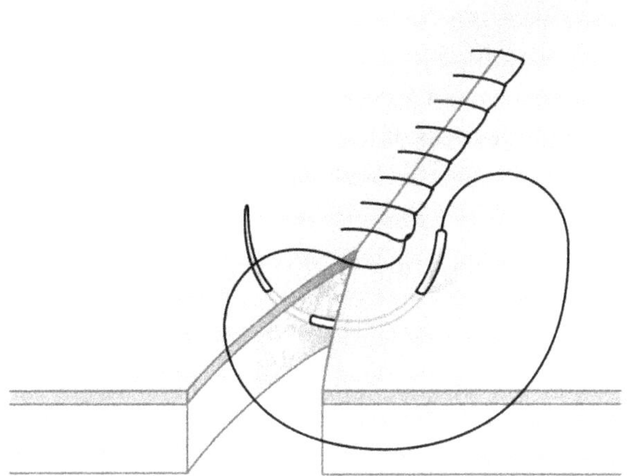

Intradermal Suture Pattern

The appositional **intradermal** (also called continuous buried cutaneous) **suture** is placed over another layer and is recommended when an alteration to the horizontal mattress suture is required. It starts off in much the same way as the interrupted buried pattern. The stitches are set in a pattern that sits at right angles to the incision line. The surgeon sets each loop of surgical thread to prevent any empty space. The surgeon fastens every fourth or fifth loop of surgical thread to the tissue on the bottom.

In completing the **continuous intradermal suture**, the final suture should be tacked down with a loop fixed to the loose end. This knot can be pulled down into the lower tissue and secured. The skin sutures which lie on top should be placed close together in such a way as to reduce the spaces left open in the epithelial closure. These sutures produce a good effect in the stitching of intradermal and subcutaneous closures. This method is an inexpensive use of suture materials. In addition, when using dissolving sutures, there is no need to remove the sutures at a later date.

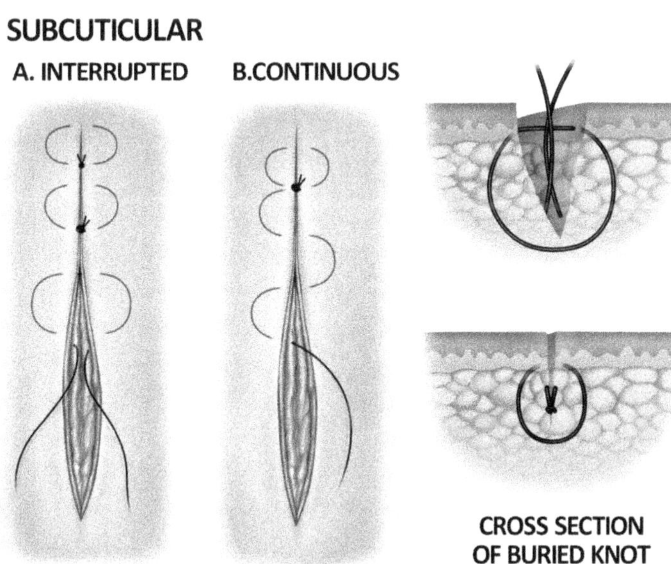

Simple Interrupted Suture Pattern

The **simple interrupted pattern** is considered appositional because it allows adjustment and regulation of the suture tension used. The stitches are about 5-10 mm apart from each other, and the skin's thickness must be considered in deciding on the distance from the edge of the incision to where the stitch is placed. The simple interrupted pattern is used to suture skin, subcutaneous tissue, fascia, vessels, nerves, the gastrointestinal tract, and the urinary tract.

The interrupted suture pattern can be applied over cutaneous sutures that are buried to strengthen and support the skin sutures. A wider stitch is used on thin skin or when cutaneous sutures are not present. The suture will be pushed through the full thickness of the tissue. However, in cases where the skin is too thick a suture will be placed partway into the tissue. This is also true when buried cutaneous sutures are applied. This partway placement is considered a split thickness approach.

Simple Interrupted Intradermal Suture Pattern

The **simple interrupted intradermal suture** is placed so that the knot is buried within the skin. This simple interrupted pattern is placed upside down into position. The pattern gains passage deep in the tissue, past the superficial subcutaneous tissue, to the dermis just below the epithelial edge. The pattern runs across the incision site and then gains passage from the dermis to the superficial subcutaneous tissue, where it leaves off. The suture is secured at the base of the tissue with two square knots. This pattern ensures contact with the protective layer of surface tissue and the lining of the organs. This is an appropriate method to use for intradermal or subcuticular closures.

Mattress Suture Patterns

Mattress sutures lower the stress placed on the incision's edge. These sutures are ideal whenever there is a high level of tension already present in the tissue. The interrupted horizontal, interrupted vertical, and continuous horizontal suture patterns are all names of specific mattress suture patterns used by a surgeon. However, mattress sutures have a propensity to evert or turn outwards from the boundaries of the tissue.

The surgeon will select an **interrupted vertical mattress** suture for use on tissue with tension. This type of suture is sturdier than the horizontal mattress suture.

The **continuous horizontal mattress** suture applies sturdy quality surgical seams over an existing suture layer. The sutures are completed by tying a loop to the loose end.

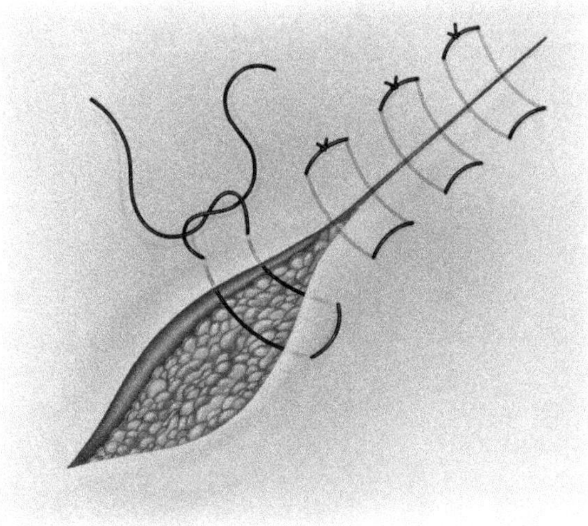

INTERRUPTED MATTRESS SUTURES

Lembert Suture Patterns

The **Lembert suture pattern** uses an inverting or reversal pattern which is best used for closures of hollow organs, such as the bladder, stomach, or uterus. The Lembert suture can be used to form either an interrupted or a continuous suture pattern. The serous membrane is the thin external lining around the internal organs of the body. The tissue, serosa to serosa, is physically brought together through the inverted Lembert suture using the interrupted pattern. The serosa is found on the inner chest, abdomen, and stomach. The surgeon places the suture so as not to block the lumen. Suture stitches are cast perpendicular to the incision line. These surgical sutures will be placed deep inside sturdy tissue. In the case of operations involving the intestines, the submucosa is included in this deeply sewn stitch. In the case of small mammals, this stitch must be modified so that the lumen of the intestines and the submucosa are part of the stitching process.

Removing Sutures

Sutures that are firmly fixed in place may cause the epithelial cells in the skin to quickly grow down the length of the stitch. The problem occurs when the cells reach the lower tissue. At that point the cells become keratinized, and redness and swelling in the form of an abscess can result. Usually, this happens with sutures that are left in the body for an excessive length of time. Thus, the surgeon will want to remove the skin sutures after 7-10 days. In cases where the sutures are buried and have resulted in tissue binding strength, only 7 days is usually required before removal. Sutures that have not succeeded in binding the skin together may need to stay in for 10-14 days. The surgeon will remove the skin sutures by grabbing the loose tab attached to the knot. The surgeon uses fingers or a hemostat to perform this task. The surgeon will pull the buried suture's knot up to expose it for clipping. The surgeon can then begin cutting and removing the clean suture material through the skin.

Other Forms of Incision Closure

Stainless steel skin staples are a simple, affordable alternative to suturing. They are quick to apply and easy to remove. They come in pouches that are sterile and should be used immediately. Unused staples can be sterilized for future use with the Sterrad Sterilizer or ethylene oxide, but should not be placed in the autoclave.

Cyanoacrylate tissue adhesives such as Vetbond are used for cutaneous wound closure. They are inexpensive, quick, and provide comparable tensile strength to sutures.

Chapter Quiz

Ready to see how well you retained what you just read? Scan the QR code to go directly to the chapter quiz interface for this study guide. If you're using a computer, simply visit the online resources page at **mometrix.com/resources719/vtne** and click the Chapter Quizzes link.

Dentistry

Transform passive reading into active learning! After immersing yourself in this chapter, put your comprehension to the test by taking a quiz. The insights you gained will stay with you longer this way. Scan the QR code to go directly to the chapter quiz interface for this study guide. If you're using a computer, simply visit the online resources page at **mometrix.com/resources719/vtne** and click the Chapter Quizzes link.

Dental Anatomy and Physiology

Anatomy of the Tooth

The **crown** of a tooth is covered by hard, white **enamel** and is the section that has erupted from the **gingiva**, or gums. Enamel covers the dense **dentin**, which forms the bulk of the tooth and protects the **pulp cavity**, which is made up of connective tissue, nerves, and blood vessels. The tooth **root** is covered by **cementum** and is the section of the tooth that remains unerupted, anchoring it to the **alveolar bone** in the mandible and maxilla via the **periodontal ligament**. The **gingival sulcus** is the space between the gingiva and the enamel. The **apical delta** is the opening in the tooth root where the nerves and blood vessels enter and exit the tooth.

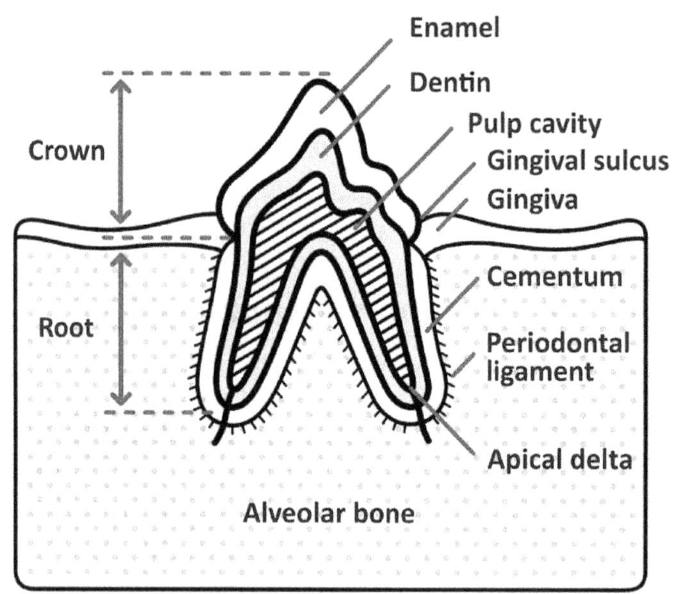

Enamel

Hydroxyapatite is the chief mineral found in the **enamel** of teeth. This mineral is one of the hardest and most plentiful found in the body. Enamel is composed of 96% mineral and 4% water and organic substances. The 2 proteins found in enamel are called amelogenins and enamelins. Enamel is the exterior layer that is used to wrap the uppermost part of the tooth or crown. Ameloblasts function to shape the enamel when the tooth is being formed. This process stops when the tooth breaks through the gums. The enamel functions to prevent bacteria from damaging the tooth. The enamel does not contain any nerve endings.

Canine tooth enamel can range in thickness from <0.1 mm to 0.6 mm. Feline tooth enamel can range in thickness from <0.1 mm to 0.3 mm. The enamel in hypsodont teeth of herbivores, such as horses and cattle, both covers and exists in complicated folds within the dentin. In this way the durability of the tooth is increased for animals that must constantly chew hard, cellulose-based foods. This folding can be used to determine an animal's age.

Dentin and Pulp

Dentin is formed by odontoblasts through dentinogenesis, is softer than enamel and cementum, and has a tendency to decay rapidly. Exposed dentin can lead to severe cavities when left untreated. The dentin provides an extra barrier to prevent bacteria from getting in the pulp. Dentin is porous and yellow. Dentin permits the movement of fluids through its pores. Dentin is composed of about 72% inorganic material, 18% organic material (mostly collagen), and 10% water. Dentin is innervated and is sensitive to heat, cold, touch, and changes in osmotic pressure. The collagen in the dentin gives the tooth the flexibility needed to absorb shock. This keeps the tooth from breaking or fracturing.

Dental pulp is located on the inside of the tooth. It is formed from connective tissue, odontoblasts, and fibroblasts and contains blood vessels, nerves, and lymphatic vessels. Exposed pulp will lead to pain, inflammation, and necrosis.

Root

Mineralized **cementum** functions as a structural system that attaches the tooth to the stabilizing periodontal ligaments. Enamel and dentin are both harder than cementum. Cementoblasts secrete the cementum into place. It is constantly reabsorbed and mended. Periodontal ligaments fasten the gingiva to the cementum. However, the gingiva cannot be readily secured back to the cementum if disturbed.

The **cementoenamel junction** is at the base of the crown where the enamel meets the cementum that envelops the tooth's root. The cementoenamel junction fastens the tooth with periodontal ligaments at the gingiva.

The **periodontal ligament** anchors each tooth in the alveolus or socket by fastening the cementum of the tooth to the alveolar bone. This support system provides the teeth with enough strength to undergo large compression forces used in chewing without damage to the bones. The teeth are not directly attached to the bone. The periodontal ligaments can absorb shock and protect the nerve endings. The sensory nerve endings located in the ligaments function as pain and pressure sensors used by the brain to respond to changing pressures during chewing, among other forces impacting the teeth.

Alveolar Bone and Gingiva

The bone enveloping and sustaining the teeth is known as the **alveolar bone**. This bone undergoes constant internal repair and regeneration.

The **gingiva** is soft mucosal tissue that envelops the jawbone, and it protects teeth from harmful bacteria. The 3 sections of the gingiva consist of the marginal gingiva, the attached gingiva, and the interdental gingiva.

The section of gingival tissue immediately beside the tooth and forming an adherent pocket is known as the **gingival sulcus**. The gingival sulcus should be probed as part of a dental examination between the marginal gingival tissue and the tooth and is typically measured at a depth of 1-3 mm in dogs. This section is measured at a depth of 0.5-1.0 mm in cats.

Dentition

Descriptive Dental Terminology

Buccal: In dentistry, refers to the surface of the tooth or gums that is closest to the cheek within the mouth (Latin *bucca*: cheek)

Distal: In dentistry, refers to the direction moving toward the last tooth in each quadrant of a dental arch

Furcation: Refers to the dividing point between the roots of a tooth that are joined at the crown

Gingival: Refers to the gingiva or gums

Incisal: In dentistry, refers to the shearing edge of an incisor

Labial: In dentistry, refers to the surface of the tooth or gums that is closest to the lips within the mouth (Latin *labium*: lip)

Lingual: In dentistry, refers to the surface of the tooth or gums that is closest to the tongue within the mouth (Latin *lingua*: tongue)

Mandibular: Pertaining to the mandible or jawbone, which holds the lower set of teeth

Maxillary: Pertaining to the maxilla, which holds the upper set of teeth

Mesial: Refers to the surfaces or objects closest to the midline of the dental arch

Occlusal: The surface of molars and premolars that functions to chew or grind food

Palatal: Refers to the region in the mouth that is closest to the palate or the roof of the mouth

Rostral: Refers to the portion relating to or oriented toward the nose of an animal

Types of Teeth

Incisors have a sharp edge that is ideal for cutting and shearing; they each have a single root. **Canines** serve to grasp food, anchoring it in the mouth or tearing it into pieces; they each have a single root.

Premolars cut, sever, and hold the animal's prey or food. They can have one root, two roots, one root fused from two roots, or three roots. The **molars** work to masticate or grind the food into a form that can be easily swallowed and are found at the back of the mouth.

The **carnassial** teeth are modified, paired molars and premolars found in carnivorous animals used to cut and tear meat. Canine and feline carnassial teeth are the fourth maxillary premolars and first mandibular molars.

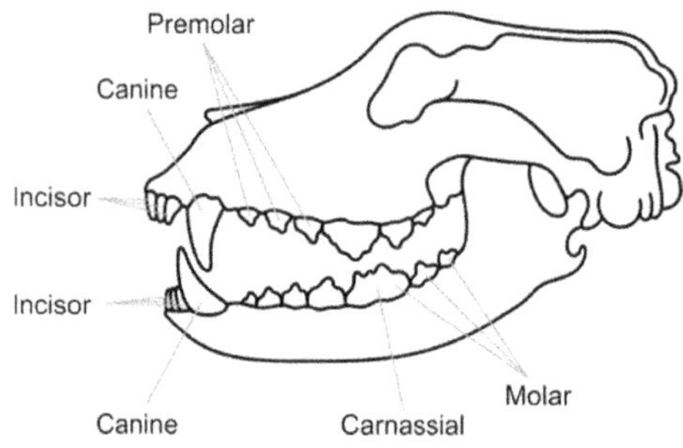

Dental Formulas by Species

Dental formulas indicate the number of different types of teeth expected for a species. **Permanent**, or adult, teeth are represented by capital letters; **deciduous**, or baby, teeth are represented by lower case letters. Incisors are represented by I or i, canines are represented by C or c, premolars are represented by P or p, and molars are represented by M or m.

$$\frac{\text{Maxillary Arcade}}{\text{Mandibular Arcade}} \qquad \frac{\text{I C P M}}{\text{I C P M}} \qquad \frac{\text{i c p m}}{\text{i c p m}}$$

These numbers represent only one half of the dental arch and can be added together and then doubled to give a total that represents all of the teeth that should be present in the mouth.

Species	Deciduous	Permanent
Canine (dog)	$\frac{3\,1\,3}{3\,1\,3} = 14$	$\frac{3\,1\,4\,2}{3\,1\,4\,3} = 21$
Feline (cat)	$\frac{3\,1\,3}{3\,1\,2} = 13$	$\frac{3\,1\,3\,1}{3\,1\,2\,1} = 15$
Equine (horse)	$\frac{3\,0\,3}{3\,0\,3} = 12$	$\frac{3\,1\,(3)4\,3}{3\,1\,3\,3} = (20)21^{*}$
Porcine (pig)	$\frac{3\,1\,3}{3\,1\,3} = 14$	$\frac{3\,1\,4\,3}{3\,1\,4\,3} = 22$
Ruminants: Bovine (cow), ovine (sheep), caprine (goat)	$\frac{0\,0\,3}{3\,1\,3} = 10$	$\frac{0^{**}\,0\,3\,3}{3\,1\,3\,3} = 16$

*__Wolf teeth__ are the small upper premolars found in most (but not all) horses that may be removed in performance horses to reduce discomfort when using a bit.

Ruminants, such as sheep, cattle, and goats, lack upper incisors and instead have a **dental pad, which works with the tongue to grasp large quantities of plant matter when eating. Additionally, their mandibular canine teeth are sometimes classified as fourth incisors.

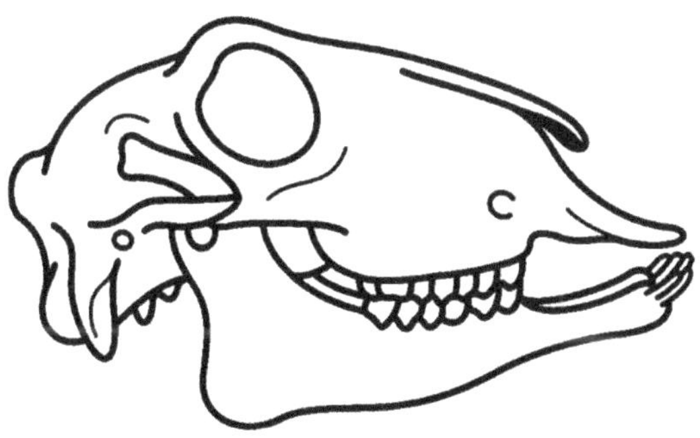

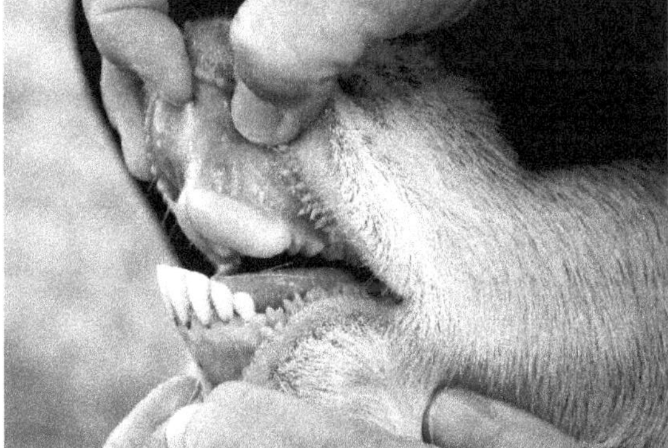

The Modified Triadan System

Veterinarians employ the **modified Triadan system** to number the teeth of any species. In this system each tooth is given a 3-digit number. The first digit indicates the quadrant. The mouth of the animal is divided into 4 quadrants or sections. For permanent or adult teeth: 1 = upper right quadrant; 2 = upper left quadrant; 3 = lower left quadrant; 4 = lower right quadrant. For deciduous or baby teeth: 5 = upper right quadrant; 6 = upper left quadrant; 7 = lower left quadrant; 8 = lower right quadrant. Note that upper teeth are also called maxillary teeth, and lower teeth are also called mandibular teeth.

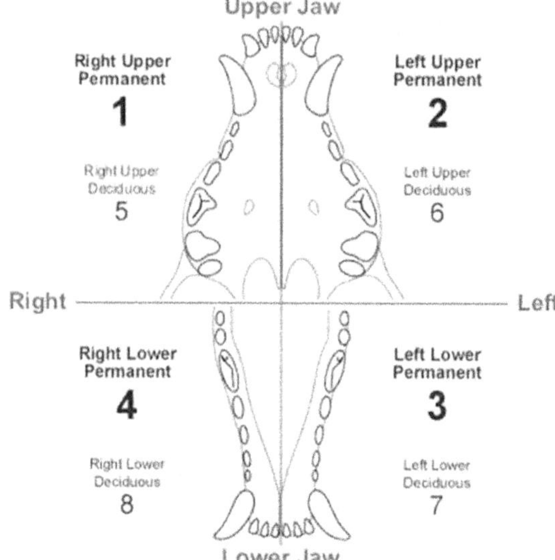

The second and third digits indicate the particular tooth in the quadrant, numbered 01-11, starting with the teeth nearest the midline and progressing distally. This system simplifies nomenclature between species. For example, in all species the first incisor is 01, canines are 04, and the first molars are 09, regardless of whether a species naturally lacks certain teeth. 108 and 208 represent the maxillary carnassial teeth in both cats and dogs.

Canine Triadan System

In small animal medicine, the use of the modified Triadan system in canines is important for communicating about and documenting the results of dental exams and procedures.

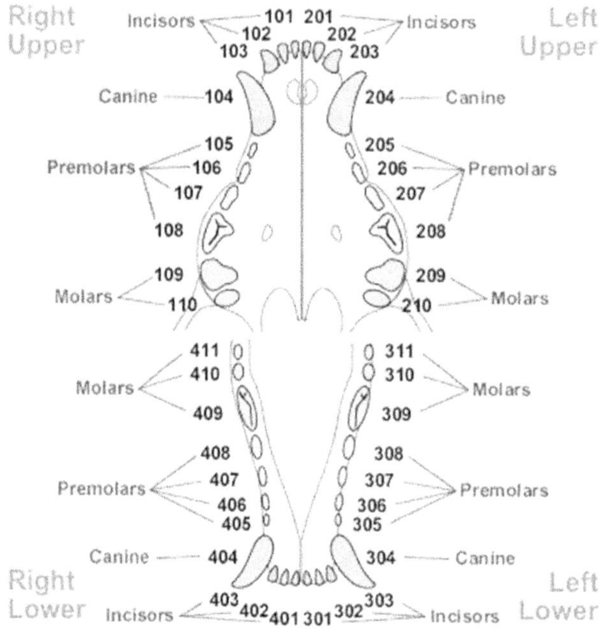

Incisors and canines (01-04) each have only one root. In the dog, premolars and molars have one, two, or three roots:

Tooth Type	1 Root	2 Roots	3 Roots
Premolars	105, 205, 305, 405	106, 107 206, 207 306, 307, 308, 309, 310 406, 407, 408, 409, 410	108, 208
Molars	311, 411	None	109, 110 209, 210

Dental Pathophysiology

Plaque and Tartar

Plaque is a mix of bacteria and their by-products, salivary components, inflammatory cells, and oral debris that can form within hours on the teeth. As the pet eats, the food particles stick in between the teeth, and once bacteria in the mouth start to digest these food particles, plaque forms. Dead bacteria and calcium in the saliva can calcify, forming a hardened form called **tartar (dental calculus)**. As plaque spreads, it leads to inflammation of the gums called gingivitis, and as plaque and tartar continue to develop underneath the gum line, they can infect the tooth root, and dental scaling will be needed to clean the teeth. In the later stages of periodontal disease, the surrounding tissues of the tooth break down and are destroyed and the bony socket holding the tooth in place becomes eroded, loosening the tooth.

Gingivitis

Gingivitis is a term referring to general inflammation of the gums. It can be localized to one tooth, or it can be widespread. It is caused by **plaque**, a buildup of food debris and bacteria. Left uncleaned, plaque hardens into tartar, making it even more difficult to keep the teeth clean of plaque. Most bacteria found in plaque are aerobic, gram-positive rods and cocci. Treatment of gingivitis may cure or alter the course of the gum's condition. Untreated, gingivitis can spread into the ligaments and bone that support the teeth and cause them to eventually fall out.

The gingivitis index is used to measure the amount of inflammation present within the animal's mouth. The designation of GI0 is given to describe normal, healthy gingival tissue. This state is characterized by fresh breath, a sharp gingival margin, pink gum coloration, and a normal gingival sulcus depth.

There are three stages of gingivitis:

Stages	Signs
GI0	None (normal, healthy gingival tissue)
GI1	Mild edema (swelling), no bleeding on probing (BOP), some color change, normal gingival sulcus depth, mild odor
GI2	Moderate edema, BOP, deep red color
GI3	Severe edema, spontaneous bleeding, early periodontitis, deep red and purple color

Ultimately, the animal can also experience periodontal **attachment loss (AL)**. This is measured by degrees. A periodontal probe is used to make an assessment of the degree of attachment loss in the animal's mouth.

Gingivitis can be prevented with proper care of the animal's teeth. This care requires daily maintenance, as plaque can build up on the teeth within a 6-hour period. Plaque is formed from organic debris and bacteria which can be transformed through a mineralization process to produce a hard deposit on the teeth after only 24-48 hours.

Periodontal Disease (PD)

Periodontal disease is the infection and subsequent inflammation of the tissues around the teeth, including gingivitis, affecting the gingiva, and periodontitis, affecting the periodontal ligament. Periodontal disease is caused by bacteria, plaque buildup, and the animal's response to the bacteria present in the mouth. Dogs and cats usually do not develop periodontal disease until after the age of 4. However, at least 85% of all dogs and cats over the age of 4 will have early periodontal disease.

The development of calculus will escalate the periodontal disease process, making it easier for bacteria and debris to accumulate around the teeth. In addition, the bacteria now accumulating will be anaerobic, gram-negative rods and various filamentous organisms. Endotoxins and exotoxins will be created. Endotoxins are released when bacteria decompose. Exotoxins that are released by bacteria can have negative impacts on the central nervous system. These toxins further damage tissues and undermine the support structure of the tooth. Periodontal disease is progressive in nature and cannot be cured. However, animals with this disease do respond positively to dental management and care.

Stages and Treatment

Periodontal disease first appears as red and swollen gingiva (gums). More advanced stages (2-4) involve **furcation exposure**: in multirooted teeth, the periodontal probe fits partially under the crown of the tooth due to the loss of alveolar bone. There are four stages of periodontal disease:

Stages	Signs	Attachment Loss (AL)
Stage 0	No disease	None
Stage 1 (PD1)	Gingivitis	None
Stage 2 (PD2)	Early periodontitis, furcation 1 exposure (probe fits less than halfway under crown)	<25%
Stage 3 (PD3)	Moderate periodontitis, furcation 2 exposure (probe extends more than halfway under crown)	25-50%
Stage 4 (PD4)	Advanced periodontitis, furcation 3 exposure (probe may pass completely under the crown)	>50%

The severity of the disease can only be diagnosed by a veterinarian. The veterinarian may employ a number of treatments in the care and management of the disease. Treatments that can have a beneficial impact on the animal include: a) complete scaling and prophy (tooth polishing), b) root planing, c) antibiotics, d) gum surgery, e) tooth extraction, f) home care, and g) products like dry food and chew toys, as recommended by the **Veterinary Oral Health Council** (VOHC).

Mobility Index (MI)

The veterinarian will employ the **mobility index** to determine the amount a tooth moves when manipulated. This can help in determining the extent of disease present.

- M0: indicates no movement (<0.2 mm)
- M1: indicates movement measured between 0.2 mm and 0.5 mm, with no axial mobility
- M2: indicates movement measured between 0.5 mm and 1.0 mm, with no axial mobility
- M3: indicates movement greater than 1.0 mm in any direction, or any axial movement. Typically, the veterinarian will recommend extraction of a tooth with an M3 designation.

Tooth Abscesses

The veterinarian should check animals with serious, progressive periodontal disease on a regular basis. Animals can develop accelerated decay and root abscesses as a result of this disease. The most common location for an abscess is the fourth maxillary premolars (108 and 208), which have three roots. The root nearest to the surface is the one most likely to become abscessed.

To develop an **abscess**, infectious bacteria must work past the gum line and into the root, a common result of serious decay or broken teeth. In situations of considerable swelling, the abscess may present as a lump underneath the skin.

An untreated abscess can lead to more systemic infection, even spreading to the sinuses or eyes. An abscess-induced **oronasal fistula** is the result of erosion between the oral cavity and the anterior respiratory tract. This fistula can allow food and fluids to enter the respiratory tract, resulting in chronic inflammation and infection. The dog may exhibit symptoms such as nasal discharge, a protuberance on top of the tooth root, sneezing, and a persistent cough.

Gingival Hyperplasia

The animal that has **gingival hyperplasia** can experience a gradual enlargement and overgrowth of the gums. The enlarged areas of the gums can trap plaque and calculus below the gum line; however, the pseudopocket formed should not automatically be assumed to be the result of attachment loss.

This condition can be attributed to genetic factors, or it can be attributed to the excessive administration of drugs. The following drugs are particularly prone to inducing this condition: diphenylhydantoin, nitrendipine, nifedipine, and cyclosporine.

Animals with this condition will exhibit gradually expanding mass or masses near the gum line, bleeding gums, and mouth tenderness. Large and giant breed dogs more commonly present with gingival hyperplasia. Boxers are also more prone to gingival hyperplasia. Other dogs associated with gingival hyperplasia include the Great Dane, Collie, Doberman Pinscher, and Dalmatian. The enlarged mass or masses can be surgically removed by the veterinarian. The application of a scalpel blade can be used as long as the animal is under anesthesia. However, this procedure may need to be repeated, as these growths can come back in the future.

Morphological Anomalies

Anodontia: This term refers to the congenital absence of teeth.

Attrition: Tooth wear caused by contact with other teeth at the occlusal or incisal surface; this may expose the dentin or pulp.

Brachygnathism: This term is used to describe the physical position of the upper jaw projecting out past the lower jaw. This malformation is due to the mandible being shorter than the maxilla. This is also known as overshot jaw or parrot mouth.

Dental interlock: A condition in which the growth of one jaw can be restricted by the eruption of deciduous teeth that have developed in an abnormal fashion. The mandible may stop developing in a normal fashion when other deciduous teeth interrupt the process. One illustration is when the upper deciduous canines emerge rostral to the lower canine teeth to "lock" or prevent the mandible's normal forward development.

Edentulous: Refers to having lost all teeth (typically later in life).

Enamel hypoplasia: This term refers to a state where tooth enamel does not form correctly or is damaged during development. Either mishap will cause portions of the enamel to be omitted or diminished. The weakened enamel may wear or chip away, leaving the dentin open to the elements. The dentin cannot hold up to oral events and exposures without proper enamel protection. Therefore, these teeth will deteriorate more quickly than teeth that have developed normally. Another name for enamel hypoplasia is distemper teeth, in reference to young dogs with enamel hypoplasia due to a distemper virus infection prior to the eruption of their permanent teeth.

Fusion: This term refers to the development of a single larger tooth from 2 tooth buds. This large tooth is developed by a joining or merging of 2 or more teeth including the crowns, roots, and dentin.

Gemination (dental): This term refers to a single root with 2 crowns. This abnormality is a result of one tooth germ that did not properly divide into 2 fully developed teeth.

Impaction: Refers to a tooth that fails to emerge from beneath the gums. It stays inside the tissue or bone and causes the animal pain.

Level bite: This term refers to a situation where the upper and lower incisor teeth meet each other end to end, rather than the upper (maxillary) incisors just overlapping the lower (mandibular) incisors as they should.

Malocclusion: This term is used to describe a condition in which the teeth in the maxilla do not make proper contact with those in the mandible when biting down.

Oligodontia: This term refers to the condition of having fewer teeth than normally found in the animal's species.

Polyodontia: This term refers to the condition of having more teeth than are normally found in the animal's species.

Posterior crossbite: A condition in which the maxilla is narrower in width than the mandible in the back, positioning the upper fourth premolar inside the lower first molar. This is a rare occurrence, particularly in dogs that have long noses.

Prognathism: This term is used to describe the physical position of the maxilla to the lower jaw. In this case, the lower jaw projects out past the maxilla or upper jaw. This is also known as "undershot" or "bulldog bite." This physical malformation is more common in brachycephalic breeds that have short, broad-shaped heads. This condition can occur in conjunction with animals that display an anterior crossbite.

Wry mouth: This term refers to the animal with half of its jaw somewhat longer on one side than on the other side. This condition is not easily treatable. In addition, this condition tends to be hereditary.

Persistent Deciduous Teeth

Occasionally, an animal's deciduous teeth will persist, which may lead to misdirected permanent teeth. Typically, this can lead to malocclusion and attrition. The double sets of teeth trap food and thus lead to dental decay. The double sets of roots prevent normal development of the tooth socket, and ultimately erode gum support around both teeth. Animals with persistent deciduous teeth may present with abnormal wear, periodontal disease, and/or premature tooth loss. It is important to extract persistent deciduous teeth early to prevent problems, though great skill is required to prevent damage to permanent teeth in the process.

Oral Neoplasia

Epulis is the most common oral tumor found in dogs; it is benign, and there are two types: fibromatous and ossifying. Common malignant canine oral tumors include: squamous cell carcinoma, fibrosarcoma, osteosarcoma, and malignant melanoma.

Squamous cell carcinoma is the most common oral tumor in cats.

Early detection of oral neoplasia is important, and oral exams should be performed as part of routine physical examinations. If a mass is detected, dental radiographs and a biopsy are important for diagnosis.

Stomatitis

Stomatitis is a condition in which the mucous membranes lining the mouth become red and irritated. This inflammation often involves cheeks, gums, tongue, lips, and the roof or floor of the mouth.

Stomatitis may form as a consequence of poor oral hygiene, iron deficiency anemia, foreign bodies, or thermal, chemical, or electrical burns (chewing on electrical cords, indiscriminate ingestions, etc.). It usually represents an inefficient immune response. Cats may contract stomatitis from coming into contact with a bacterial plaque that induces hypersensitivity or an allergic reaction. Animals having stomatitis may exhibit a number of symptoms, including a change in behavior, severe pain, irritability, aggressiveness or depression, excessive drooling, or changes in appetite. The appetite changes may be attributed to problems associated with chewing and eating.

The veterinarian will check for a series of multiple lesions around a tooth or an entire gum line. The lesions appear as broken or infected skin. The veterinarian who detects such lesions can diagnose the patient with stomatitis, indicating inflammation in the animal's mouth.

Feline Lymphocytic-Plasmacytic Stomatitis (LPS)

Cats are susceptible to a serious condition known as feline lymphocytic-plasmacytic stomatitis (LPS). This disease is associated with an irregular and severe immune reaction to the presence of bacteria-bearing plaque. There is no direct research that identifies any specific cause for the condition. However, specialty-bred cats like Siamese, Himalayans, and Abyssinians seem to contract the disease more often than other cats. Typically, the disease will quickly progress to include the following symptoms: intensely red and swollen gums, inflamed lesions located along the back side of the throat or esophagus, difficulty chewing, loss of appetite, and significant weight loss. The entire oral cavity may eventually become painfully inflamed. The animal will stop grooming itself and will have an unkempt and untidy appearance. The veterinarian can perform an oral biopsy to confirm the diagnosis. The diagnosis may lead to the decision to remove some or all of the cat's teeth. Any teeth remaining in the cat's mouth should be cleaned daily.

Feline Odontoclastic Resorption Lesions

Feline odontoclastic resorption lesions (FORL) are common observations made when treating cats (nearly 60% are affected). Other names for FORL are feline cervical lesions, neck lesions, or enamel erosions. These lesions should not be mistaken for caries. The lesion originates at the CEJ (the tooth's cemento-enamel joint). There will be evidence of missing enamel. The granulation tissue (fibrous connective tissue found in healing wounds) inside the lesions has small lumps with a rough, grainy texture. Cells inside of the lesions differentiate into odontoclasts along the periodontal ligament, causing dentin and root replacement resorption as they attack and take in the nutrients or chemicals found in the dentin and enamel. The lesions will work into the pulp. The outward appearance of the tooth can be misleading, as the root may be small or nonexistent. There may also be one or more lesions on either the lingual or the buccal side of the tooth. These lesions should be considered progressive, though not all lesions are visible.

Signs and Diagnosis

The reason an animal develops feline odontoclastic resorption lesions (FORLs) is not known, though it is common in purebreds including: Persians, Abyssinians, Siamese, Russian Blue, Scottish Fold, and Oriental Shorthairs.

Clinical signs include evidence of oral pain, including change in appetite, change in food preference, decreased self-grooming, difficulty chewing, irritability, aggressiveness, tenderness in the jaws, bleeding around the mouth, and/or excessive salivation.

Lesions may be detected underneath sections of plaque or inflamed gums. Therefore, it is advised to remove the plaque to increase the chance of detection. Dental radiographs can then be obtained to isolate neck lesions and determine lesion severity.

Instruments & Equipment

Dental Hand Instruments

The veterinarian will utilize 2 varieties of hand-held instruments in dental work. These instruments are categorized as cutting or non-cutting implements. The **cutting instruments** are fashioned with the following:

the cutting edge, the blade, the shank, and the handle. The **non-cutting instruments** are fashioned with the following: the point or face, the nib, the shank, and the handle. The shank is found on both varieties of instruments. It functions to connect the handle of the instrument to the working end: the blade of the cutting instrument or the nib on the non-cutting instrument.

The veterinarian will grasp the handle utilizing an adapted pencil grip. This allows the middle finger to remain at rest along the shank. The middle finger can feel vibrations that flow through the instrument when it is moved over a rough surface. This movement is directed with the additional support provided by the middle finger. A fulcrum (i.e., a point of rest, typically on an adjacent jaw) provides a steady handhold on the instrument. This fulcrum can also help direct the movements of the instrument with more precision. The third or fourth finger can be used to hold the fulcrum.

Periodontal Probe

A **periodontal probe** is a non-cutting instrument. The periodontal probe is shaped in a form that is extended, slender, and curved along one end. The veterinarian will use the probe to determine the depth of the gingival sulcus to help determine the presence and progression of periodontal disease.

The probe has tiny marks etched in millimeters on the blunt end. It is placed parallel to the long axis of the tooth, and with slight pressure it is run around the tooth to measure the pocket depth. The pocket depth is the distance between the base of the pocket and the gingival margin. In dogs, it should not exceed 3 mm, and in cats, 0.5-1.0 mm is normal. If there is gum recession, it can be measured with the periodontal probe. Gum recession is important to document at each annual dental cleaning and to keep in the patient's record to see trends and diagnose stages of periodontal disease.

Shepherd's Hook

The **shepherd's hook** is also known as the **explorer**; it is used to examine the surface of the tooth with its flexible steel tip that can detect any abnormalities, such as a furcation, and is used to investigate the condition of the tooth's enamel. The veterinarian will also check out any decay or broken teeth that are found in the animal's mouth. The tool can be applied with a light touch which does not hurt the gums. The explorer can be beneficial in exposing any subgingival calculus or loose teeth. Cats can also be examined with the explorer. In particular, the explorer can help detect external feline odontoclastic resorption lesions, found in approximately 28-67% of all cats.

Sickle Scaler

Scalers have sharp tips and edges and are used to remove supragingival (above the gum line) calculus from the teeth. The **sickle scaler** is fashioned in the form of a triangle. This instrument has 2 cutting edges with a sharp tip. The straight shank can be applied to the anterior or front teeth. The contra-angle shank can be applied to the posterior or back teeth. The sickle scaler should be pulled in a direction away from the gum line. The cutting edge of the sickle shank should be positioned just beneath the raised strip of the calculus. This will allow the calculus or tartar to be scraped away from the tooth without harming the gingiva.

Curette Scaler

The **curette scaler** is fashioned in the form of a spoon and has two sharp edges, a blunt tip, and a curved back, and it is used to remove calculus from under the gumline (subgingival) on the root surface and on the gingival tissue on the opposing side (gingival curettage). The architecture of the curette scaler utilizes a half circle in cross section. The curette scaler comes in 2 forms, the universal and the area-specific.

It is also useful for root planing and for removing the soft tissue found in the periodontal pocket. The veterinarian will position the cutting edge adjacent to the tooth, and the handle should be held in a parallel direction towards the root. The curette scaler should pull away from the root of the tooth as it moves, and multiple strokes may be necessary to remove the calculus. This is done until the tooth's surface begins to appear shiny and even.

Elevators

A **periosteal elevator** is used to lift the gum tissue to help remove some of the alveolar bone in an extraction with the flat side of the blade pressing against the tooth's surface and the curved side against the soft tissue to decrease tearing. **Dental elevators** are used by placing the concave side of the instrument along the tooth's surface and the curved side between the tooth and the alveolar bone to stretch and tear the periodontal ligament in order to loosen the tooth for easier extraction.

Power Scalers

Ultrasonic scalers are the most popular type of power scaler, and they remove supragingival gross calculus or tartar. A gentle pressure on the tooth is all that is necessary. This light touch will ensure that heat is not allowed to become intense. Heat can cause the enamel to become rutted, which can result in injury to the pulp. The area beneath the gum line should not be treated because of the likelihood of heat buildup. This is caused by the inability of the tip to be cooled off by water when under the gum line. The application of an abundant supply of water is recommended. The water keeps the teeth cool in the ultrasonic cleaning process. The water should be demineralized or filtered to reduce problematic buildup in the tubing. The veterinarian should only work for about 5 seconds on each tooth. The tips require replacement on a regular basis. The tips should be checked for proper length, as they have a tendency to wear and shorten with use. This will reduce the efficiency of the equipment. The patient should be given an oral rinse frequently. It should be a disinfectant, preferably a 0.12% chlorhexidine solution.

Ultrasonic Scaler Tips

Veterinarians will employ ultrasonic scalers as an efficient method to remove calculus from the surface of the tooth. The instruments function with a vibration that moves along the end of the scalers at a frequency rate of 20-45 kHz or 20,000-45,000 cycles per second; this is an ultrasonic frequency rate. The instruments are available with a variety of power ratings. The tips can be oval or egg-shaped, formed as a bowed line, or in the shape of a number 8. There are 3 tips available: magnetostrictive, piezoelectric, or sonic. The magnetostrictive tip pulsates at a frequency of 18-29 kHz in an oval pattern. The piezoelectric tip keeps a linear pattern and pulsates at 40 kHz. The piezoelectric tip is the tool of choice, as its linear vibration does not produce a high degree of trauma or stress in the patient. The sonic tip can pulsate with a frequency of up to 18 cycles per second. It operates on an oval-shaped pattern. The units function at a lower temperature, giving off little heat. Some commercial units work better than others.

Air-Driven and Roto-Pro Bur Scalers

The veterinarian might employ the use of a low-speed handpiece, high-speed handpiece, or a three-way air and water syringe when using a basic air-driven scaler. The more complex units will have a variety of available options, including piezoelectric scalers, sonic scaler outlets, suction, fiberoptic illumination, extra electrical outlets, and electrosurgical outlets. Compressors will be required to supply the air. However, this can be alleviated by the use of compressed air tanks. Air can be supplied by low-noise, oil-cooled compressors or by noisier oil-free dental compressors. The oil-free dental compressor is more expensive. The maintenance of the compressor requires a weekly check on the oil level. The oil must be changed at least every 6 months.

Depending on the need for the mechanical scalers, a roto-pro bur scaler may be the best tool for the job. It can operate at 300,000-400,000 rpm. The mechanical scaler is beneficial in the removal of tartar and calculus that is deeply built up on the teeth; however, caution should be used due to the risk of injury to the enamel, dentin, and soft tissue.

Caring for High-Speed Handpieces

The **high-speed handpiece** must be properly maintained so that it avoids malfunction and sticking. The spray nozzle is the front of the handpiece head with a small hole where the water sprays out onto the teeth. This water line can become clogged, so a gauge wire can be inserted into the hole to loosen debris if needed. It should also be oiled after each use to prevent overheating or sticking. The rubber gasket on the bottom of the handpiece helps make a seal so that water and air will not leak out; this gasket needs to be replaced when it becomes worn. The head of the handpiece contains a turbine that spins, and when a lot of debris accumulates inside, it will make the turbine stick, which makes it difficult to remove the dental burs. If the turbine begins to stick, it must be removed, and the head chamber should be cleaned out with a swab of alcohol and then oiled.

Maintaining Low-Speed Handpieces

The **low-speed handpiece** should be cleaned daily with hot water and a nonabrasive cleaner on the outside of the handpiece. The handpiece should be lubricated daily by rotating the pins on the bottom of the handpiece and placing oil in the smaller of the holes, called the air inlet, then running the handpiece to distribute the oil for a few seconds. Every week, the nose cone, which is the removable part of the handpiece that holds the motor, the chuck housing ring that locks and unlocks the handpiece so the prophy angle can be set in place, and the speed direction ring located in the bottom of the handpiece that changes the rotation direction to forward or reverse and controls the handpiece speed should all be lubricated.

Dental Machine Maintenance

There are a few components to the **dental machine** that need to be properly maintained in order for it to work properly. First, the scaler tips must be regularly checked for wear before they are used and changed out if there is more than 2 mm of wear. The high- and low-speed handpieces must be lubricated and cleaned only with alcohol after use. Lubricating the high- and low-speed handpieces prevents them from sticking. The compressor will need to be drained after each use to get rid of the extra moisture and pressure buildup. Always use distilled water for the dental machine because tap water will cause clogging, corrode the valves in the dental system, and introduce bacteria.

Controlling Oral and Environmental Bacteria

Staff should seek to control **cross-contamination** that may negatively impact the health of patients, coworkers, or themselves. Cross-contamination prevention requires the staff to take measures in advance to provide protection from any contaminants. The staff should only use equipment and implements that have been completely sterilized after being thoroughly washed and rinsed with a detergent-based solution to remove all gross fragments. The implements and detergent are placed within an ultrasonic bath and covered, while sharp and hinged instruments are given a surgical milk wash to remove any contaminants hiding within their crevices.

The **autoclave** is incorporated in the next part of the sterilization process. The use of autoclave film or envelopes will reduce the time needed for the autoclave process. However, for those items that cannot be placed in the autoclave, it is recommended to use plastic infection barriers. Staff members should follow the directions suggested by the manufacturer of the product to ensure that sterilization procedures are maintained to prevent any sterile areas from becoming contaminated.

Oral Examinations and Treatment

Routine Dental Cleanings

It is important for dog and cat owners to bring their pet into the veterinarian for an annual examination; this will include a full oral exam, consisting of checking for any fractures, furcations, oral lesions, ulcers, periodontal disease, as well as gingivitis. After a dog or cat turns 1 or 2 years of age, it is time for them to have their first **dental prophylaxis** (dental cleaning to halt the progression of periodontal disease and gingivitis) if their teeth have started to develop tartar. A routine dental cleaning includes dental radiographs, ultrasonic scaling of the teeth to remove any calculus, and polishing to smooth over where the scaling took place. While the pet is under anesthesia, a thorough oral exam is performed, including checking pocket depths and assessing any tooth resorption or abnormalities seen on radiographs. Dental disease can cause pain, tooth loss, and bad breath. Any bacteria caught under the gums can travel to the vital organs such as the heart, kidneys, and liver.

Dental Exams

The veterinarian will need to find out about the patient's history in the initial steps of the examination, and then closely inspect the animal's face and head for symmetry during the routine physical exam. The nasal and ocular regions should be inspected for any secretions, lumps, or swollen areas as much as the patient will allow. The lips, mouth, tongue, teeth, and gums should also be checked, if possible. Note that many animals are not accustomed to oral examination, and veterinary technicians assessing oral health should be extremely careful, even if there are no bite warnings in the patient file.

Concerning findings may trigger the need for further examination or dental procedures under anesthesia.

Dental Charts

The veterinarian should check the patient's file and dental chart at the outset of each visit. A dental chart is the written record of every visit that the patient has made, and the design and layout of the chart will be determined by the facility's selection among the chart formats available. The chart normally represents the mouth with a picture of the full dentition of the patient, and there is an area on the dental chart for notes, diagnosis, and the preferred treatment plan. The written record should be organized in such a way as to give sufficient space to document the condition of the teeth. This section should include a listing of all known calculus, caries, fractures, gingivitis index, malocclusions, resorptive lesions, and oral lesions.

Charting is normally the first step to the dental cleaning process. If there is a suspected extraction, that tooth will require less scaling; therefore, less anesthesia time will be needed. The degree of calculus and plaque will be noted in the chart as well as any missing or fractured teeth. Worn teeth can be notated either by attrition (tooth-on-tooth contact) or abrasion (tooth-on-object contact). Important abnormalities to include in the dental chart would be tooth mobility, pocket depth measured by the periodontal probe, degree of gingivitis (0–3), and stage of periodontal disease. Any furcation exposure, abnormal bite, and tooth resorptions should be noted as well.

The chart in the animal's permanent record should make note of any dates that the animal received dental care. In addition, the chart should describe the treatment and prognosis given at the time of the visit. The veterinarian will rely on the accuracy of this record in treating the patient on the next visit. The veterinarian will need to make an assessment of the overall treatment success or failure in comparison with the state of the mouth on the initial visit.

Technician Safety

There are certain procedures that the dental technician should use for protection against injury during a dental examination. The equipment that provides the most protection against bacteria includes a surgical mask, goggles or face shield, and disposable gloves. Further reduction of bacterial aerosolization can be accomplished by an application (by rinsing or brushing) of spray in the patient's mouth. This spray consists of a solution that is 0.12% chlorhexidine.

In addition, the technician should work on the animal from a seated position. This position reduces stress on the technician's back. The animal should be at a height where the technician's forearms and wrists can rest on the table. The technician's knees should be able to fit comfortably under the table that the animal is resting upon. The technician's thighs should be in a horizontal position facing the table. The technician's hand should be able to rest on the surface of the table to gain support.

The dental examination should be performed in a well-lit area. The best lighting conditions include head-mounted halogen lights or a directional light mounted to the ceiling.

Patient Safety

The patient should be intubated with an appropriately sized endotracheal tube (ET), which should be adequately cuffed to prevent aspiration. The table should be inclined and the patient should be in lateral recumbency, with the head lower than the tail, promoting fluid drainage from the mouth.

Mouth gags are used to prop open the patient's mouth during a dental procedure. Using spring-loaded mouth gags between the canine teeth to prop the mouth open is not recommended for cats because they produce a constant pressure that can cause bulging of the soft tissues between the mandible and the tympanic bulla. The force from the mouth gag can also compress the maxillary arteries, which are a cat's main route of blood supply to the retina and the brain, which can cause temporary blindness. Another option to hold the mouth open would be to cut off the end of a 25-gauge needle cover and place it between the upper and lower canines. The **temporomandibular joint** is subject to harm if a properly sized mouth gag is not applied during the examination.

The patient should have its eyes covered to prevent accidental ocular injury.

Positioning Patients

The handling of the animal requires precise, deliberate movements. One such movement involves lifting the animal by the sternum. This cuts down on the likelihood of the animal experiencing gastric torsion. In addition, it is not a good idea to turn the animal an excessive number of times as this increases the likelihood of more stress. The turning of the patient should be conducted in such a way that the sternum is rolled under. Large-breed animals are particularly susceptible to harm if turning is not done correctly.

The veterinarian should finish the dental procedure on one side of the mouth before moving on to the other side. The labial surfaces of the teeth should be scaled and polished first, followed by palatal and lingual surfaces. The veterinarian will finish one side before the animal is turned for work on the other side of the mouth. The scaling and polishing should then be completed on the remaining labial, palatal, and lingual sections of the mouth.

Hypothermia

Hypothermia is a risk with dental patients, so body temperature should be monitored throughout the procedure. The patient's head will be consistently doused in water during the cleaning, and extractions can add to this exposure, making the patient colder. Wet towels must be consistently exchanged for dry ones under the patient's head. The patient can have a heat pad placed underneath its body to minimize the possibility of hypothermia. Another method to maintain body temperature involves the use of a circulating water blanket.

Under Anesthesia

Once under anesthesia and positioned properly, a more thorough oral exam and dental cleaning can occur. The gingival sulcus will need to be measured around the perimeter of the tooth. The normal measurement for canines is 0-3 mm, for felines it is 0-1 mm. The veterinarian should apply the scaler above and below the gingiva. Minuscule ruts created by the scaling process will require a thorough polishing to even out the teeth and remove any plaque. The veterinarian will then wipe down the teeth. The teeth should be allowed to air dry. The veterinarian should then place fluoride solution on the teeth, which should remain on the teeth for the recommended time period. The veterinarian should record the services performed on the teeth at the time of each patient's visit.

Occlusion Assessment

Normal occlusion is the act of bringing the upper and lower teeth to a closed position or bite. The normal bite that is recommended for cats and dogs is a scissor bite. In general, a scissor bite means that the upper carnassial teeth overlap the lower carnassials. A scissor bite is also described as a closing of the lower incisors just behind the upper incisors, along with the closing of the lower canines between the upper incisors and canines, without touching each other—this bite pattern differs some in dogs. The canine teeth and the maxillary fourth premolar teeth tend to be at greater risk of fracture than other teeth. Thus, they deserve careful and regular examination.

Scaling & Polishing

Scaling is the process of removing calculus and plaque from the teeth, which will usually leave grooves on the teeth. The application of a mechanical scaler eliminates supragingival calculus and plaque. A hand curette removes any residual subgingival calculus that is left on the teeth. Cats require a light touch, as they have delicate teeth that can be broken or cracked with little difficulty.

Polishing will take off any plaque not removed in the scaling process. A low-speed handpiece is used with prophy paste, which will reduce the heat generated by the friction of polishing. With pressure, the veterinarian will polish all surfaces of the teeth that have been scaled. Use light pressure for only three seconds on the crowns of all teeth starting at the most caudal teeth, ending with the incisors. The veterinarian should work on the surfaces of the supra- and subgingival regions. Polishing will leave a smooth surface on all teeth, preventing plaque and bacteria from adhering to the rough, grooved surfaces created by scaling. After polishing, use the rinse handpiece to rinse excess prophy paste from the mouth.

The polishing handpiece can cause thermal damage and enamel loss to the tooth if held in place for too long with too much pressure.

Cats are cleaned with a Cavi-jet type system. This system has small prophy cups which are appropriate for the smaller teeth found in cats.

Applying Fluoride to the Patient's Teeth

A fluoride treatment is spread over the teeth as soon as the teeth have been thoroughly polished. This topical solution should be left on the teeth for up to 4 minutes. The residual topical fluoride is wiped from the teeth after that time. Some prophy paste already has a fluoride base, alleviating the need for an additional treatment with fluoride. However, most veterinarians prefer the second application of fluoride so as to increase the protection offered to the patient.

Fluoride offers protection to the teeth in the form of an antibacterial agent. Fluoride also desensitizes the teeth to feelings of pain from cold, heat, or touch. Fluoride increases the defensive ability of the enamel by fostering the tooth's mineralization development. The fluoride left in the animal's saliva will be absorbed in the spots on the tooth surface that are absent of minerals. These bare spots will also entice other minerals to the tooth's surface, like calcium. Fluoride is turned into a substance known as fluorapatite when it becomes part of the tooth in this absorption process. Fluorapatite is more resistant to acids than hydroxyapatite, and will not dissolve easily.

Characteristics and Benefits of Local Anesthesia for Animal Dental Procedures

Local anesthesia can be given when there is no evidence of infections or abscesses. Local anesthesia is usually short in duration but can be effective for a period of 6-8 hours. Amide agents, derived from ammonia, can begin working after 3-5 minutes. The anesthesia is best administered via the nerves entering and exiting the bony foramina. The veterinarian should take precautions to prevent injury to the nerves when giving this drug through an injection.

Epinephrine is found in some types of anesthesia. This drug is a **synthetic form of adrenaline** that works to relax the airways and constrict the blood vessels. However, epinephrine is not recommended for use on some patients due to certain associated risks. Thus, the type of anesthesia should be selected in conjunction with the needs of the individual patient.

The benefits surrounding the use of local anesthesia include: a) a lower rate of postoperative discomfort; b) induced loss of sensitivity to pain can be sustained and adjusted at lower levels; and c) fewer complications in the recovery period.

Tooth Extraction

Administering Nerve Blocks Prior to Tooth Extraction

Four **nerve blocks** can be used in dogs to provide a local block prior to extractions. These include the infraorbital, maxillary, middle mental, and inferior alveolar. In cats and brachycephalic dogs, the infraorbital foramen is too short, allowing for the whole maxilla on the corresponding side to be affected so that the nerve block is not used. The infraorbital nerve block (rostral maxillary) provides analgesia to the incisors, canine, and first three premolars on that side, along with the soft tissue and adjacent maxillary bone. The maxillary nerve block affects the branches of the maxillary nerve including the infraorbital nerve, pterygopalatine nerve, and palatine nerves. The bones, teeth, and soft tissues of the maxilla will be blocked. The middle mental nerve block (rostral mandibular) affects the canine, incisors, and soft tissues and bone of the corresponding side. The inferior alveolar nerve block (caudal mandibular) blocks all of the mandibular teeth, bone, and soft tissues on the corresponding side rostral (toward the nose) to the injection.

Tools Used for Extractions

The dental instruments that will be needed for a tooth extraction will depend upon which tooth is being extracted. Single-rooted teeth such as incisors and canines will require an appropriately sized elevator, forceps, a blade, and small sutures (4-0). Canine tooth extractions will require the use of a periosteal elevator to lift the flap if the tooth is well attached, then a tapered fissure bur will be used to cut around the tooth. An elevator will then be used to loosen the tooth, and forceps are used to extract the root. A bone rasp can be used to remove any remaining bone pieces.

In order to extract multirooted teeth, a flap is created with the use of an elevator and a surgical blade. The high-speed handpiece will be used to drill the bone with a round bur from the alveolar crest, and then a tapered fissure bur will be used to cut the tooth in two so that each root is separate. Extraction forceps are used to grip and remove the tooth after it has been loosened and can also be used to crack off heavy calculus. **Root tip picks** are used to stretch and break the periodontal ligament to obtain a fractured root tip if necessary. Forceps will be used to pull out the roots, and a small suture will be used to close the area.

Radiographs will be needed for all pre- and post-extraction films.

Floating a Horse's Teeth

Floating is the process of filing the occlusal surfaces of equine teeth in order to make the horse's bite level and consistent. Equine oral exams should be performed annually to assess if floating is needed.

Unlike humans, an adult horse's teeth continue to grow throughout its lifetime. However, the upper jaw's structure causes the narrower, lower jaw to move in a sideways direction when the horse is eating. Thus, the horse will grind its food using a slanting chewing motion. The effect can produce pointed edges on the horse's teeth. The condition may become bad enough to cut at the horse's cheeks and interfere with the horse's eating, and the horse may even accidentally drop food and lose weight if the problem is severe. Consequently, the veterinarian will check the condition of the horse's mouth, including symptoms such as halitosis, lacerations in the mouth, and difficulty eating as noted by an inability to keep hold of its food, the presence of head tilts when wearing a bit, and undigested food present in the horse's fecal matter. All of these symptoms could lead the veterinarian to suggest that floating a horse's teeth is necessary.

Dental Radiography

Digital Dental Radiography

Dental radiographs assist a veterinarian in assessing an animal's dental needs based on the condition of the teeth and the presence of fractures, tooth root abscesses, tooth resorption, bone or soft-tissue tumors, bone loss, retained deciduous teeth, and impacted teeth. In addition, the radiograph can give the veterinarian the ability to judge the severity of any intraoral neoplasia present. The veterinarian can use the x-ray to count the teeth, even unerupted teeth, in the mouth. Any periapical abscesses present within the mouth are also exposed by the x-ray images. Common findings seen on dental radiographs include fractures, tooth resorption, oral masses, and pockets greater than 3 mm in dogs and greater than 2 mm in cats.

It is also recommended to take radiographs before and after tooth extraction to ensure that the entire root has been extracted and that the surrounding bone is intact.

The veterinarian will recommend the practice of obtaining scheduled dental radiographs for young animals. This routine practice should provide the veterinarian and other caregivers a means of reviewing the permanent dentition recorded in the animal's charts. An animal with periodontal disease should be scheduled for radiographs at a rate of every 12-24 months.

Digital sensors are used in place of traditional film, and they come in sizes comparable to the traditional 0, 1, and 2 options. A larger size 4 film was required for large-breed dogs, and an indirect digital imaging system now allows for radiographs of the larger teeth. Digital radiograph technology significantly decreases radiation exposure.

Views and Positioning Techniques

Dental radiographs need to include the entire crown and root of each tooth to allow for an accurate diagnosis. A full-mouth set of radiographs consists of rostral maxillary and mandibular views as well as right and left maxillary and mandibular views. The maxillary canines should be imaged on their own separate oblique views to prevent superimposition of the first and second premolars on the canine roots.

Any film placed in an animal's mouth should be held firmly in place with a section of gauze that has been pressed between the upper part of the film and the teeth's occlusal surfaces. This particular placement allows the veterinarian to target specific areas in the mouth, like the mandibular molars or the premolars.

Dental Radiography Techniques

Parallel technique is used for imaging the caudal mandibular premolars and molars. For the parallel technique, the patient is in dorsal or lateral recumbency, the sensor is placed parallel to the long axis of the tooth, and the x-ray head will be perpendicular to the tooth and the sensor. The image may also include other related structures found in the animal's mouth, and this technique results in minimal distortion in the resulting radiographs.

Bisecting angle technique is used for all maxillary teeth and rostral mandibular teeth. For the bisecting angle technique, the patient is in sternal or lateral recumbency for the maxillary teeth and dorsal recumbency for imaging the mandibular teeth. The sensor is placed in the mouth under the root and tooth being imaged, and then the x-ray head is angled such that the beam will be perpendicular to the line that bisects the angle created between the long axis of the tooth and the sensor. Distortion will appear as either elongation (object appears longer) or foreshortening (object appears shorter).

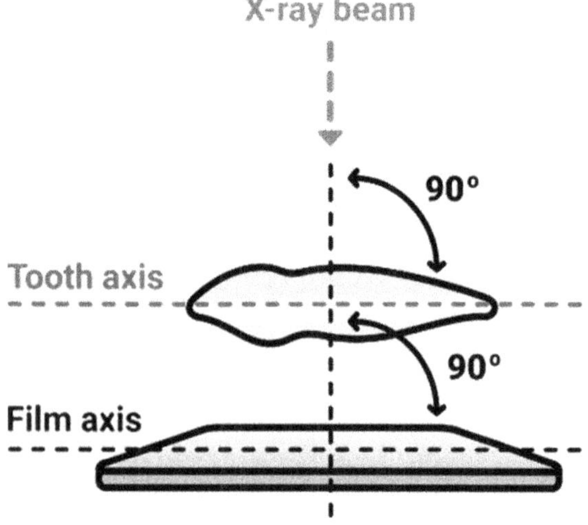

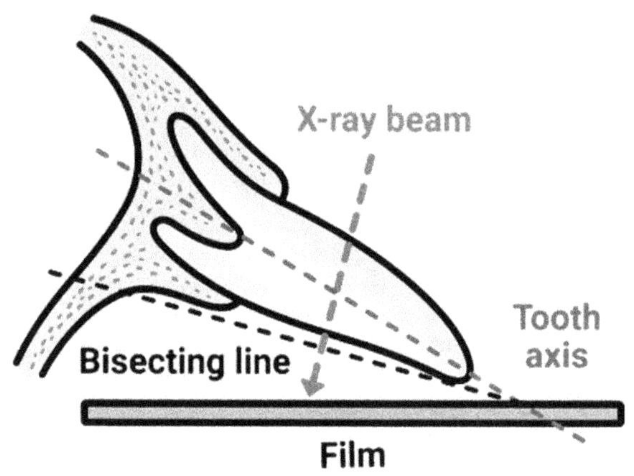

Tube Shift Technique

The **tube shift technique** is applicable for obtaining radiographs in conjunction with the bisecting angle technique. The tube shift technique can be referred to as the localization technique, the buccal object rule, or "SLOB." All of these refer to the same technique. The acronym SLOB indicates the following: S for same; L for lingual; O for opposite; and B for buccal. Two radiographs capture the image of the target and the reference object. Lingual to the reference point are those objects that have the appearance of moving in a similar direction to the direction in which the tube head was aligned. Buccal to the reference object are those objects that have the appearance of moving in the direction opposite to the direction in which the tube was aligned.

Chapter Quiz

Ready to see how well you retained what you just read? Scan the QR code to go directly to the chapter quiz interface for this study guide. If you're using a computer, simply visit the online resources page at **mometrix.com/resources719/vtne** and click the Chapter Quizzes link.

Laboratory Procedures

Transform passive reading into active learning! After immersing yourself in this chapter, put your comprehension to the test by taking a quiz. The insights you gained will stay with you longer this way. Scan the QR code to go directly to the chapter quiz interface for this study guide. If you're using a computer, simply visit the online resources page at **mometrix.com/resources719/vtne** and click the Chapter Quizzes link.

Clinical Hematology

Hematology is the study of the blood's **morphology** (shape) and the quantity of the cellular components of blood: **erythrocytes** (red blood cells, or RBCs), **leukocytes** (white blood cells, or WBCs), and **thrombocytes** (platelets). Abnormalities of these characteristics indicate disease conditions. These cellular components are suspended in **plasma**, the liquid component of blood.

When venous blood is collected for hematological evaluation, it should be placed in the purple-top, ethylenediaminetetraacetic acid (**EDTA**) tube. An anticoagulant, EDTA has a low propensity to cause changes in the structure of an organism.

Complete Blood Count

A **complete blood count (CBC)** gives information on the patient's RBCs, WBCs, and platelets.

Information provided by the CBC about RBCs includes the **packed cell volume (PCV)** or **hematocrit** results, which indicate the proportion of RBCs to whole blood volume, and the **hemoglobin**, indicating whole lysed blood concentration. Anemia is a deficiency of healthy RBCs; polycythemia is an elevation of the number of RBCs above normal, which may be relative or absolute. A CBC also reports erythrocyte size and appearance.

A CBC shows the total number of WBCs along with the numbers of certain types of WBCs including eosinophils, neutrophils, monocytes, lymphocytes, and basophils. An abnormal increase or decrease in WBCs can indicate severe infection. Leukocyte appearance is also noted.

The CBC gives platelet count, size, and appearance. If platelet numbers are reading low on the CBC, indicating a clotting disorder, it may be caused by an immune disorder or a serious systemic illness.

Erythrocytes

Normal mammalian erythrocytes lack a cell nucleus; they carry oxygen throughout the body by way of the protein hemoglobin.

Erythrocyte indices are established by red blood cell (RBC) counts, hemoglobin (HGB) content, and packed cell volume (PCV) or hematocrit (HCT). These amounts will be automatically added to the outcomes derived from the electronic counting tools. Erythrocyte indices can be applied to identify various types of anemias or blood deficiencies.

Erythrocyte Total Numbers

One important measure of **erythrocytes** is the total count of cells found in a given sample. The cells can be counted using a tool that is operated manually or mechanically. The tool will require calibration based upon cell size. The size of the cell may vary based upon the kind of animal from which the sample was taken. These calibrations are critical in the settings used for automatic counters. One type of manual counter is known as a **hemocytometer**. It is not as accurate in obtaining a cell count as an automated counter, but it is economical and readily available for use. Both the manual counter and the automated counter require a diluted sample. RBC indices can be obtained from the total erythrocyte numbers compared to the PCV.

Neubauer Hemacytometer Method

The **Neubauer hemacytometer method** is a manual means of determining the number of red blood cells (among other cells). The veterinarian will normally apply the **Unopette system** in the preparation of the sample to be tested, requiring that the calibrated blood sample be diluted or weakened with acetic acid at a dilution ratio of 1:100 to reduce the number of cells that require counting.

The red blood cells, or RBCs, require a ten-minute period to hemolyze following the dilution process. Next, the hemolyzed RBCs are placed into the hemocytometer chamber. This chamber has nine compartments which have been separated by a counting mechanism. Each compartment is occupied by a specified quantity of cells. These cells can be measured under a microscope at 10x objective magnification to determine the exact quantity present.

Packed Cell Volume

Packed cell volume (PCV), also referred to as **hematocrit (HCT)** or **erythrocyte volume fraction (EVF)**, is a measure of the percentage volume of whole blood that consists solely of red blood cells (RBCs or erythrocytes).

A normal PCV is between 35% and 45% in canines and between 25% and 45% in felines. An abnormally low PCV reading, also known as **anemia**, could result from hemorrhage possibly from ulcers or trauma; **hemolysis**, the destruction of RBCs, possibly from an enlarged spleen; or lack of RBC production from bone marrow, as in cases of cancer. An increased PCV reading normally results from dehydration or an increase in RBC production.

Performing and Evaluating a PCV

The materials needed to perform a PCV are two microhematocrit tubes, a clay stopper, a PCV analyzer card, a microhematocrit centrifuge, and a microscope. Insert one end of the microhematocrit tube slightly into an anticoagulated blood sample so the blood flows into the tube. Place a finger at the top of the hematocrit tube and insert the other end of the hematocrit tube into the clay to plug it. Repeat with the second tube. Place them into the microhematocrit centrifuge opposite from each other. Once the tubes are spun down, line up the bottom of the blood in the microhematocrit tube with the bottom of the card reader. The area in the microhematocrit tube where whole blood stops and plasma starts is where you get your reading; log that number as the PCV value.

The **plasma fraction** (i.e., separated portion) of the hematocrit tube is suitable for screening for microfilariae. This screening is accomplished by direct microscopic examination of the "buffy coat" (middle white blood cell layer) and plasma fractions for evidence of microfilaria and other blood-borne parasitic infestations. Another diagnostic consideration is the color and clarity of the plasma.

Mean Corpuscular Volume

To calculate **mean corpuscular volume** (MCV), the PCV percentage, measured in units of L/L (i.e., liters of RBCs obtained divided by the total whole blood volume in liters) is divided by the total RBC count. The outcome of this calculation is multiplied by 1,000. The result of this final calculation is given in terms of SI units; it indicates the average volume of a red blood cell in the sample, measured in **femtoliters** (fL, which is 10^{-15} liters).

$$MCV\ (\text{fL}) = \frac{PCV \times 1{,}000}{RBC}$$

Hemoglobin

Hemoglobin, abbreviated as Hb or Hgb, is an iron-containing protein found in red blood cells. Hemoglobin functions to carry oxygen from the lungs to tissues within the body. This allows hemoglobin to assist with the acid/base balance of the blood. Hemoglobin can be measured by means of photometric methods or automated cell counters. These measurements are recorded in g/dL or g/L. A rapid qualitative assessment takes the animal's Hb by computing one-third of the PCV.

Mean Corpuscular Hemoglobin

The **mean corpuscular hemoglobin** (MCH), sometimes called mean cell hemoglobin, is the average mass of hemoglobin found in a sample per red blood cell.

The MCH can be calculated by dividing the Hb concentration by the total RBC multiplied by 10. The result is reported in picograms (pg, which is 10^{-12} grams).

$$MCH\ (\text{pg}) = \frac{Hb \times 10}{RBC}$$

The measurements associated with Hb and RBC counts are not considered to be as precise as those used to determine the measurement of PCV (packed cell volume). Thus, the mean corpuscular hemoglobin index is considered to be a less than precise, but still useful, reference.

Mean Corpuscular Hemoglobin Concentration

The **mean corpuscular hemoglobin concentration** (MCHC) represents the average concentration of hemoglobin (Hb) in a given volume of packed red blood cells. The MCHC is derived by taking the Hb concentration and dividing it by the PCV (packed cell volume) and multiplying by 100.

$$MCHC\ (g/L) = \frac{Hb\ concentration\ (g/L)}{PCV}$$

The MCHC will also indicate the average shade of red for the red blood cells: a lower value indicates cells that appear paler. MCHC is reported in units of g/dL. This calculation does not employ the total RBC count. Therefore, this measurement can be considered to be one of the most precise, in terms of RBC indices.

Blood Smear

To obtain a hematology sample for a blood smear, draw 2 mL of blood and place into an EDTA (anticoagulant) purple-top tube. The supplies needed to create a good **blood smear** are two glass slides with a frosted edge, a microscope, immersion oil, and the blood sample. Place a small drop of blood (usually one drop from a 1 mL syringe will be sufficient) on one of the slides right under the frosted edge. The second slide is the spreader slide. Hold the spreader slide at about a 45-degree angle in front of the blood sample on the sample slide. Bring the spreader slide up to meet the drop of blood (still at a 45-degree angle), and allow the blood drop to spread along the short edge of the spreader slide. Next, push the spreader slide in the opposite direction quickly and gently, dragging the blood across the sample slide in a single motion to create a perfect smear. The blood smear is done correctly if it has a feathered edge on the end. The slide should air dry and then be fixed and stained.

Blood Smear Evaluation

Once the slide is prepared for a **differential blood smear**, it is stained and then examined under 100x magnification with immersion oil. Three portions are evaluated, including RBC morphology, WBC differential count, and an estimated platelet count.

First, examine the RBCs and note any abnormalities in size, shape, or color as well as any inclusions (Heinz bodies or Howell-Jolly bodies).

Using a manual counter, the technician will perform the WBC differential and count the monocytes, lymphocytes, neutrophils, eosinophils, and basophils starting from one side of the slide on the start of the monolayer moving to the other side of the slide. Then, move up and repeat (the "battlement pattern") until you have counted 100 WBCs. To get the absolute value of each WBC type, the total counted for that specific WBC (e.g., eosinophils) is multiplied by the total WBC count.

Last, the platelets are estimated by examining 10 fields in the same pattern as the WBC differential count and counting all the platelets in each field. Then add all of the platelet counts together from all 10 fields and divide by 10. Take that result and multiply by 20,000 to get the estimated platelet number per microliter of blood.

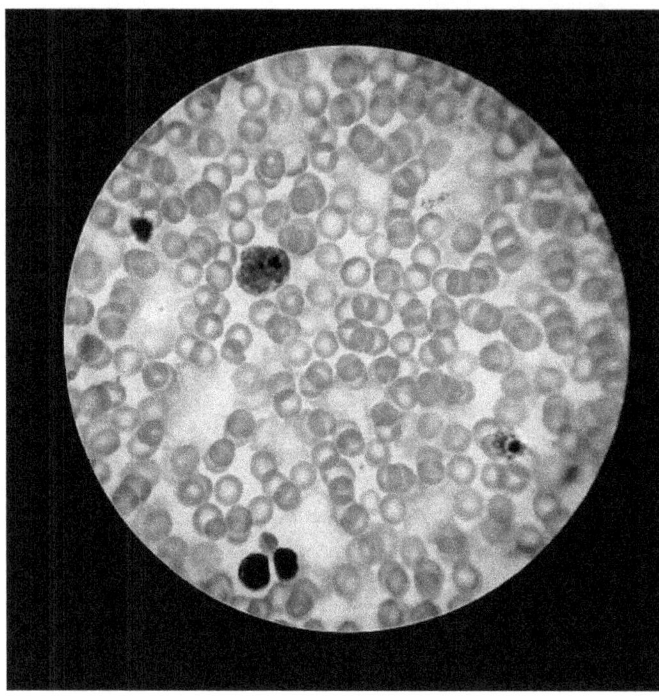

Erythrocyte Size Variations

Mature erythrocytes come in many sizes. Well-developed, mature erythrocytes generally have a uniform, average size referred to as **normocytic**. **Macrocytic** RBCs are unusually large; cells that are smaller than average are referred to as **microcytic**. Typically, the size can be attributed to the type of animal from which the erythrocyte was taken.

Smaller erythrocytes may be caused by vitamin or mineral deficiencies, genetic traits, or certain iatrogenic conditions. They also are associated with a diminished mean corpuscular volume (MCV) and mean corpuscular hemoglobin concentration (MCHC), causing them to be **hypochromic** (paler than normal). **Anisocytosis** describes substantial discrepancies in RBC size. The size of the RBCs observed should be compared with the size of RBCs normally found in the animal's species. The veterinarian will note the presence of larger, normal, or smaller sizes using the terms mild, moderate, or marked to indicate observed severity.

Erythrocyte Color Variations

Fully developed cells with a normal amount of hemoglobin are known as **normochromic** cells. Cells with an inadequate concentration of hemoglobin are called **hypochromic** cells. Normochromic cells will turn a pinkish color when a stain has been applied; hypochromic cells will be a much paler shade of pink. A mammal's normochromic erythrocyte cell has a whitish, innermost area, due to its biconcave formation and lack of a nucleus and cell organelles. However, reptiles, birds, and amphibians have nucleated red blood cells.

Macrocytic erythrocytes may be mistaken for hypochromic cells. Both are characterized by large widths. However, the distinction can be evident when hypochromia and microcytosis are both found in the same sample. This is further confirmed by MCV results.

A **torocyte** is a red blood cell with an abrupt transition from pale center to the red hemoglobin-rich ring of the outer cell circumference. Sometimes referred to as a "punched out" cell, this presentation is typically induced by poor slide smear technique. However, it should be noted that horses, cattle, and some other animals have naturally low central pallor, making observation of this condition more difficult.

ERYTHROCYTE ABNORMALITIES

Poikilocytosis describes a 10% or more increase in the number of abnormally shaped red blood cells.

Codocytes and **leptocytes** are erythrocytes that have undergone a surface volume change resulting in excess cell membrane. Codocytes are sometimes referred to as "target cells" for their dark circular "target" appearance, which may be due to cell membrane collapse secondary to very low hemoglobin content. Other suspected causes include increased cholesterol and lecithin content, bile insufficiency, liver disease, splenectomy, or anemia. **Leptocytes** describe abnormally thin, flattened red blood cells, and they are sometimes referred to as Mexican hat cells due to a central rounded area of pigmented material, a clear unpigmented mid-zone, and an outer pigmented cell rim. This form may be attributed to a reduction in hemoglobin volume or to an increase in the surface area of the cell membrane. Leptocytes are found in cases of regenerative anemia.

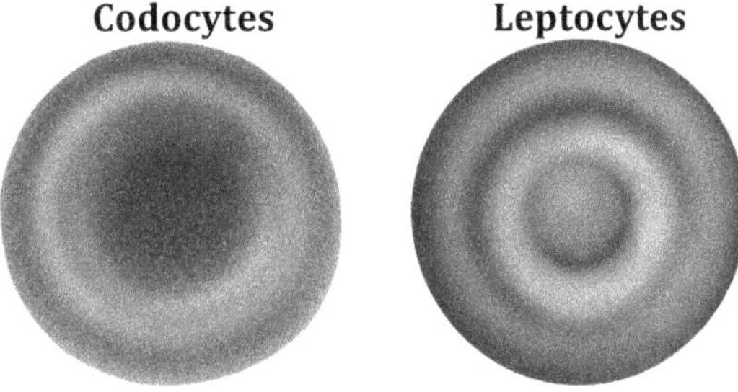

Ovalocytes (or **elliptocytes**) are cigar- or egg-shaped erythrocytes; their elliptical form can be attributed to a flaw in the membrane. They can be found in animals that have any of a number of types of anemia. The center of the cell has the typical erythrocytic light or pale color.

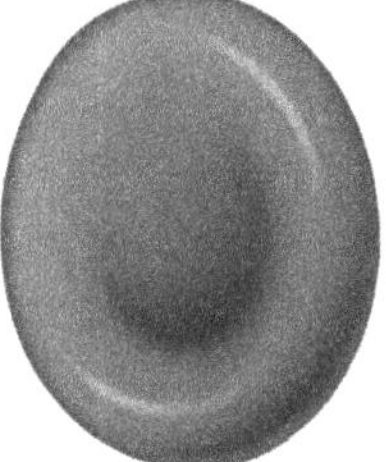

Schistocytes are fragmented RBCs of varying shapes: horn-like keratocytes, triangle-shaped triangulocytes, and helmet-shaped cells. Typically, the fragmentation occurs when erythrocytes are cut by fibrin strands lining micro-vessels. True schistocytes are not the softer-edged "bite cells" which occur when the spleen ingests abnormal hemoglobin (i.e., a Heinz body), leaving a bitten-apple appearance (although they are often lumped together). Schistocytes are seen in burns, uremia, various hemolytic anemias, and in disseminated intravascular coagulation (DIC) disorders.

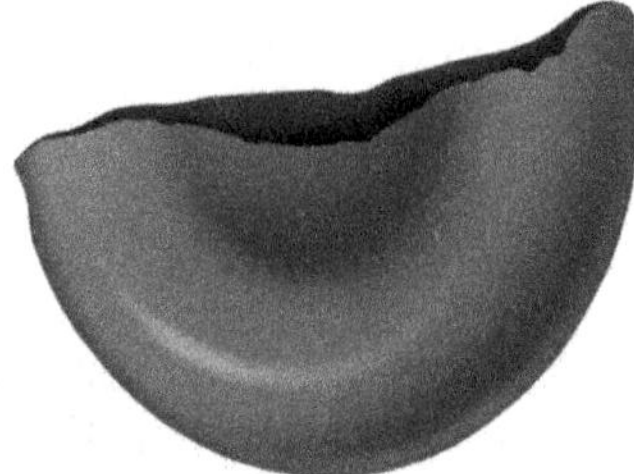

Spherocytes are red blood cells that have a round, spherical form instead of the biconcave disk shape of a normal RBC. Although typically involved in immune-related hemolytic anemias, other causes include defective membrane assembly and traumatic or toxic injury to the erythrocytes. Spherocytes are two-thirds the diameter of a normal RBC, with a decreased surface area. Their hemoglobin is denser and stains a deeper red, and the cell lacks a central pallor. They are more readily seen in dogs than many other animals that already have smaller erythrocytes with less central pallor (cats, horses, etc.). However, in thick areas of a dog's blood smear all the RBCs may resemble spherocytes. Therefore, clinicians must focus on the monolayer areas of the blood film.

Stomatocytes present with an abnormal-appearing center. Rather than the circular pale center of a normal erythrocyte, the pale center of a stomatocyte is rod-shaped, or even smile-shaped, in appearance. An inherited disorder has been linked to the presence of stomatocyte cells in dogs, and liver disease may also predispose the animal to the condition.

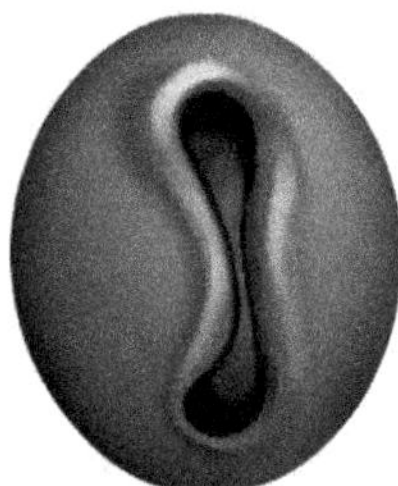

Spiculated Erythrocytes

Spiculated cells include acanthocytes and echinocytes. **Acanthocytes** are cells exhibiting obvious blunt protrusions extending out from the cell wall. These types of cells have an inconsistent shape. Acanthocyte cells are also called "spur cells." Acanthocytosis is caused when RBC membranes contain excess cholesterol as compared to phospholipids. It may be caused by high blood cholesterol and/or abnormal plasma lipoproteins.

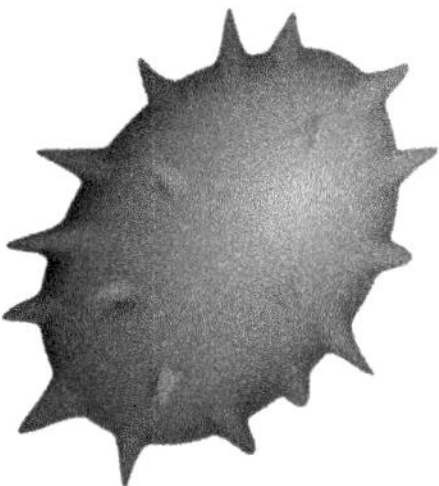

Echinocytes (or "burr cells") have copious amounts of little spicules (micro-spikes) protruding from a roughly spherical surface. Burr cells are found in animals with renal disease. However, the blood cells of a horse may exhibit these characteristics after vigorous exercise. Canines with lymphosarcoma and renal disease may also exhibit burr cells. Other causes of echinocytosis include: uremia, pyruvate kinase deficiency, liver disease, low potassium or low ATP in red cells, hypomagnesemia, hypophosphatemia, high calcium in RBCs, the absence of a spleen, hyperlipidemia, myeloproliferative disorders, and heparin therapy. Also, specimen handling errors such as procuring a blood smear immediately after a transfusion, or artifact due to improper drying, may cause the condition.

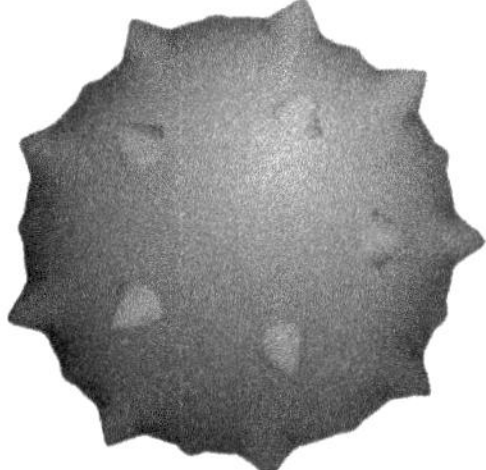

Other Erythrocyte Abnormalities

Agglutination refers to erythrocytes that are clustered together without any clear structural constriction. This type of cell formation can be detected by noticing a grainy appearance on the slide. The veterinarian will not be able to continue with an automated RBC counting or sizing when agglutination has been detected. This phenomenon can be associated with the presence of an antibody or in situations of immune disease.

Basophilic stippling is the granulated appearance of ribosomal RNA clusters found in certain erythrocytes. They can be easily observed through the use of **New Methylene Blue stain**, which makes the RNA appear as tiny, blue-colored granules inside the red blood cells or erythrocytes. This basophilic stippling is a result of ineffective heme formation, often due to various pathologies, including some anemias found in cattle, sheep, and felines and lead poisoning in certain animals. However, it is also characteristic of active erythropoiesis in sheep and cattle.

Blister cell (also known as **pyknocyte** or **hemighost**) refers to an RBC where a blister or a vacuole has formed and is absent of any hemoglobin content. This is often a result of oxidation damage on the cell's surface potentially due to iron deficiency anemia. Later rupture or removal of the blister by the spleen may result in a keratocyte, or "horn cell." However, if the cell forms only one slim horn-like protrusion, it is sometimes called an "apple stem" cell.

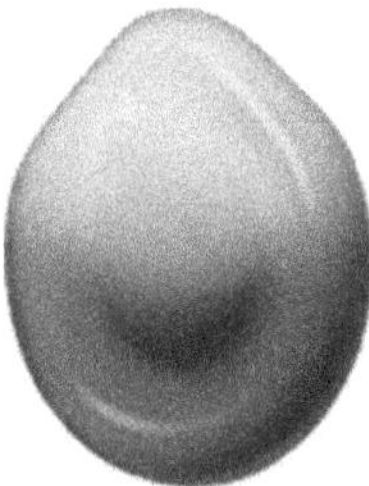

Crenation describes the process where cells contract due to a lack of water. Crenated cells, with their characteristic notched or scalloped edges, can be seen when RBCs are allowed to dry on a blood film (smear). This slow drying process will produce visible barbs on the film.

Eccentrocytes are RBCs that have been subject to the harmful effects of oxidation, resulting in adhesion of the cell membranes from opposing sides of the cell. The hemoglobin is thus forced to one side of the cell, causing the RBC to appear semi-circular in form. Eccentrocytes are associated with fragmented anemia, keratocytes, and schistocytes. Often presented as synonymous with blister cells (with both undergoing oxidative damage, etc.), it appears they differ in the membranous adhesions as opposed to the blister-like vacuole development. Causes include onion and garlic ingestion (in dogs, cats, etc.), and the administration of oxidant drugs.

Ghost cells are RBCs that have lysed in a hypotonic solution, spilling out hemoglobin contents. Over time a ghost cell will resume its normal disk shape and will likely have retained at least some of its prior hemoglobin contents. Thus, when stained it appears as a very pale, ghost-like cell.

Howell-Jolly bodies are defined as erythrocytes that did not entirely expel their nuclear DNA, now visible as purple-blue basophilic inclusions upon staining. These inoperative, basophilic DNA fragments are stored in the cell and appear dark and circular. The inclusion shape will be circular. In addition, non-refractive qualities are apparent when the microscope is out of focus. The presence of these Howell-Jolly bodies can be found in cases associated with splenectomy, regenerative anemia, or spleen disorders. It should be noted, however, that most cats and horses will have about 1% of all their RBCs as Howell-Jolly bodies.

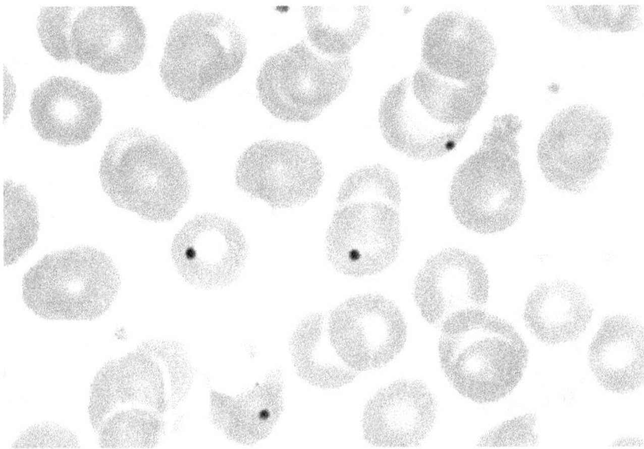

Heinz bodies (or Heinz-Ehrlich bodies) are small inclusions of **denatured hemoglobin** found within RBCs. Heinz bodies can be viewed with Wright's or Diff-Quick stains. However, an easier observation can be made with New Methylene Blue (NMB) stain. Heinz bodies are associated with the use of oxidant drugs, lymphosarcoma, and hyperthyroidism, as well as with the consumption of onions by dogs, cats, and certain primates. Heinz bodies are frequently found in felines. An abrupt rise in the number of Heinz bodies in a feline can indicate diabetes mellitus.

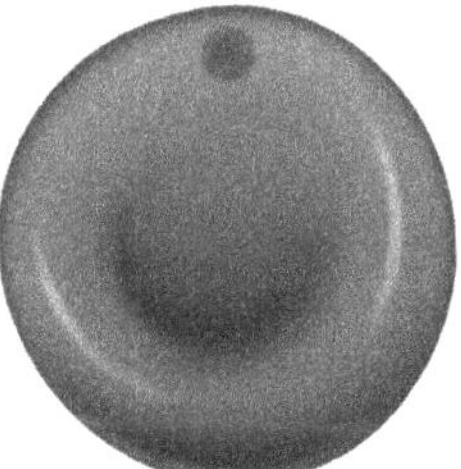

In most animals, **nucleated red blood cells** (nRBCs) are younger, smaller red blood cells that have retained their nucleus. The nRBCs have a dark staining nucleus and a bluish-red cytoplasm and are of significance if there are more than 5 in a 100 WBC count. Normally, nRBCs are not found in mammalian peripheral blood films and tend to indicate serious bone marrow stress, from hemolytic anemia to metastatic cancer. An increase in nRBCs in the blood indicates hyperproduction of RBCs, not allowing them to mature before they are released into the bloodstream. However, nRBCs are normal in some non-mammalian species, including birds, reptiles, fish, and amphibians, which have well developed nRBCs with an elliptical shape.

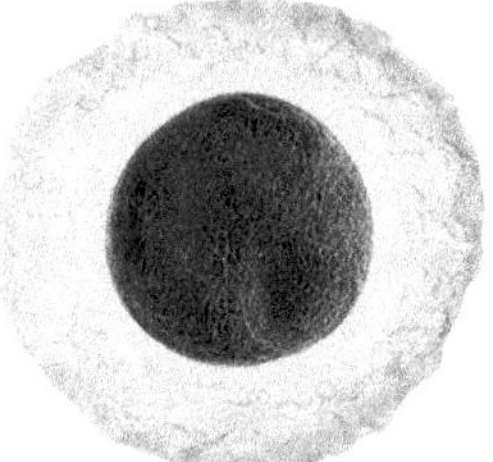

Rouleaux are erythrocytes that are gathered in chains or stacks—not unlike stacks of coins. In such formations, the cells are not free to readily absorb and carry oxygen. It is a precursor to many serious diseases, including inflammatory or plasma protein transformations. However, a certain degree of rouleaux is expected in horses.

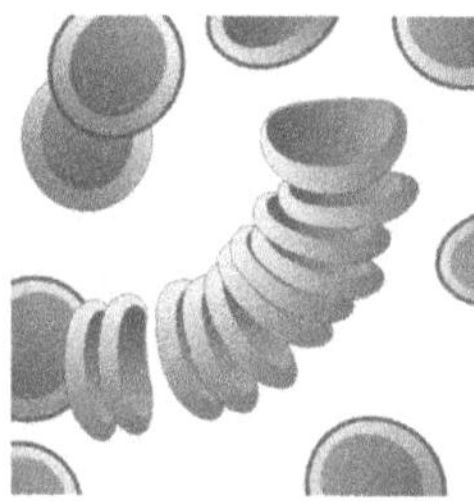

Reticulocyte Count

Reticulocytes are immature red blood cells, and they are visible only when properly stained. Wright's stain gives a bluish-gray color to immature RBCs, indicating the presence of cytoplasmic RNA. If stained with NMB (New Methylene Blue), the ribosomal RNA becomes directly visible and reticulocytes are more easily counted.

Cells or cell components that are stainable with more than one format of stain (i.e., Wright's alcohol-soluble and NMB's water-soluble stains) are referred to as "polychromatophilic." Thus, a few drops of blood and NMB stain are blended together in like amounts. The NMB/blood mix is checked to obtain the quantity of reticulocytes visible. The results are extrapolated to produce a percentage of reticulocytes per 1,000 RBCs. This percentage can be noted as an absolute count when measured as reticulocytes per milliliter. Reassessments may be needed, as automated counts routinely miscount reticulocytes by as much as 20%.

Reticulocyte Production Index

In most animals, reticulocytes should constitute less than 1% of all RBCs. However, situations such as blood loss, disease-shortened RBC life, general anemia, and low oxygen intake can all cause the reticulocyte count to rise, known as **reticulocytosis**. In situations of anemia (low RBC count) reticulocytes, as a percentage, can appear artificially high.

To correct for this, the **Reticulocyte Production Index** (RPI, or "corrected reticulocyte count") was created, with "normal" usually defined as 30-45, depending on animal type:

$$\text{RPI} = \text{Reticulocyte Count} \times (\text{hematocrit} \div \text{normal hematocrit})$$

If the count is 100,000 mm^3 or higher, the anemia is likely of the hyperproliferative type (hemolytic anemia, anemia from blood loss, etc.). If it is under 100,000 mm^3, the anemia may be hypoproliferative (iron, B12, or folic deficiency, suppressed bone marrow, etc.). It should be noted that this assessment may not be valid in a horse, as horses do not discharge reticulocytes into the circulation directly from the bone marrow except in cases of severe chronic anemia.

The Reticulocyte Production Index (RPI) determines how rapidly reticulocytes are released into the bloodstream; deviations from normal can be indicative of certain health problems.

Leukocytes

Neutrophils, sometimes referred to as the first responders, are the first white blood cells (WBCs) to arrive at the site of inflammation and will continue to come to the site as long as the inflammation lasts. Neutrophils will engulf microorganisms and destroy them; they also signal the other WBCs to the site. **Eosinophils** are slightly larger than neutrophils and have segmented nuclei with eosinophilic cytoplasmic granules. They are often seen associated with mast cells, allergies, parasitic disease, and fungal infections. **Lymphocytes** arrive at the site of inflammation a few days after it started. They have a round nucleus that is about the same size as an RBC. There are two types of lymphocytes: T cells and B cells. T and B cells spring into action when they come across antigens. **Monocytes** remove damaged cells and microorganisms and are usually plentiful during inflammation. **Basophils** increase due to an allergic or parasitic response, but they are normally very scarce.

STAINED LEUKOCYTES

There are many kinds of leukocytes that can be differentiated by staining, with the best methods employing the largest occupied section of the film. Pay attention to patterns of blood dispersion across the stained region, understanding that a monolayer arrangement of the cells will yield the best results. Feathered edges are not useful in detection. The form and structure of the leukocyte must be examined. There are 5 types of leukocytes, in 2 main groups: **polymorphonuclear** leukocytes (also granulocytes—characterized by stain-revealed granules in the cytoplasm), including neutrophils, eosinophils, and basophils; and **mononuclear** leukocytes (non-granular), including monocytes and lymphocytes. **Banded cells** are granulocytes in an immature state. They may be elongated and narrow, with non-segmented nuclei. Neutrophils may be referred to as "toxic" when they undergo morphologic changes (shape, color, etc.). The degree (based on numbers of cells affected and changes incurred) is labeled as mild, moderate, or marked. Severe toxic change is indicated when toxic granulation, diffuse cytoplasmic basophilia, or cytoplasmic vacuolation are present.

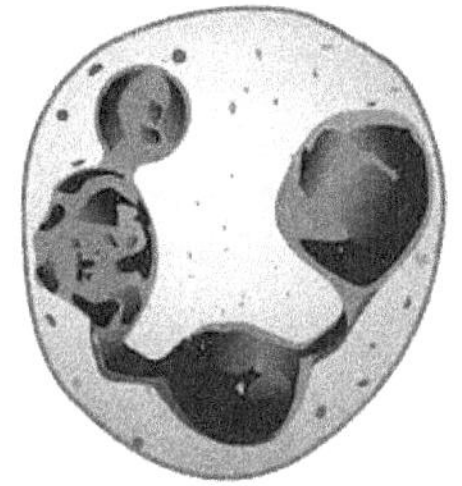

Neutrophil

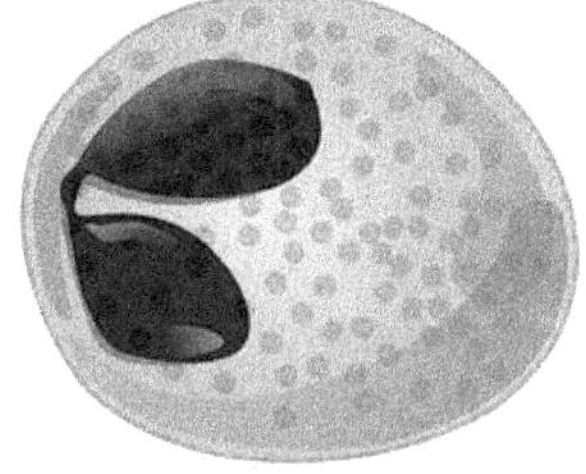

Eosinophil

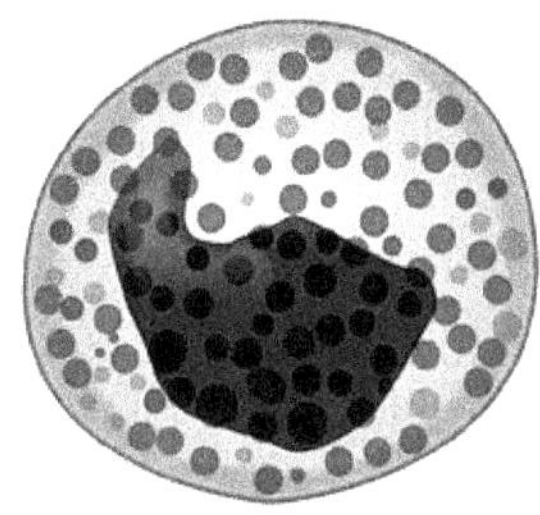

Basophil

Neutrophils and **lymphocytes** are the most common leukocytes. The largest WBCs are monocytes, staining with a gray-blue cytoplasm. Monocytes are found in peripheral blood. Eosinophils are granular cells with cytoplasm of a unique red-purple stain. Basophils are almost never found in peripheral blood. Their cytoplasm is distinguished with a blue or blue-black stain.

HEMATOLOGY LOGISTICS

Blood smears should be prepared immediately after the sample is collected to minimize cell deterioration, and they should be stored at room temperature until sent to the reference lab. **Ethylenediaminetetraacetic acid** (EDTA) is the anticoagulant of choice for a complete blood cell count because it best preserves the cellular components of the blood and prevents platelet aggregation. EDTA samples do need to be inverted multiple times, and they must be kept in the refrigerator until shipping. Blood for coagulation testing should be collected into a blue-top tube that contains sodium citrate and then centrifuged for 5 minutes. After the sodium citrate tube is spun down in the centrifuge, the plasma should be removed and transferred to a clean tube without anticoagulant and kept frozen until it is analyzed. Whole blood samples should not be frozen because this causes cell lysis and gross hemolysis, which interferes with testing.

SENDING BLOOD SAMPLES TO AN OUTSIDE LAB

When sending out a blood sample, it is important that the sample is collected into the correct blood tube and that it has the correct corresponding documentation. The tube must be labeled with the patient's name, client's name, date, clinic name, and the test to be run. There will be a corresponding form from the reference lab that will be filled out with the same information along with the age of the patient, sex (including if the pet is neutered or spayed), if the patient has fasted, and the doctor's name. The reference form will normally list a variety of tests that they have available, and the one requested needs to be marked. Always use a pen with black or blue ink when labeling sample tubes and forms. The sample tube is then placed into the bag provided by the reference lab along with the form.

Maintaining Hematology Samples

Patients should be prepared in advance when conducting blood work. Most tests require the patient to have **fasted** (gone without food) prior to taking the sample. The technician collecting the sample should be familiar with 1) the correct sizes of needles to be used, 2) the proper dimension of dry syringe needed, 3) the appropriate evacuation tubes to prevent hemolysis and clotting, and 4) the volume of blood needed for testing.

Hemolysis is the rupturing and destruction of red blood cells. Hemolysis often arises from improper specimen collection. Contamination, poor line connections, incorrect tube mixing or tube filling, and incorrect needle size may all cause hemolysis.

Serum is the post-clotted liquid part of blood that is used to conduct certain tests. Serum will often be beneficial in preventing unwanted chemical interactions. Tests requiring whole blood or plasma samples should be mixed with an anticoagulant when collected. However, the technician should verify that the tests being conducted will not be hindered by the presence of the anticoagulant. The technician should compare the normal values for a given test procedure to each sample collected in the laboratory. Conventional laboratory quality control procedures should be maintained.

Storing Hematology Samples

Hematology samples, including plasma, serum, and whole blood, must be kept in the refrigerator until they are sent to the lab, and they should be shipped with cold packs. Blood cytology slides should be kept out of the refrigerator to avoid lysing of cells. To obtain a blood sample for clotting factors, a sodium citrate (anticoagulant) blue-top tube would be used. Draw enough blood for the coagulation profile, spin the sample down in the centrifuge, and draw off the serum to place in a red-top tube. Either store the sodium citrate sample in the freezer, or send it to the lab within a half an hour of obtaining it. All samples must be clearly labeled with the patient's name, client's last name, and date, and all necessary paperwork must be sent with the sample to the laboratory.

Clinical Biochemistry

Plasma

Whole blood is formulated from a mixture of fluid and cellular substances. **Plasma** is the yellowish fluid that contains blood proteins and lipid particles in the bloodstream. Plasma makes up 55% of total blood volume. Blood plasma can be broken down into the following substances and amounts: 90% water and 10% dissolved proteins, hormones, lipids, enzymes, salts, carbohydrates, vitamins, and waste materials. Cellular components suspended within the plasma are erythrocytes, leukocytes, and thrombocytes (also called platelets). **Anticoagulants** can be added to plasma to prevent clotting, which is necessary when plasma is separated from whole blood.

To obtain a plasma sample, 3 mL of blood will be drawn and placed into a green-top heparinized (anticoagulant) tube.

Anticoagulants

Many kinds of blood tubes are utilized in the serum separation process. These tubes have been specifically designed to perform a unique function. Whole blood and plasma require a tube containing an anticoagulant. However, the technician should be aware that some types of anticoagulants in plasma can hinder the results of certain tests. Thus, the technician should be aware of the type of anticoagulant found in each tube.

For instance, heparin is derived from a salt of sodium, potassium, lithium, or ammonium and is often the best choice to use in plasma samples due to its low propensity to alter the chemical analysis done in tests. The measurement for a supplement of this anticoagulant is given at 20 units of heparin per milliliter of blood. EDTA is not a good choice when used for plasma-based tests that require chemical analysis. Finally, sodium fluoride is a glucose preservative with additional anticoagulant properties.

Serum

Serum is plasma after coagulation has already occurred. It is collected via a centrifugation or separation process that removes the clotted and solid materials from the residual fluid.

To obtain a **serum sample**, 3 mL of blood (which normally produces ~1 mL of serum) must be drawn and placed into a serum separator tube then allowed to clot. The sample is spun down in a centrifuge, and the serum should be drawn off of the sample within an hour and placed into a red-top tube.

Serum Abnormalities

Hemolytic serum will appear pink or reddish in color. This RBC rupture could be **iatrogenic**, caused by staff handling samples improperly. However, in other instances hemolysis may occur for reasons outside of staff control. Regardless, the technician should be aware that higher levels of phosphorus, potassium, total protein, and aspartate aminotransferase can be found in tests performed on hemolytic serum.

Serum that is a yellowish color, a symptom known as **jaundice** or **icterus**, may be indicative of a serious problem in the animal. **Icteric serum** could indicate the presence of liver disease, bile obstruction, or excessive hemolysis; it has a tendency to produce high bilirubin readings during the chemical analysis of the specimen. Other aspects of the test results may be impacted by these increased levels.

Lipemic serum has high triglyceride or lipid levels caused by poor diet or disease. Lipemic serum has a murky or opaque appearance, due to the high concentration of suspended fat present. It may hinder accurate chemical analysis in some tests performed. Blood samples from animals that are prone to have lipemic serum should be collected after a fast of 12 hours or more, so as to reduce the likelihood of a lipemic serum specimen.

Separating Serum from Whole Blood Samples

A blood sample should be allowed to reach room temperature before attempting to separate serum from a whole blood sample. The blood requires about 20-30 minutes for complete clotting. The next step requires a wooden applicator stick, which is used around the rim or inside edge to separate the clot from the sides of the tube. Next, the blood goes through a centrifugation process set at 2,000-3,000 rpm for 10 minutes. The speed and time should be carefully monitored to prevent hemolysis from occurring, which is problematic and caused by prolonged centrifugation. Next, the serum at the top of the tube is poured into another container. Another method allows the serum to be removed with a pipette or a small tube that draws the liquid out from the centrifuged tube. The liquid or serum in the pipette should also be transferred into another tube. The carefully marked tube should be placed in a refrigerator or freezer, depending upon the subsequent need.

Total Serum Protein

The **Goldberg refractometer** is a device which can gauge **total serum protein (TSP)** levels and can be obtained from the American Optical Company in Greenwich, CT. This instrument is beneficial in screening a variety of metabolic processes, including electrolytes, lipids, hemolysis, urea, and glucose. These measurements gained in the screening process can point to other conditions in the patient. Other tests may be necessary to obtain more accurate results.

The **Biuret method** is also used to determine the total amount of serum protein in a sample. This method can be employed in both wet and dry chemical analysis. This method requires that an automated or computerized serum analyzer be used. An analyzer applies a total dye binding process to calculate the serum proteins present in the serum.

The sample collected should be non-hemolyzed and non-lipemic. The serum or plasma samples can be collected with EDTA or heparin preservatives, but heparin will produce a measurement that is somewhat lower. Of additional note, proteins can be denatured or changed on a molecular level when detergent or UV light is introduced, so detergent and UV light should be kept away from the sample.

TSP Variations

Protein levels in serum are calculated based upon the amount of albumin and globulin found in the blood. Albumin and globulin are the two primary kinds of protein contained in the blood. The amount of serum globulins can be compared to the amount of serum albumin. While there is generally slightly more albumin, the ratio should be close to 1:1. Any substantial variation could be indicative of other health problems.

Serum protein changes may be shock-induced. Further, high albumin levels may be caused by severe dehydration. **High globulin** levels may be caused by many things, including: diseases of the blood (leukemia, hemolytic anemia, etc.), autoimmune diseases, and certain kidney and liver diseases. **Low albumin levels** may be caused by: malnutrition, severe burns, other kidney and liver diseases, gastrointestinal malabsorption syndromes, Hodgkin's lymphoma, uncontrolled diabetes, hyperthyroidism, or heart failure. Thus, each serum protein level must be checked to explore many aspects of an animal's health. However, pregnancy, injuries, infections, chronic illness, and certain medications may also affect blood protein levels.

Serum Albumin

Animals may sometimes present with one or more diseases that will contribute to altered albumin or globulin concentration. However, it is important to note that, generally, the total serum protein (TSP) will remain the same. The reason that the TSP level does not change is because globulin levels tend to rise as the albumin level lowers. Even so, certain infections, stressors, malnutrition, and other factors can sometimes affect TSP levels (usually then seen as an overall decrease). The serum albumin levels can be calculated by applying the albumin dye binding technique.

An animal suffering from shock may experience a rise in albumin levels. More frequently, the animal will have a lower albumin count due to the presence of other conditions, including acute liver disease, starvation or undernourishment, malabsorption, enteritis, colitis, parasites, pregnancy and lactation, persistent fever, improperly managed or untreated diabetes, shock, nephritis or nephrosis, ascites, and loss or reduction in blood volume.

Globulin

The **globulin** level can be used to derive the albumin level by subtraction. The globulin level is determined by subtracting the albumin level from the TSP level. **Electrophoresis** involves the electrically induced movement of molecular particles. It can also be applied to protein molecules, such as globulin or albumin. Electrophoresis is a technique used to divide globulin from albumin. **Fibrinogen** is a soluble protein that allows blood to clot. Fibrinogens are also present in the globulin fraction. Fibrinogen can occasionally be calculated from the total protein present. The amount of fibrinogen equals approximately 4 g/L of the total plasma protein fraction. This measurement requires a plasma base.

Electrophoresis can reveal any comparatively larger or smaller quantitative differences in protein particles. Upon separation, observation, and measurement, these differences may indicate the presence of particular diseases in the animal. However, each species of animal should only be compared with normal levels in relation to that specific species.

Globulin levels may be raised when antigenic stimulation occurs. In addition, other factors, including inflammation or infections, neoplasia, or abnormal immunoglobulin production can contribute to this rise in levels.

Urea

In aquatic organisms, the most common form of nitrogen waste (a product of protein metabolism) is ammonia. In birds and reptiles, nitrogen waste is excreted as uric acid. In mammals, nitrogen waste is excreted as urea.

Urea (or carbamide) is a nitrogenous byproduct of protein breakdown, and it must be eliminated from the body. Urea also helps produce an important countercurrent system in the kidneys. This system allows for crucial reabsorption of water and essential ions. Specifically, as some urea is reabsorbed it raises the osmolarity in the kidney. The greater the osmolarity, the more water that will be reabsorbed. This is important for maintaining both blood pressure and a proper concentration of sodium ions in the blood plasma. Thus, the tubules in the kidneys work to reabsorb up to 40% of the urea being processed (the remainder is excreted in urine and sweat). The level of excreted urea is one measure of the health of the kidney's glomerular filtration system.

Urea Nitrogen

Serum samples allow the technician to perform **urea nitrogen (UN)** or **serum urea nitrogen (SUN)** tests on an animal. Plasma samples measuring UN require anticoagulants heparin or EDTA. These samples are taken with ammonium oxalate, which creates an artificial rise in the **blood urea nitrogen (BUN)** level. Likewise, plasma samples taken with fluoride will artificially lower the BUN levels.

A rise in serum urea nitrogen levels can be attributed to a number of factors beyond kidney function alone: dehydration and heart failure can both result in elevated BUN. Further, urea excretion levels can be impacted by non-renal factors such as an increase in protein consumption, medications such as corticosteroids, and fever. However, the kidneys are nevertheless impacted by various pre-renal, post-renal, and non-renal factors. Shock can be considered either a pre-renal or a post-renal factor. Other post-renal problems may involve a blockage of the ureters, bladder, or urethra.

Animals that have anorexia, liver disease, or renal tubular damage may exhibit lower levels of urea excretion. Urea levels that are high can be instrumental in the diagnosis of a low- or nonfunctioning kidney.

Serum Creatinine

A primary source of cellular energy is the aerobic breakdown of ATP (Adenosine-5'-triphosphate) to ADP (Adenosine diphosphate), by which energy is released. When sufficient oxygen is not available for this normal energy production process, the body draws upon stores of creatine phosphate (or phosphocreatine) found in the muscles and brain. This molecule is used to anaerobically generate ATP from ADP in situations of intense energy demands or low oxygen availability. A byproduct of this process is **creatinine**.

The **glomeruli** in the kidneys filter almost all creatinine out of the blood. Therefore, an animal that has high blood serum levels of creatinine usually has low or non-functioning glomeruli.

Other factors that can lead to a high serum creatinine include dehydration and other pre-renal or post-renal causes. Thus, the technician should collect a serum or plasma sample for necessary testing. However, the technician should be aware that hemolyzed serum samples can impact the results of this test. **Hyperbilirubinemia** (high bilirubin levels) may also provide misleading results.

Serum Alanine Aminotransferase

The enzyme **alanine aminotransferase (ALT)** is also known as **serum glutamic pyruvate transaminase (SGPT)** and **alanine transaminase**. ALT/SGPT enzymes are specific to liver and muscle tissue. Injury to any of these cells releases this enzyme into the bloodstream. Therefore, knowing where this enzyme is most active can reveal where tissue damage may be occurring in the body when the levels of this enzyme are elevated.

It has been noted that more than 90% of all ALT activity is found in the hepatocytes of dogs, cats, rats, rabbits, and primates. Thus, in these animals, an elevated level of ALT is generally diagnostic of liver disease. Therefore, the ALT level in these animals is measured whenever the status of the liver's function is in question.

However, birds, horses, pigs, and ruminants have a much lower level of hepatocellular ALT activity. In these animals, ALT enzymes are more active in various muscle tissues. Therefore, increased levels of serum ALT in these animals are typically indicative of skeletal muscle injury or necrosis, rather than liver disease.

Measuring ALT

The level of ALT can be measured in both plasma and serum samples. There may be a high ALT level measured in initial tests that lowers when further tests are performed over time. That might indicate either that the first test was simply out of the norm, or that a transiently injurious event occurred that is quickly resolving. Unfortunately, when the levels increase or remain high over time, it is likely that a serious disease is involved. In animals in which ALT enzymes are more active in the liver, the veterinarian will need to explore the liver's functioning capacity and health. In animals where ALT enzymes are more active in muscle tissues, the veterinarian will look to skeletal muscles for sources of disease and damage.

In some cases canines are given medications that can unintentionally and artificially increase ALT levels. However, medications are less likely to produce this side effect in cats.

Serum Alkaline Phosphatase

Practically all the organic tissues within the body are constructed with the involvement of the enzyme alkaline phosphatase, which catalyzes and synthesizes phosphoric acid. **Alkaline phosphatase (ALP)** is produced primarily in the liver and bone, with some made in the intestines and kidneys, and by the placenta during pregnancy. ALP is usually found in low quantities in the serum.

Elevated ALP levels may indicate: intrahepatic or post-hepatic cholestasis, medication-induced liver damage, bone tumors, osteomalacia, parathyroid hormone overproduction, etc. The rise in ALP levels will not usually be linked to reduced rates of enzyme metabolism and discharge, rather, elevated ALP levels can usually be attributed to a rise in production of ALP. Young animals may have a rise in ALP that can be linked to bone growth. Older animals may have elevated levels from a bone injury or obstructive liver disease. Anticonvulsants and glucocorticoids will cause this rise for about 2 weeks after the drug has been given to the patient.

Serum Gamma-glutamyltransferase

Gamma-glutamyltransferase (GGT) is an enzyme found in the liver, pancreas, and kidney. High concentrations of GGT in the serum likely indicate liver dysfunction. In particular, the liver disease known as cholestasis is often suspected when GGT levels are high. However, there can be other liver diseases that can contribute to the higher GGT levels. Therefore, both ALT and GGT should be monitored in the smaller-sized animals. A rise in both ALT and GGT levels should initiate active exploration of potential causes of liver disease in the small animal.

Another type of disease found in small animals that elevates GGT enzymes is fatty liver disease. Any medication side effects that can cause increased levels of GGT should be ruled out when determining a differential diagnosis.

Serum Aspartate Aminotransferase

The enzyme **aspartate aminotransferase (AST)** is also known as aspartate transaminase, formerly known as serum glutamic oxaloacetic transaminase (SGOT). AST enzymes, along with other enzymes, facilitate many intracellular processes and functions. Thus, they are only found in the bloodstream when cellular damage has released them into extracellular fluids, by which they are drawn into the vascular circulation.

The level of AST has not been linked with any particular organ in the body. However, this enzyme has been linked to various tissues of the body, including cardiac muscle, diaphragmatic muscle, skeletal muscle, and the liver. Therefore, whenever these tissues sustain any injury, a rise in AST levels in the serum or plasma can be expected. The significance of high levels of **aspartate aminotransferase (AST)** in serum can be linked to a number of potential health issues, including an impairment of the liver, destruction of red blood cells, or damaged heart or skeletal muscle tissue.

AST Testing

AST levels are determined using a plasma or serum sample that is not hemolyzed or lipemic. The specimen should be properly centrifuged, allowing the AST to be separated from the red blood cells. This will give a more accurate reading of the AST level.

The results of the AST analysis alone are not definitive: the ALT and AST tests should be used in conjunction when considering a diagnosis, particularly when assessing the liver. Other contributing factors could be linked to the rise in AST levels, as changes in these enzymatic levels are not diagnostically definitive.

Serum Sodium

Sodium is essential to sustaining osmotic pressures and fluid balances within the body. Sodium is key to the extracellular positive ion attraction that primes the sodium-potassium-ATPase pump responsible for moving vital nutrients and materials into and out of cell structures.

Patients will not normally have a high level of sodium in their blood serum. When a high level is noted, then the patient may suffer from **hypernatremia**. However, this may occur in part because the patient is dehydrated. Problems associated with **hyponatremia** include kidney failure, vomiting or diarrhea in association with diuretics, disproportionate ADH, congestive heart failure, and water toxicity.

Patients with sodium imbalances should have their fluid intake monitored to prevent them from ingesting more liquids than needed. The veterinarian should use a non-hemolyzed serum specimen for the serum sodium test. Plasma samples can be tested, provided they are collected with lithium or ammonium heparin. However, both serum and plasma specimens must be centrifuged to remove cellular components from the residual fluid used for testing.

Serum Potassium

The **potassium** cation (positively charged ion) contributes to sustaining the fluid and electrolyte balance within the body. This balance is maintained by fluid dynamics, 90% of which take place within the cells of the body.

The normal range of both serum and plasma potassium levels is roughly 3.5-5.5 mEq/L, depending on species, and they are the same whether reported as milliequivalents per liter (mEq/L) or millimoles per liter (mmol/L). Higher levels of serum potassium are indicative of a number of potential concerning conditions. These conditions include adrenal cortical hypofunction, acidosis, and late-stage renal failure. A high potassium level is referred to as **hyperkalemia**.

An abnormally low level of serum potassium is referred to as **hypokalemia**. Conditions that are attributed to hypokalemia include alkalosis, insulin therapy, and fluid loss associated with diuretics, vomiting, and diarrhea.

The best test results are generally obtained with a plasma sample. However, the sample may be either non-hemolyzed serum or heparinized plasma. Blood cells must be separated from the fluids within 2 hours or the testing values may be altered. This is particularly critical when analyzing samples taken from cattle and horses, as their blood cells continue to release potassium over time.

Serum Chloride

The kidneys are responsible for controlling the levels of **chloride** ions found in the body.

Hyperchloremia is the term used to describe an abnormally high serum chloride level. The patient with hyperchloremia may have serious health issues, including metabolic acidosis or renal tubular acidosis and overactive parathyroid glands.

The patient with **hypochloremia**, an abnormally low level of serum chloride, may have other issues, including vomiting, anorexia, malnutrition, and diabetes insipidus.

A blood sample for testing should be non-hemolyzed serum or heparinized plasma. Blood cells must be separated from the plasma or serum promptly in order to avoid illegitimate test results.

Serum Calcium

Calcium is the principal element found in the body's skeletal system. Approximately 99% of all calcium found in the body is contained within the bones. The remaining calcium is employed to help move inorganic ions and fluids throughout the body. Calcium is needed in the function of cell membranes, blood coagulation, muscle contraction and nerve impulse transmission, as well as in the activation of certain enzymes.

Parathyroid hormone (PTH), calcitonin, and vitamin D work together to control the calcium and phosphorus levels within the body. Serum protein, albumin levels, and serum calcium levels should all be appraised simultaneously. This gives the veterinarian the opportunity to observe how the serum calcium levels fluctuate together with the protein and albumin levels.

An irregular rise in serum calcium is referred to as **hypercalcemia**, which can point to other serious conditions, including pseudohyperparathyroidism, hyperparathyroidism, excessive vitamin D intake, and cancerous bony metastases. An abnormally low level of serum calcium is called **hypocalcemia**, which can point to serious conditions such as malabsorption, eclampsia, pancreatic necrosis, hypoalbuminemia, and hypoparathyroidism.

Milk Fever

Low levels of serum calcium in ruminants may indicate gastrointestinal stasis. Female cows, dogs, sheep, and horses may experience calcium-related peri- or post-parturient health events with the onset of lactation, as the demands of milk production for nursing overwhelm the body's calcium supplies. It is often called parturient paresis or milk fever, but may also be referred to as puerperal hypocalcemia, hypocalcemic tetany, or milk or lactation tetany. To test for calcium disorders, the veterinarian should obtain a non-hemolyzed serum or heparinized plasma sample.

Serum Phosphorus

Phosphorus is another important bodily element. The skeleton contains 80% of the body's phosphorus. **Parathyroid hormone** (PTH) helps regulate the balance of both calcium and phosphorus.

Serum phosphorus levels should be monitored along with serum calcium levels due to the inverse relation that these substances have to each other. **Hyperphosphatemia** is an abnormally high level of phosphorus which can point to kidney failure, anuria, and hypoparathyroidism. It can be induced by ingestion of an excessive amount of vitamin D, or poisoning with ethylene glycol. Abnormally low serum phosphorus is called **hypophosphatemia**. It can sometimes arise from a diet low in phosphorus and may be related to primary hyperparathyroidism, malabsorption, hyperinsulinism, diabetes mellitus, lymphosarcoma, and hyperadrenocorticism. Non-hemolyzed serum or heparinized plasma is needed for laboratory testing.

Blood Glucose

Hyperglycemia is indicated when an animal has a high level of glucose present in the bloodstream. This is often an indication of **diabetes mellitus**. The pancreas secretes hormones (including insulin), glucagon, and somatostatin into the bloodstream. **Insulin** is responsible for moving glucose out of the blood and into the cells, where it is burned for energy. Diabetes mellitus occurs when the pancreas produces insufficient insulin, thus allowing glucose levels in the blood to rise.

However, there are other diseases and factors unrelated to the pancreas that can produce this same condition. For example, cats can experience high levels of stress when going for a vet clinic visit, which may induce abnormally high glucose levels, known as **stress-induced hyperglycemia**. Other abnormal readings can be attributed to conditions such as malabsorption, chronic liver disease, etc. Thus, the technician may want to conduct a more definitive glucose tolerance test to gauge how well the animal makes use of carbohydrates and sugars over a longer period of time.

Serum/Plasma Glucose Testing

The technician should take precautions when collecting samples for the purpose of **glucose testing**. These precautions should include special handling methods to prevent any variability in the blood glucose levels measured. One precaution involves separation of the cellular components in blood from the plasma or serum to prevent continued metabolic interactions from occurring; if continued interaction is permitted, the glucose in the blood will continue to be used up at a rate of 7-10% for every hour that contact is maintained. Thus, the technician should divide the plasma or serum from the cellular components almost immediately.

Further, cats and dogs should not be fed for a period of 16-24 hours prior to phlebotomy (blood drawing), to obtain the more definitive fasted glucose level. This fasting period is not necessary for ruminant animals. Serum is the preferred blood sample. However, the technician should be aware that serum will test at a 5% higher glucose level. Again, the technician should place the sample in the centrifuge without delay. If delays are unavoidable, then the technician should use fluoride, which requires one hour to stop the red blood cells from further metabolizing the glucose.

Bilirubin in the Liver

Bilirubin is a byproduct of the metabolism of hemoglobin. Hemoglobin is broken down into heme and globin by the mononuclear phagocytic system (sometimes called the reticuloendothelial system). Heme is then further broken down into bilirubin. The liver functions to modify byproducts and toxins such as bilirubin, reducing them into a form that can be readily excreted from the body.

Bilirubin not yet modified by the liver is called unconjugated or indirect bilirubin. Bilirubin that has been modified has been attached to a glucuronide (creating glucuronic acid), allowing it to be excreted in the bile. This bilirubin is called conjugated or direct bilirubin. Added together, indirect and direct bilirubin serum levels provide a total bilirubin measure.

If bilirubin builds up faster than the liver can metabolize it, or if the liver is not functioning properly, a condition called **hyperbilirubinemia** may develop. When the concentrations of bilirubin are particularly high, it can discolor the skin, mucous membranes, and whites of the eyes to make them appear yellowish—a condition called **jaundice** (from the French word jaune, meaning yellow). In such situations, the liver's own enzymes are sometimes measured to determine whether or not the liver is functioning properly.

Unconjugated and Conjugated Bilirubin

Bilirubin levels can be measured in either blood plasma or serum. Total and direct levels of bilirubin can be measured specifically in the blood. The level of unconjugated bilirubin is the difference between these two. When bilirubin levels are high (due either to liver damage or rapid RBC hemolysis), significant amounts of bilirubin may pass into the urine (instead of being excreted largely through the bile, passing through the bile ducts and into the intestines). In the intestines, direct bilirubin is further broken down by bacteria into a substance called **urobilinogen**, which ultimately gives stool its normal yellowish-brown color. All bilirubin in the urine is of the direct or conjugated form, as indirect or unconjugated bilirubin is not water soluble and thus cannot readily pass out of the body.

Prehepatic jaundice is defined as the liver's failure to process unconjugated bilirubin. Hepatic jaundice and post-hepatic jaundice are directly linked with a rise in conjugated bilirubin levels. **Post-hepatic jaundice** typically involves partial or full obstruction of the biliary and cystic ducts (cholestasis), which keeps the conjugated bilirubin from leaving.

Detecting Bilirubin

Diazo reagent is used in plasma or serum analysis to detect the presence of bilirubin. Ictotest tablets have a form of diazo reagent and are employed to identify the presence of bilirubin in the urine. Ictotest tablets are able to detect as little as 0.05-0.1 mg of bilirubin/dL, and thus are very unlikely to produce false negative results. When the urine is diluted by known increments and re-tested in a serial fashion, the analysis may reveal semi-quantitative results. The rate of the color formation (blue to purple) and the color intensity are both proportional to the amount of bilirubin in the urine. A pink or red color indicates a negative result.

Reagent strips like Ictostix and Multistix can also be employed in testing. These reagent strips also contain a form of diazo reagent. However, the Ictotest tablet is more useful, due to its higher sensitivity to bilirubin in urine. False-negative results may occur if a test sample has been left out too long, as bilirubin rapidly breaks down, especially with exposure to light. False-negative results may also occur if the urine contains large quantities of ascorbic acid or nitrites (released via bacterial growth). In addition, some medications can result in a false-positive reading.

Serum Cholesterol

Cholesterol is a steroid alcohol created through a liver synthesis process. **Hypothyroidism** can result from higher levels of serum cholesterol in an animal. Hypothyroidism is a deficiency in thyroid hormone production. High cholesterol levels may also indicate lipemia. **Lipemia** is an unusually high level of lipids or fats in the blood. Higher levels of cholesterol may indicate diabetes mellitus, hyperadrenocorticism, nephrotic syndrome, certain liver diseases, bile duct obstruction, or pregnancy complications.

The test for serum cholesterol levels cannot be used alone to diagnose liver dysfunction but should be used in combination with other diagnostic indices and liver function tests. Prior to collecting a blood specimen, the patient should not be fed for a number of hours so a more accurate base level can be determined. A non-hemolyzed serum or heparinized plasma sample should be utilized for testing.

Serum Bile Acid

Bile is produced by the liver and is very important in the digestive process. Bile acids are both hydrophobic (lipid, or fat soluble) and hydrophilic (polar, or water soluble), so bile is able to break down water-insoluble fats in a water-saturated environment (i.e., the intestinal tract).

Bile is synthesized from cholesterol—more than half of which comes from diet, with the remainder created by synthesis in the body (in the liver, intestines, and other cells). Bile is stored in the gall bladder in humans and most domestic animals, except in horses and rats.

Usually, serum bile acid levels are low. This is due to the body's bile reabsorption process in the ileum or lower small intestines and the filtration of blood through the liver. Low serum bile acid levels **post-prandially** (after a meal) may indicate ileal dysfunction. An animal with ileal or post-jejunal small intestinal disease will have a lower serum bile acid level.

High levels are indicative of liver disease (even when other liver function tests may appear normal) and hepatocytic inability to filter bile. Postponed emptying of the stomach and fasting will lower these levels.

Sorbitol Dehydrogenase

Sorbitol dehydrogenase (SDH) is an enzyme produced in liver cells. In veterinary applications, SDH has been found to be a particularly effective indicator of acute hepatocellular (liver cell) damage and disease. It also has a high sensitivity to toxins, and thus is a very early indicator of toxin- or medication-induced liver damage.

Likewise, necrosis (the death of cells) in the liver can be associated with higher levels of SDH in the serum. Necrosis is a result of injury or disease in the patient.

SDH levels should be analyzed to determine if a large animal has liver disease. The SDH test is more appropriate for use with larger animals than is ALT testing. However, the SDH enzyme is known to be unstable and can lose its ability to react after about 8 hours. Therefore, the sample should be analyzed as soon as possible after collection. The practice of sending samples to outside labs to be analyzed may be problematic if the tests are thereby delayed. Thus, using a local laboratory or one within the clinic may alleviate this problem.

Serum Amylase

Amylase is a digestive enzyme that functions to break down carbohydrates and starches into sugars, which first occurs in the saliva. It is also found in the pancreas, where it catabolizes stored glycogen into glucose.

There are a number of factors that may precipitate a rise in serum amylase levels: acute, chronic, and obstructive pancreatitis; hyperadrenocorticism; upper gastrointestinal inflammation; obstructions in the digestive system; or kidney failure.

Some tests are adapted from those originally intended for humans, which may require some revision to be successfully applied in animal populations. Serum amylase testing is one of these. The serum should be diluted with a prescribed amount of normal saline prior to running the test; this will compensate for the higher rate of serum amylase activity found in animals as compared to humans.

Maltose does not impact the test results. Therefore, dogs are good candidates for **amyloclastic** tests. However, the same tests used for humans or dogs are not always compatible in testing cats. The tests will require non-lipemic serum or heparinized plasma samples to produce accurate amylase results. Hemolysis present in the samples can cause the amylase rates to artificially rise.

Serum Lipase

The enzyme **lipase** works to digest the long-chain fatty acids that constitute lipids. This process produces reduced fatty acids and alcohols. Normally, only a small amount of lipase can be detected in the serum. High serum lipase levels may indicate: acute or chronic pancreatitis, kidney failure, hyperadrenocorticism, dexamethasone treatment, and bile tract disease. Colorimetric and dry chemistry kits can be used to make an initial assessment regarding lipase levels. However, it is a tedious measurement process.

If a veterinarian believes an animal's symptoms point to acute pancreatitis, serum amylase and lipase tests should be conducted on the patient. However, a cat with pancreatitis should not be diagnosed solely on the basis of serum lipase levels. The serum lipase levels in cats can be low despite the presence of disease in the animal.

Regardless, the testing sample collected should be non-hemolyzed and non-lipemic serum or heparinized plasma.

Serum Trypsin-Like Immunoreactivity Test

Animals with **exocrine pancreatic insufficiency (EPI)** do not secrete sufficient digestive enzymes to properly digest their food, and diagnosis can be difficult. Serum **trypsin-like immunoreactivity (TLI)** is considered the definitive testing standard for an EPI diagnosis. The test measures the levels of certain enzymes in the blood (trypsin, trypsinogen, and particularly TLI).

The digestive enzyme **trypsin** breaks down proteins, is normally retained in the pancreas, and only enters the bloodstream if the pancreas is inflamed. The pancreas also produces a forerunner enzyme known as trypsinogen, though very little is normally found in the circulatory system. TLI is able to detect both of these enzymes, and thus has a high rate of success in identifying canine EPI. The enzymes should be analyzed with a ligand assay technique, and the animal should not be fed for a period of 12 hours prior to sample collection. 5.2-35 μg/L is a normal canine TLI range (12-82 μg/L for cats). TLIs lower than 2.5 μg/L are indicative of EPI (8 μg/L for cats). Chronic pancreatitis can also result from EPI. Juvenile atrophy and pancreatic hypoplasia are also linked to EPI or exocrine pancreatic insufficiency.

ACTH Stimulation Test

An **ACTH stimulation test** is run to detect Cushing's disease. **Adrenocorticotropic hormone (ACTH)** is the hormone produced by the pituitary gland that signals to the adrenal glands how much cortisol to produce. As the blood cortisol level increases, the pituitary gland will decrease ACTH hormone production. With the ACTH stimulation test, a baseline blood cortisol will be drawn and then an injection of synthetic ACTH given intravenously. Another blood sample is taken an hour after the injection and compared to the baseline sample. The ACTH stimulation test will indicate if the patient has Cushing's disease. A dog with Cushing's disease will show an increase in cortisol production in the hour after the blood sample because the body is not being alerted to the slow cortisol production.

Low-Dose Dexamethasone Suppression (LDDS) Test

A common test used to diagnose Cushing's disease is the **low-dose dexamethasone suppression (LDDS)** test. With this test, a sample of blood is drawn to determine the dog's baseline cortisol level, and then a small dexamethasone (synthetic cortisol) injection is given to the dog intravenously. Another blood sample is taken at 4 and 8 hours after the dexamethasone injection was given to measure the dog's cortisol levels. As blood cortisol levels increase after the dexamethasone injection is given, the pituitary gland should be lowering the production of ACTH (the hormone that stimulates the adrenal glands to produce cortisol), and there should be a drop in cortisol levels in the blood in the post-dexamethasone blood samples. The LDDS test can tell you if Cushing's is of pituitary or adrenal origin. If there is a pituitary tumor, there will be a slight decrease in cortisol production noticed in the 4- and 8-hour post-dexamethasone samples. If there is an adrenal tumor present, then there will be no reduction in blood cortisol at either the 4- or 8-hour blood sample.

Testing for Non-Plasma Specific Enzymes

There are particular enzymes that are not normally present in either plasma or serum. The presence of such enzymes may indicate destruction of tissue cells, intensified tissue cell production, barriers in the excretory path, or poor circulation.

A **non-plasma specific enzyme test kit** will consist of the following items: substrates, coenzymes, and cofactors. The enzymes should be analyzed at specified temperatures. Particular care should be taken in sample collection, especially regarding samples that contain anticoagulants.

The international unit (IU) of measure is used to display the quantitative measurements obtained through enzyme analysis and is the standardized index used for this practice.

In general, the older unit indices are no longer used. However, occasional deviations from this reporting standard may still occur, whether due to specific machine calibration, operator preference, or residual operating policy. Regardless, the laboratory has the responsibility to include any laboratory-specific reference ranges and standards with any enzyme level reports issued from that facility.

Clinical Cytology

Cytology Staining

There are 3 types of **Romanowsky stains** employed in the examination of cytology samples: **Wright's**, **Giemsa** and **Diff-Quik**. There is a noticeable variation in the staining quality of these products. Therefore, a single type of stain should be used consistently to reduce the likelihood of misinterpretations due to the stain style and quality variations.

The **new methylene blue (NMB) stain** is used to examine cell nuclei, mast cell granules, and most infectious organisms and agents. However, there are limitations associated with its use. NMB should only be applied to the examination of nucleated cells, bacteria, fungi, and mast cells. This stain may be applied directly to a slide that has been allowed to dry in the air.

Bacterial agents may be classified by the employment of a Gram staining solution. Pink coloration indicates cells and bacteria that are Gram-negative; the purple color indicates a Gram-positive result.

A hematoxylin/eosin stain may be used in the examination of histological studies, particularly stains that can expose the nuclear detail of the sample. These solutions are known as Papanicolaou stains.

Fine Needle Aspiration

To obtain a **fine needle aspirate**, you will need a 25-gauge needle and a 10 mL syringe. Insert the needle into the cutaneous or subcutaneous mass or lesion, apply a small amount of suction through the syringe, and redirect a few times inside the mass while suctioning back to get a good-sized sample. Release the syringe plunger to release the suction, and then pull the syringe with the needle out of the lesion. Remove the syringe from the needle, pull back the plunger to fill the syringe with air, and then replace the needle. Push the plunger to express the sample onto a clean slide (it should be just small enough to be in the needle and not the syringe). Too much force or pressure will rupture the cells, so obtain and prepare the sample gently. Air-dry the sample on the slide. Once dried, the sample must be stained using either a modified Wright or rapid stain. Once the slide is stained, examine it under 40x magnification; place a drop of immersion oil on the sample spot identified under 40x; then move to 100x for evaluation.

Highly cellular fluids obtained via fine needle aspiration (FNA) can be smeared directly onto a slide, whereas low-cellularity fluids should be centrifuged first to concentrate the cells to create a more adequate smear.

Impression Smears

Cells to be examined under a microscope may be collected with **impression smears**, which can be used for cutaneous or subcutaneous tissues. Likewise, some tissues removed by surgical procedures can be used to make imprints. The veterinarian will need to expose the center of the mass by making a cut with a small surface area, and the excess fluid and blood should be blotted clean. Imprints are taken by touching a fresh microscope slide to the cut surface and lifting it away directly. Multiple imprints can be taken per microscope slide.

This technique is best for epithelial cells, lymph nodes, splenic tissue, mast cell tumors, and other tissues that exfoliate cells easily.

Scraping

For tissues that do not exfoliate cells readily, samples can be collected via **scraping**, which employs a sterile scalpel blade to mildly scrape on a freshly cut tissue surface. This scraping is streaked smoothly on a slide for examination. It is then air-dried before staining and examination under a microscope. As these samples are considered "dirty," they should be stained so as not to contaminate the staining liquid.

When collecting samples from sensitive areas, such as a corneal lesion, an anesthetic may be applied first.

Swabbing

For the **swab technique**, a cotton swab is used to gather the cutaneous or subcutaneous cell samples by rubbing it gently over the target area, and then applying the resulting sample to a microscope slide or culture dish for further evaluation.

A swab is particularly helpful when applied in the gathering of cell samples used for diagnosing problems associated with exposed mucous membranes, such as the vagina, or the ears. Such samples are collected to analyze the estrous cycle stage using uterine and vaginal discharges. The veterinarian will use a speculum when gathering vaginal samples.

The swab technique is also useful in the examination of **fistulated lesions** (lesions that create an abnormal passageway), which require cleaning of the fistula before and after the sample is collected.

Fluid Aspiration

There are a multitude of names for **fluid aspiration** (withdrawing fluid by suction, i.e., a syringe), largely based on the aspiration sites: **abdominocentesis** (abdominal), **thoracocentesis** (chest), **cystocentesis** (bladder), **cerebrospinal fluid tap** (CSF tap), and **arthrocentesis** (joints).

The veterinarian will clean the site with a surgical scrub before taking a sample. This is required for all samples dispatched for microbiology testing and is essential to maintain proper aseptic conditions. The animal should be restrained in a standing position during these procedures except during cystocentesis and CSF tap. Cystocentesis requires that the animal be placed in dorsal or lateral recumbency; the animal must be placed in a lateral recumbency position when a CSF aspiration is required.

The aspirated fluid will be cultured to check for bacteria or centrifuged for inspection of the sediment.

Fluid Sample Characteristics

Fluid samples should be examined for color, odor, and turbidity. **Turbidity** refers to the opaque qualities found in the fluid, such as particles and sediment. The total nucleated cell count (TNCC) and total protein should be noted to help further categorize the type of fluid sample taken.

There are 3 types of fluid: **transudates, exudates**, and **modified transudates**. The fluid samples categorized as transudates are those that are found to have less than 500/mL of TNCC in conjunction with a total protein level measuring less than 3 g/dL (typically, extracellular fluids that have filtered through membranous tissues). Transudates are further categorized when the sample lacks color, as with ascites. **Ascites** is described as fluid in the abdominal region. The fluid samples categorized as modified transudates include total protein counts between 2.5 and 7.5 g/dL. Modified transudates have an opaque or pink coloration. The exudate samples that have total protein counts higher than 3 g/dL should be noted as indicative of inflammation.

Sending Samples to a Reference Lab

Samples that will be sent out to a reference lab must be air-dried and labeled with the patient's name, the client's name, and the date; then they are placed into a slide holder to be shipped along with the reference lab form.

A tissue sample such as a **biopsy** or **mass** that has been removed from a patient is sent out to a reference lab for histopathology. The sample is placed into an appropriately sized formalin jar, labeled with the patient's name, client's name, type of specimen, date, and clinic name. A corresponding reference lab form will be filled out that will include all of that same information plus the location of where the mass was on the patient and the size and diameter of the tissue that was excised.

Pulmonary Cytology

Pulmonary lesions can be examined using fine needle aspiration, though it may cause pneumothorax or hemorrhage; thus, caution and careful post-aspiration follow-up are important. The other technique involves a scraping and/or impression taken of any suspicious-looking tissue during a procedure for biopsy.

The veterinarian may also compare normal cells with those taken in a tracheal wash. The cancerous cells associated with the lung include **carcinoma** and **adenocarcinoma**. Inflammation found in the lungs can be a result of the following: bacterial infection with *Mycobacterium spp.*, fungal infections with *Cryptococcus spp.* or *Blastomyces spp.*, parasites such as *Toxoplasma spp.* or *Pneumocystis spp.*, viral infection, neoplasia, or trauma.

Splenic Cytology

The veterinarian may apply fine needle aspiration or biopsy collection techniques in gathering cells from the spleen. However, splenic tissue is fragile, so great care should be taken to prevent tears or bleeding in the tissue.

Splenic hyperplasia may be the result of bacterial, viral, or fungal infections, parasites, or immune-mediated conditions; it can also be attributed to extramedullary hematopoiesis, hemangiosarcoma, or fibrosarcoma, which commonly affect the spleen. Splenic cytology results should be analyzed alongside other clinical signs to make a diagnosis.

Neutrophils and Necrosis

Exfoliative cytology (cells shed from body surfaces) may reveal neutrophils that are comparable in appearance to the neutrophils located in peripheral blood. These observations can be found by examining neutrophils under a microscope. **Hypersegmented neutrophils** may have 5 or 6 sections or lobes. Other neutrophils may be undergoing pyknosis, which is the degeneration of chromatin in a cell nucleus when undergoing cellular death or apoptosis. Still other neutrophils may be undergoing **karyolysis**, the digestion of chromatin in the nucleus by way of the enzyme DNase. This digested material is known as **karyorrhexis**, the fragmented particles of the cell's nucleus undergoing necrosis. **Necrosis** is the death and decay of parts of cells or whole cells in a patient's tissues or organs. The detection of necrosis can indicate injury or disease, such as cancer or other decay-inducing processes.

Mesothelial Cells and Mast Cells Found

Mesothelial cells form **mesodermal tissue**, which provides the interior lining of a body cavity or the covering of an embryo. This lining is specifically found on pleural, peritoneal, and visceral surfaces within the body. Mesothelial cells generally have a circular shape and a single nucleus. However, some mesothelial cells are known to be multinucleated. In addition, these cells contain a network structure of nuclear chromatin and slightly basophilic cytoplasm. The basophilic descriptor indicates that the cytoplasm has little difficulty in being stained with ordinary dyes.

Some cells function to remove unwanted or phagocytic debris. They can be identified by looking at the cells with cytoplasm, nucleoli, or a corona.

Mast cells have a distinctive shape and color. These cells have either round or elliptically formed nuclei. In addition, there is a bluish-purple coloration found in a majority of the cytoplasmic granules.

Lymphocytes, Plasma Cells, Erythrocytes, and Eosinophils

Exfoliative cytology (cells shed or gathered from body surfaces, as opposed to body fluids) can reveal cells and changes not always available via peripheral vascular fluids.

Lymphocytes and **eosinophils** are white blood cells that present similarly, as when found in peripheral blood. However, plasma cells will be visible as **elliptical cells** with an abnormal nucleus, basophilic cytoplasm, and perinuclear clear zone. **Erythrocytes** (RBCs) can sometimes be observed in the interior of phagocytic cells; this is especially true in macrophages found in the exfoliative sample. **Macrophages** are large white blood cells that are critical in the protection against infections in the body. These sizeable cells come from the monocytes found in peripheral blood. The nucleus in the macrophages will have an elliptical shape. These cells are pleomorphic: they present in two different forms throughout the overall life cycle. **Exfoliative cell chromatin** will form chromosomes that have the appearance of lace. The chromatin may also form denser or more condensed molecules. If staining turns the cytoplasm blue, then the vacuole should be checked for phagocytic debris. This is indicative of a macrophage, which can have one or more nuclei and vary in size.

Neoplasia Cytology

Cytological samples can explore and confirm or reject the presence of a **malignancy**. Specifically, the changes in the cell nucleus can determine if a malignancy is present. For example, the coarse chromatin pattern in a cell nucleus bears distinctive markings resembling a cord or rope, and variations may indicate disease.

A particularly concerning pattern of nucleus deformity is called **nuclear molding**, which occurs when the nucleus in one cell spontaneously changes to a deformed state in response to other deformed nuclei in the same cell, or to match the deformed nuclei of neighboring cells. If a cell contains two or more nuclei, it is considered **multinucleated**.

The size, shape, and number of nucleoli in cells should be noted when assessing malignancy. **Anisonucleosis** is the term used to describe an inconsistency found in the size and profile of the nucleoli indicating nuclear injury.

Round or oval nuclear shapes are usually normal. However, pointed shapes indicate angular nucleoli. **Macronucleoli** are nucleoli that are larger than normal and may point to a malignancy. The existence of a multitude of nucleoli also suggests that a malignancy is present.

Anisokaryosis, N:C Ratio, and Mitotic Activity

Malignancy is a term given to describe a cancerous growth. **Metastasis** describes a cancer that spreads to other parts of the body. This growth can be detected through changes that occur in the nucleus of a cell in a cytological sample. For example, a sizeable variation can be found in the measurement of a cancerous cell's nucleus. This difference can be beyond that which is normally anticipated for the tissue type involved. Nucleus size variation is a condition known as **anisokaryosis**.

The normal **cellular N:C**, or nucleus to cell cytoplasm ratio, is typically in the range of 1:3 to 1:8. Higher N:C ratios may indicate malignancy. Normally, cells will divide mitotically and split evenly into two cells. When cells do not split evenly, malignancy may be suspected.

Clinical Urinalysis

Urine samples should be analyzed within 30 minutes of collection (especially for crystal evaluations), or the sample should be refrigerated (allowable for up to 24 hours and acceptable for pH and specific gravity evaluation). If urine cytology is necessary but cannot be performed right away, 10% formalin should be added.

The following may induce or indicate degradation of urine samples: a rise in ammonia levels; the presence of hemolyzed erythrocytes (as opposed to intact red blood cells); a pH level which allows bacteria to grow; lower levels of bilirubin, glucose, ketones, leukocytes, and urobilinogen; the disappearance of casts; an alteration in crystals; a darker discoloration; the appearance of nitrites; a harsher smell; a lower or higher concentration of protein; or an opaque, muddy appearance.

Samples collected by owners are often unreliable, and efforts should be made to retrieve samples in the clinic by cystocentesis, urethral catheterization, or clean-catch voiding.

Urine Color

The color of normal urine ranges from pale yellow to a pale yellowish-brown. The color is directly related to the presence of **urochromes**, which are responsible for the yellow pigment found in urine. The **specific gravity** (the ratio of the liquid's density as compared with water, abbreviated SG) is responsible for the intensity of color. Urine with a lower SG will appear lighter in color than urine with a higher SG. In addition, bile pigments are associated with colorations noted as yellowish-brown or greenish, and urine containing bile pigments will froth when shaken.

The presence of RBCs is indicated by a reddish urine tint, called **hematuria**. Hemoglobin is abbreviated as Hb, and, when present in urine, causes a reddish-brown tint, known as **hemoglobinuria**. **Myoglobinuria** is indicated by brown-tinted urine.

Urine Transparency

The transparency of urine samples is defined in 3 levels or degrees: clear, cloudy, and flocculent. Most animals when healthy produce **clear**, transparent urine. However, the horse, rabbit, hamster, and gerbil do not. Healthy equine urine contains mucus and calcium carbonate crystals; normal rabbit, hamster, and gerbil urine contains calcium salts. The presence of these components will produce a cloudy, though transparent, urine.

Cloudy urine can be created from RBCs, WBCs, epithelial cells, crystals, bacteria, casts, mucus, semen, or lipids. In addition, bacteria or crystals present in the urine can turn voided, standing urine a cloudy color. This is a problem associated with bacterial proliferation and crystal formation that can occur when urine is not stored correctly after collection. Thus, samples should generally be tested promptly to avoid these problematic changes.

The term **flocculent** describes urine that appears pathologic, containing easily visible particles, mucus, and other debris—often due to the presence of crystals and/or infection.

Urine Volume

The volume of urine output is controlled by 5 variables:

- The amount of water that the animal drinks
- The temperatures within the animal's environment
- The animal's physical activity levels
- The animal's size
- The animal's genus or species

Pollakiuria describes frequent urination; this is not to be mistaken with **polyuria** (voiding excessive quantities of urine), often found in patients with undiagnosed diabetes. Other conditions associated with polyuria include nephritis and **polydipsia** (abnormal thirst). Patients that are in shock, dehydrated, conserving water, or in kidney failure will not produce normal amounts of urine, and consequently will not have a desire to urinate as much. **Oliguria** (abnormally small amounts of urine production) is a result of these declining conditions. If the patient becomes unable to urinate, then a diagnosis of **anuria** can be made; anuria can be a direct result of renal shutdown or an obstruction which prevents urine from passing out of the body.

Urine Concentration

The water deprivation/urine concentration test is given to an animal that has been gradually denied water over a period of 3-5 days on an escalating basis. This test will allow the urine to be assessed for the concentration of endogenous **antidiuretic hormone (ADH)**. ADH is released by dehydrated animals to increase renal reabsorption of water, so as to better conserve what little water is remaining in the body. The gradual restriction of water over a 72-hour period should produce the desired ADH release effect. The animal is expected to lose about 5% of total weight due to dehydration.

The reference measurement is given as the specific gravity of urine at a normal concentration. This measurement is 1.025 for normal levels of ADH. Insufficient ADH or tubular dysfunction may be detected when the test indicates that ADH concentrations are low. Previously dehydrated animals should not be given this test. Azotemic animals (those with preexisting high serum urea levels) should also not be given this test.

Urine Odor

Urine is typically associated with some unpleasant smells. Odor should not be used to directly derive a diagnosis; certain animals like cats, mice, goats, and pigs can put off quite a pungent odor when urinating. However, odor may indicate bacterial infection, excess ammonia, or the presence of ketones (indicated by a sweet, fruity smell). Bacterial proliferation may also emerge in standing, improperly stored urine, and high levels of bacteria can intensify the overall strength of the smell. A strong ammonia smell can also indicate a rise in bacteria levels. Ketones may signify diabetes mellitus, pregnancy toxemia in sheep, or acetonemia in cows.

Urine Chemistry

Specific Gravity

Non-centrifuged, room temperature samples are required to perform urine chemistry and specific gravity analysis.

Specific gravity (SG) gives the ratio of the density of urine in relation to the density of distilled water; it is a measure of how efficiently the kidneys concentrate urine. The kidneys function to remove waste products through the urine as well as regulate the body's fluid balance.

Different species of animals will have different urine SG values:

- The average SG value for a dog is 1.025, ranging from 1.001-1.060.
- The average SG value for a cat is 1.030, ranging from 1.001-1.080.
- The average SG value for a horse is 1.035.
- The average SG value for cattle and swine is 1.015.
- The average SG for sheep is 1.030.

If the specific gravity is too high, abnormal amounts of water are being eliminated through the urine; higher levels of SG are attributed to animals suffering from dehydration, shock, or acute renal disease. Specific gravity that is too low can be attributed to larger volumes of water intake or renal disease.

The devices used to measure SG include a refractometer, urinometer, or reagent test strips.

Measuring Specific Gravity

Urine specific gravity is most commonly measured by using a **refractometer**. A drop of urine is placed on the prism of the refractometer. The lid is closed over the drop of urine, and by looking through the eyepiece and holding it up to point at the light, you can read the specific gravity reading on the right side.

A larger urine sample is required to use the **urinometer**, which is calibrated at room temperature. The urinometer is placed inside the container holding the urine, and it floats upright with the assistance of a weighted bulb. The urinometer has a scale attached to the bulb, which can be read when the index has stopped moving. The SG is read at the meniscus or upper curvature of the surface of the urine.

The least reliable (but often quick and useful) urine testing involves the use of **reagent strips**. These strips offer inconsistent results when the reading of the SG is over 1.030. The reagent strip is set in the urine until it becomes totally soaked and changes colors. The color of the strip will then be matched with a color scale to determine the approximate SG of the sample.

Proteinuria

Protein is normally absent or present only in trace amounts in the urine. **Proteinuria** can indicate disease in the animal and is associated with excessive quantities of protein or protein metabolites within the urine. A reagent strip is used to determine the level of protein within the urine by comparing the urine-soaked strip's colors with a color chart. However, these results can be inconsistent. Furthermore, false positives, false negatives, and human error are all complications associated with the use of reagent strips.

Proteinuria is often associated with urogenital system malfunctions, and urine protein levels should be considered in conjunction with any blood found in the urine. In addition, any microscopic residue should be taken into account. Very alkaline urine may produce a false-positive protein reading. If the specific gravity is very low, a false-negative reading may occur. Further, reagent strips tend to react to albumin and less to globulin. Where urine protein levels are excessive, a sulfosalicylic acid turbidity test (sensitive to both albumin and globulin) may be helpful.

GLUCOSURIA

Urine glucose levels should also be measured. **Glycosuria** is the presence of sugars in the urine; **glucosuria** is the presence of glucose in the urine. Glucosuria can be a sign of diabetes. Further, elevated urine glucose can occur if the kidneys are unable to properly reabsorb glucose in the renal tubules, indicating that the patient may be developing renal disease.

Normal urine glucose levels are 170-180 mg/dL. A Clinitest or Ames reagent strip can test the levels of glucose in the urine. Reagent strips are useful in the identification of glucose. However, reagent tablets are able to identify all of the various forms of sugars.

A patient with high urine glucose may have an insulin deficiency in the form of **diabetes mellitus**, which usually presents with a history of hyperglycemia alongside the glucosuria. Thus, the precise measurement of blood glucose levels can provide warning of the onset of diabetes mellitus. However, it is important to also recognize that glucosuria can be caused by many other factors, including anxiety, nervous tension, agitation, intravenous fluids containing glucose, and other additional diseases.

KETONURIA

Ketones are organic compounds such as acetone, acetoacetic acid (also called diacetic acid), and beta-hydroxybutyric acid. The body produces acetone and beta-hydroxybutyric acid through **catabolism** (breaking down fats and/or muscles in the body for energy). In this process, initially, fat in the body is converted into energy. The metabolic processing of fat creates ketones. Small amounts of ketones in the body and bloodstream are normal, but large amounts can be toxic to the animal. Rapid fat metabolism can lead to **ketonuria** and lower carbohydrate metabolism, which can occur simultaneously or as a single process.

Hyperglycemia (high glucose levels in the blood) is attributed to an inadequate absorption of glucose. This condition can be exacerbated by a high carbohydrate diet. Hyperglycemia can contribute to ketosis, especially in large mammals.

Ketostix, Acetest, and Ames are reagent strips or tablets used to test for the presence of ketones in the urine, especially acetoacetic acid. Ketone concentration and reagent strip color strengths are comparative.

BILIRUBINURIA

Urine normally contains some bile pigments, including conjugated **bilirubin** and a tiny amount of **urobilinogen** that has been synthesized by bacteria within the intestines. A reactive test pad can yield a positive bilirubin reading in feline urine. However, these pads are not recommended for dogs because both false-positive and false-negative results are common.

Bilirubinuria can be attributed to biliary obstruction, hepatic infections, toxicity, and hemolytic anemia. Urine samples should be protected from the light, as prolonged exposure may cause a false-negative result due to bilirubin oxidation.

UROBILINOGENURIA

Urobilinogen test pads have been found unreliable for both dogs and cats. In these situations, bile pigments can be successfully measured using reagent test strips.

Urobilinogen is produced by bacteria in the intestines. The bacteria utilize conjugated bilirubin to produce urobilinogen. Insignificant levels of urobilinogen are released in the urine.

Cats and dogs are the only animals that are subjected to routine urobilinogen testing. Abnormally high levels of urobilinogen are indicative of hepatocellular disease. Lower levels may indicate that there is a barrier in the bile ducts. It is common for normal dogs to have no or very low amounts of urobilinogen in the urine. The urine urobilinogen analysis requires a urine sample to be analyzed promptly to prevent any urobilinogen from being changed into urobilin, which is not identifiable in the analysis used to detect urobilinogen.

HEMATURIA

Hematuria gives the urine a reddish-to-black cloudy tint. When numerous erythrocytes are present in the sediment (5 or more per HPF), the following conditions may be present: trauma, calculi, urogenital tract infection, and benign or malignant neoplasia. Reagent test strips or tablets and examination under the microscope are used when trying to determine if RBCs are in the urine. The physical exam, medical history, and reason for presentation should be considered in determining the differential diagnosis.

A fresh sample is required to further assess the urine for leukocytes with a microscope. The use of leukocyte test pads is not recommended, as these pads will frequently result in a false-positive in cats and a false-negative in dogs.

MYOGLOBINURIA AND HEMOGLOBINURIA

Myoglobinuria may cause urine to have a brownish tint; occult blood in the urine indicates a disease condition that is often hard to identify. **Hemoglobinuria** is sometimes linked to intravascular hemolysis or the destruction of red blood cells and the release of hemoglobin; urine will appear amber to red and, though transparent, will retain its color after centrifugation. Muscle disease is often linked to hemoglobinuria and myoglobinuria.

URINE SEDIMENT

Sample preparation for microscopic evaluation of urine sediment requires the specimen be blended to distribute sample contents, then poured into a centrifuge tube with a conical tip. The centrifuge is run at 1,500-2,000 rpm for 3-5 minutes. Carefully remove approximately 0.3 mL of residual supernatant. The sediment is next dispersed within the residual liquid in a suspended form. The microscope slide receives 2-3 drops of liquid for visual examination.

The slide may or may not be stained for a microscopic urine examination, which occurs first under reduced illumination with a setting of 10x magnification (i.e., a low-power field objective). This allows the slide to be scanned over its complete coverslip area, and allows for the identification of most crystals, casts, squamous cells, and other large objects. These objects are reported according to the number of each type found per low power field (LPF).

The setting is then changed to 40x, or a high-power field objective, to examine crystals, cells, sperm, and bacteria. The types of cells identified are recorded as the number of each type found per high power field (HPF).

RBCS AND WBCS IN URINE SEDIMENT

Red blood cells appear pale yellow and are smaller than **white blood cells**. More than five RBCs per high-power field (HPF) is abnormal. WBCs in a urine sediment appear 1.5 times larger than RBCs and are mostly neutrophils that are spherical and granulated. More than five WBCs/HPF indicates inflammation and infection.

Urine sediment typically has a small number of leukocytes present. When leukocytes are numerous, then the condition of **pyuria** (pus in the urine) and/or **leukocyturia** (white blood cells in the urine) is indicated. This can be due to an active inflammatory disease in the urogenital tract. A thorough physical examination is important, and an additional urine specimen should be collected when more than a few leukocytes (5-8) per high power field (HPF) are observed. Any bacteria observed should also be noted.

EPITHELIAL CELLS

There are three kinds of **epithelial cells** associated with urine sediment:

Squamous epithelial cells originate from epithelial membranes in the urethra, vagina, and vulva. They are the largest type of cells found in urine sediment with a flat, uneven shape, sharply defined edges, and a small, round nucleus. The presence of squamous epithelial cells in urine sediment is not typically a clinically significant finding. However, these cells are not normally found in samples taken using cystocentesis or catheterization.

Transitional epithelial cells derive from the bladder, ureters, and renal pelvis, and more than one/HPF is a significant finding indicating inflammation and cystitis. Transitional cells vary in diameter, have an eccentric nucleus, and are pear shaped with a granular cytoplasm. The caudate (the cell's tail) and the cytoplasm both appear granulated.

Renal epithelial cells originate from the renal tubules and are not normally found in large quantities in urine sediment. Renal cells are somewhat larger in size than white blood cells. The renal cell has a circular shape and a sizeable nucleus, and somewhat resembles the appearance of WBCs. **Renal tubule disease** can be diagnosed when these cells are found in large quantities in the urine.

Types of Casts

Casts are formed in the distal renal tubules or distal nephron and appear cylindrical with parallel sides and have rounded or blunt ends. Any structure that may be present at the time that the cast is formed will embed itself into the cast (RBCs, WBCs, or renal cells) and can indicate renal degeneration, irritation, and chronic nephritis. Cast types include:

- **RBC casts**, which may indicate bleeding from within the nephron.
- **WBC casts**, which may indicate inflammation of the renal tubules.
- **Hyaline casts**, which are protein precipitants and may appear in large numbers with fever or renal disease. **Hyaline** casts are found in the least severe cases of renal irritation.
- **Granular casts**, which may indicate renal disease if found in large numbers.
- Epithelial casts, which are associated with acute nephritis and renal tubule degeneration.
- **Fatty casts** are uncommon, but they are found in cases of diabetes mellitus in dogs and renal disease in cats.
- **Waxy casts**, which may indicate acute levels of tubular degeneration.

Struvite Crystals

Struvite crystals (triple phosphate crystals or magnesium ammonium phosphate crystals) are commonly found in a healthy canine or feline urinalysis and are normally not an issue unless there is also a bacterial urinary tract infection. If there is no bacterial infection, struvite is not related to struvite **urolith** (bladder stone) formation. Typically, the triple phosphate crystals are observed in alkaline urine. However, triple phosphate crystals may be visible in modestly acidic samples of urine, as well.

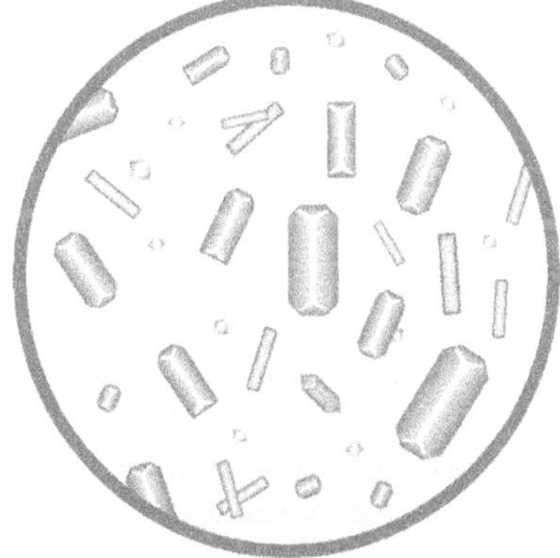

The name of these triple phosphate crystals is associated with their characteristic three- to six-sided prism shape. The crystals have no color. Struvite crystals look like coffin lids under the microscope.

Bilirubin, Calcium Carbonate, and Amorphous Crystals

Bilirubin crystals are small, yellowish, and appear granular or needle-like. They are relatively normal in canine urinalysis; however, the presence of bilirubin crystals in the urine of cats, equids, bovids, or camelids may be indicative of hepatic dysfunction.

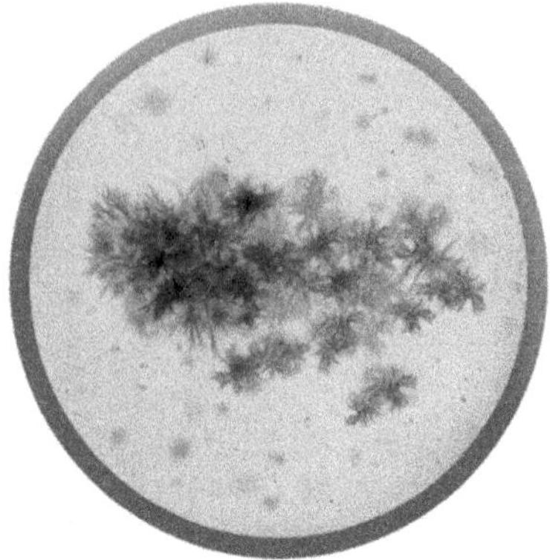

Calcium carbonate crystals are circular or oval with radial markings. These crystals have no color or appear yellowish. The presence of calcium carbonate crystals in the urine of horses, rabbits, goats, and cattle is quite common. They do not occur in the urine of dogs and cats.

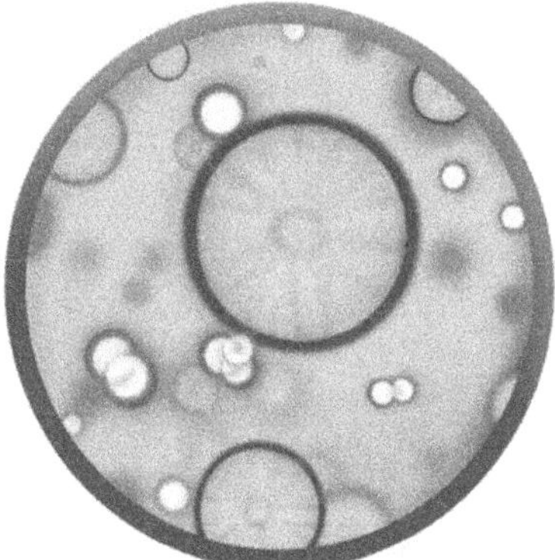

Amorphous phosphates are observed in alkaline urine samples, while **amorphous urates** are observed in acidic urine samples. These two types of crystals look like a precipitation with a grainy texture. In addition, these slightly brownish or yellowish crystals tend to appear in clusters but without any specific shape (hence *amorphous*).

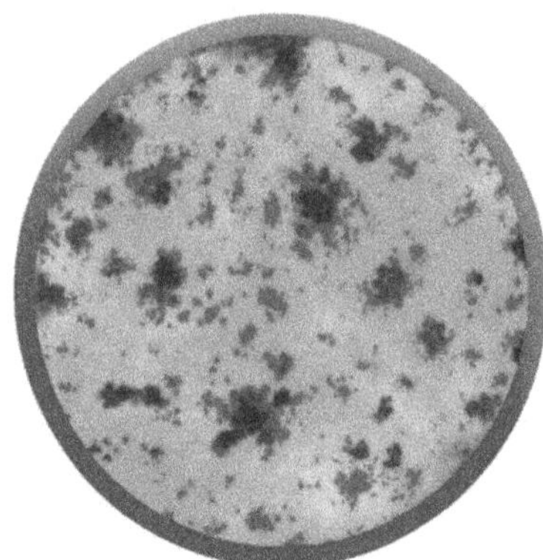

CALCIUM OXALATE CRYSTALS

Calcium oxalate crystals may result in the formation of calcium oxalate uroliths especially when there is a large amount of these crystals. **Calcium oxalate dihydrate crystals** look like little envelopes and occur in normal urine of any pH:

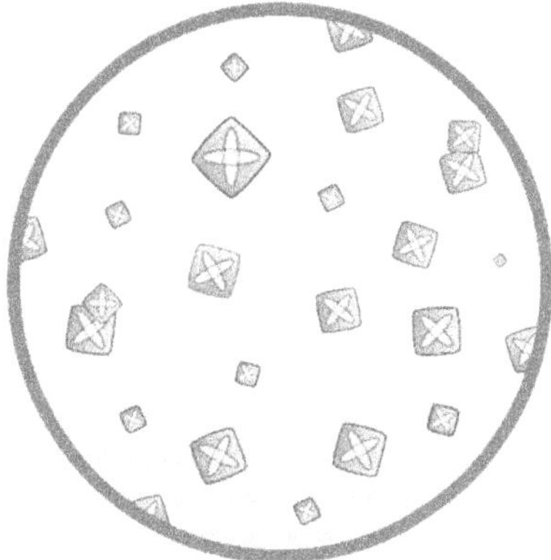

Calcium oxalate monohydrate crystals look like dumbbells, and while they are normal in horses, they do not normally occur in healthy cats or dogs:

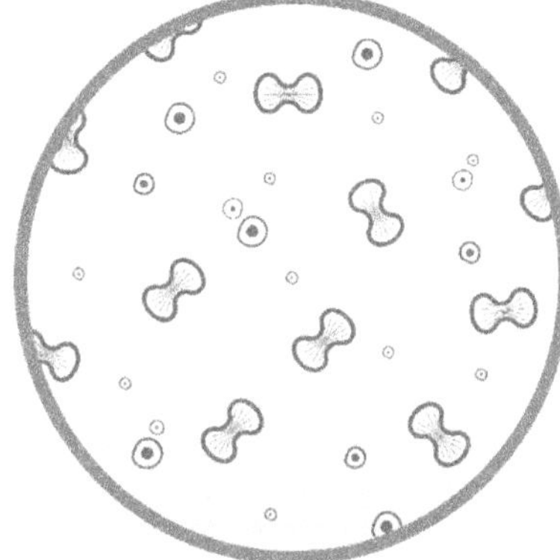

In cases of ethylene glycol toxicity, a different form of calcium oxalate monohydrate crystal appears; these crystals look like colorless picket fence posts and are found in neutral to acidic urine.

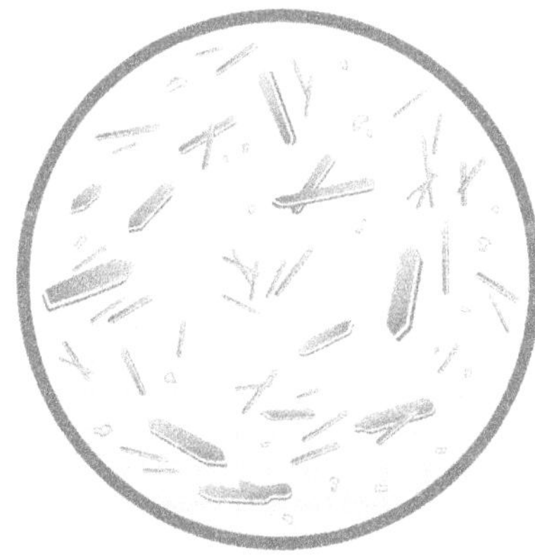

Clinical Parasitology

Endoparasites: Fecal Samples

Fecal samples are ideally examined for parasite eggs as quickly as possible, but they can be kept in the fridge for up to a week. When collecting from a litter box, owners should ensure the sample comes from the correct pet if multiple cats are using the litter box, and the sample must be fresh and not hard. If Giardia is suspected, then the sample must be obtained directly from the rectum for the SNAP test, and because trophozoites will not survive storage, a fecal flotation sample must be evaluated right away.

Samples should be stored in tightly sealed containers and labeled with the following information: collection date, site from which the specimen was acquired, the animal owner's name, the species of the animal, an identification number for the animal and/or the name of the animal, the referring veterinarian, the address of the clinic, and the telephone number.

The fecal sample can be sent for outside laboratory testing in its pure form or mixed with a solution of 10% formalin at a ratio of 1:3. The use of a diluted alcohol or formalin solution is recommended to preserve whole parasites or segments of parasites for proper laboratory microscopic examination, identification, and relative concentration or "parasitic load" indices.

Direct Smear Method

The **direct smear method** is also used to determine the presence of fecal protozoa. The direct smear method can aid in a rough calculation of the number of parasites present within the body. The direct smear method requires microscope slides, coverslips, and applicator sticks. Lugol's iodine or methylene blue stain may be used, but neither is required. Fresh fecal matter is also required (at or near body temperature and ideally less than an hour old). **Trophozoites** in older specimens will lose motility, degenerate, and become very difficult if not impossible to recognize.

A single drop of saline solution (not water, which may rupture trophozoites) should be placed alongside an equal amount of feces on the surface of the slide. If stain is to be applied, then it should be added at this time. Blend the feces and saline solution with an applicator stick. This blend is thinly spread across the flat surface of the glass plate or slide. The larger pieces of feces are removed for uniform magnification and ease in slide viewing. Parasite eggs can be viewed with a 10x magnification objective. Protozoal organisms can be viewed using a 40x magnification objective.

Standard Vial Gravitation Flotation Technique

The **standard vial gravitation flotation technique** is used to find parasitic eggs in fecal matter. The cost of this test is fairly low, which is an added benefit. However, this test may also be inaccurate, with false-negative results not uncommon. The accuracy can be jeopardized by numerous variables in the testing process. The primary variable is the relative specific gravity of the flotation solution chosen. With the density of water as the reference point, a solution of higher specific gravity should cause parasite eggs or oocysts to float to the surface as the eggs have a lower specific gravity than the floating solution. However, different parasites have oocysts of varying specific gravity, and thus flotation may not always occur. Further, old fecal samples may experience egg degradation and altered flotation patterns, and poor straining strategies may trap eggs and remove them from the flotation solution.

Fecal Flotation Technique

Sugar, sodium nitrate, and zinc sulfate are common flotation media. The standard vial gravitation technique requires a paper cup filled with about 60 mL of floating solution. Then, 2–4 grams of feces are placed into the solution using a tongue depressor. The solution and the feces are then blended together thoroughly.

This churned mixture is poured into a glass vial, which is filled to the top until a **positive meniscus** (upward curving solution surface) is formed. The parasite eggs or oocysts should float since they have a lower specific gravity than the flotation solution. Try not to overfill the tube because floated eggs can be lost once the cover slip is put on and fecal material spills over. A coverslip or cover glass is positioned on top of the vial, making contact with the meniscus. Then, the eggs are permitted to float to the surface of the vial.

Let the tube with the cover slip on it sit for 10 minutes, and then remove the cover slip and place it on a microscope slide with the liquid sample side down. Examine the entire area under the microscope at 10x magnification.

Initial Stages of the Baermann Technique

The **Baermann technique** examines fecal matter for parasites and parasitic ova and larvae. It requires a paper cup, disposable cellulose tissue or Kimwipe, elastic band, sedimentation jar, long Pasteur pipette with a bulb, and a dissecting microscope. A small amount of feces collected in the paper cup is examined for the presence of the lungworm. A Kimwipe or a disposable cellulose tissue is placed on the cup as a cover. This cover is held in place with an elastic band.

A small hole is made in the underside of the cup containing a fecal specimen. Warm water is used to fill a sedimentation jar halfway. Then, the cup should be submerged with the Kimwipe or cellulose tissue-end placed face down in the water. All of the tissue should be in the water. The sample requires submersion in this manner for 12-18 hours.

Then, at least 3-4 samples of water should be collected from the underside of the sedimentation jar using a long Pasteur pipette with bulb. The samples should be inspected under a dissecting microscope for larval movement.

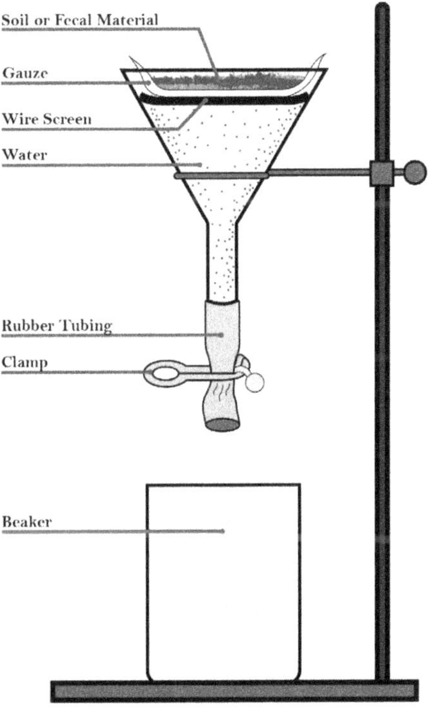

Strongylus Vulgaris

Strongylus vulgaris is an equine intestinal worm that can be up to 25 mm long and resides in the large intestine of a horse. The prepatent period of the equine worm can range from about 6-12 months in duration. Non-infective eggs are discharged in the feces when a host animal defecates. Following excretion, the eggs go through a developmental process in stages.

The eggs move from first stage larvae, or the L1 stage, to the second or L2 stage without becoming infective. This is followed by the third or L3 stage. It is in this last stage of development that the larvae become infective. After the L3 stage and upon ingestion, the larva sheds its protective sheath or covering (called "ex-sheathing"). This allows the larvae to migrate and eventually to pierce the walls of the intestines at or below the cecum. The cecum is the first intestinal pouch, at the point of which the large intestine originates.

Once the *Strongylus vulgaris* larva has penetrated the intestinal wall, it travels further until it enters the submucosa. The **submucosa** is the layer of connective tissue directly beneath the mucous membrane of the intestine.

Diagnosis and Treatment

Horses that have been infected by the equine worm will experience a range of clinical signs. The signs of infection include colic, fever, diarrhea, weight loss, and death. **Colic** is a pain that occurs in the abdominal region, typically due to spasm, obstruction, or distention of the viscera.

A *Strongylus vulgaris* infection can be detected via the fecal flotation method. The larvae in stages 1 and 2 can be killed easily. At these stages the larvae exist largely in residual manure. Thus, the spreading and breaking up of manure is an effective deterrent to the growth and development of the larva. There is also treatment available for larvae that reach stage 3 and then become adult worms. Treatment can be found in the form of antiparasitic medications that can be administered to the horse.

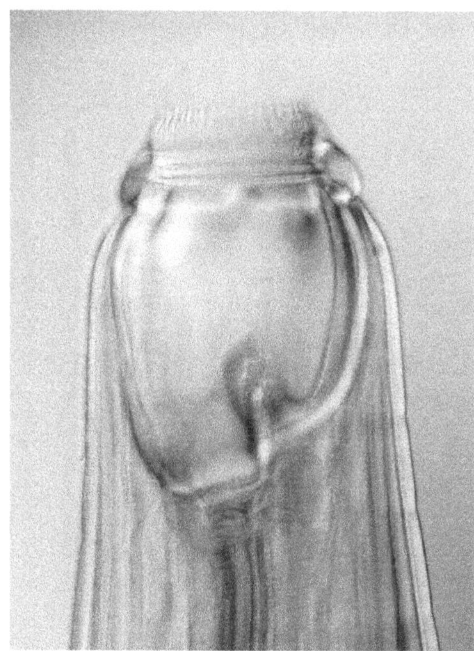

Coccidiosis

The canine or feline with *Isospora spp.* coccidiosis has been infected by the consumption of the parasite's eggs. The most prominent symptoms are frequent and excessive bowel movements consisting of watery diarrhea. The severity of the diarrhea may be indicative of the acuteness of the infection. Because of the copious fluids expelled in an effort to flush the parasites out, the animal experiencing acute symptoms may be in danger of dehydration and death.

The fecal material contains active eggs or oocysts that have been excreted with the feces from the infected animal's body. Upon proper examination, it will be noted that the infected stool contains many clear, spherical to ellipsoid, thin-walled oocysts that can best be detected by the fecal flotation method. Once coccidiosis is confirmed, the disease should be properly treated with medications and appropriate follow-up medical care.

Preventive care is also highly recommended, and involves the removal of feces from the animal's surrounding area, as the continuing presence of infected fecal matter can increase risk of recurrent infection.

Isospora spp.

Isospora spp. are sporozoan intestinal parasites of the order Coccidia. As coccidians, they are spore-forming single-celled (protozoan) parasites that reproduce in the small intestine of cats and dogs. Diseases that occur as a result of these protozoa fall under the descriptive header of coccidiosis.

Puppies and kittens that range in age from birth to 6 months of age are susceptible to the disease. Adult animals that have a suppressed immune system or experience high levels of stress can also be susceptible to this disease. The prepatent period, the time of infestation to maturation, can range from 4-12 days. Puppies or kittens are usually around the age of 2 weeks or more when they contract coccidiosis. This disease can be detected by the fecal flotation method.

Feline Roundworm

Toxocara cati (feline roundworm) has a complex life cycle. Infection occurs through eating an infected host (rodents, beetles, earthworms), through ingesting infected maternal milk, or by direct ingestion of eggs (via vomitus, fecal matter, etc.). The ingested eggs hatch inside the cat's small intestine. From there, the larvae enter the circulatory system and migrate to the pulmonary system, where they are coughed up and swallowed. There, the larvae mature and reproduce more eggs to be discharged from the body in the feces.

The development period outside of the body lasts for about 10-14 days, at which point the eggs are actively infective. Kittens can be infected by drinking the infected milk of a mother cat. *Toxocara cati* may sometimes be visible in the vomit of an animal. The recommended treatment for roundworm or *Toxocara cati* is the use of an appropriate medical deworming agent.

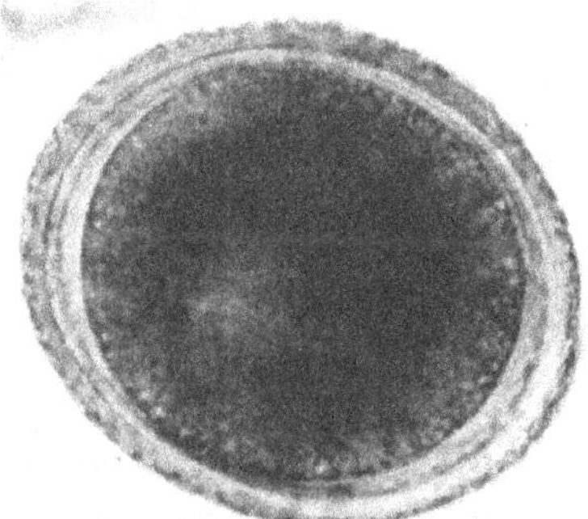

Diagnosis and Treatment

It takes about 8 weeks from initial infection until this parasite can be detected through clinical means. The fecal flotation method can be used to expose the dark brown, thick-walled, pitted eggs of *Toxocara cati*. However, the eggs are not always present in the feces, so false negatives are possible.

Laboratory and physical symptoms of *Toxocara cati* for **visceral (intestinal) larva migrans** include: hypereosinophilia, hepatosplenomegaly, pneumonitis, fever, and hyperglobulinemia. Laboratory and physical symptoms of *Toxocara cati* for **ocular (eye) larva migrans (endophthalmitis)** include: leukocoria, loss of vision in the affected eye, eye pain, and strabismus. Cats are the primary host, but humans can become infected.

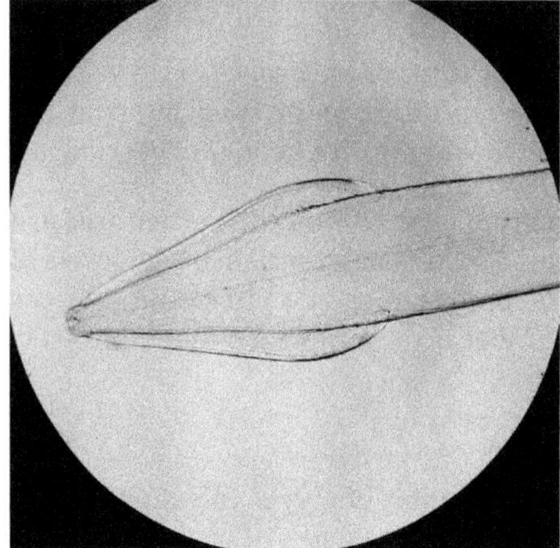

Whipworm

Trichuris vulpis, or whipworm, is a type of nematode or roundworm that can be found in human and canine intestines. The whipworm, named for its whip-like shape, resides in the cecum and large intestines of canines. The prepatent period (from infestation to maturation) is about 3 months.

An animal is infected by whipworm through the consumption of infective eggs, which may persist in the environment for several years. Once they hatch, larvae develop in the small intestine; adults live in the cecum (the first section of the large intestine). *Trichuris vulpis* attaches itself to the intestinal wall. Once attached, the whipworm feeds on blood, epithelium, and fluids drawn through the intestinal wall and capillary penetration. Clinical signs of infection include bloody diarrhea, dehydration, and weight loss.

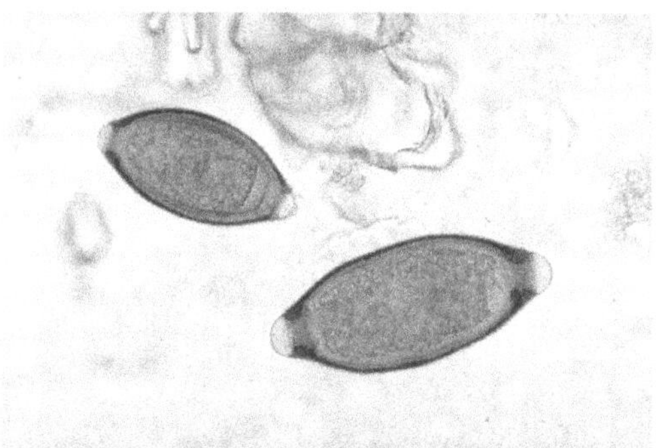

Diagnosis and Treatment

Trichuris vulpis is detected by fecal flotation. The animal may experience a range of symptoms depending upon the quantity of worms present in the animal.

The immature larvae may be resistant to certain medical interventions. However, most medications are effective in the treatment of adult whipworms, though the course of treatment may take several months. This allows all the larvae to mature so that they can be effectively eradicated as adults. Preventive care is recommended and involves the removal of feces from the animal's environment. The presence of fecal matter increases the risk of re-infection as it may have active eggs that have been excreted by an infected animal.

GIARDIASIS

Giardia duodenalis, or **Giardia**, is a single-celled protozoan which is transmitted fecal-orally. Infection occurs when the host ingests dormant cysts found in contaminated water or food. As the cysts can survive for months in a moist environment—even in cold, clean-appearing water, including water treated for city drinking—infections are difficult to avoid. Once ingested, the *Giardia* parasite fastens itself to the surface of an animal's small intestines, along which they can move freely.

Giardia can infect a number of mammals, including dogs, cats, cattle, horses, sheep, goats, and pigs. Infected animals develop severe symptoms of diarrhea. The prepatent period, the time period from initial infestation to reproductive maturity, for Giardia is 7-10 days. *Giardia duodenalis* has 2 basic life cycle states: trophozoite and cystic. In the metabolically active (feeding) stage the Giardia protozoa are known as **trophozoites**. Possessing a flagellum, the trophozoite is motile—meaning it can move freely as it seeks nourishment. The other life cycle state is the non-motile **cystic** stage. At the conclusion of the trophozoite life stage, the protozoa rapidly replicate via binary fission, and then transform themselves into inactive cysts. Upon expulsion from the host, the cysts quickly become infective and can survive in any moist environment for several months.

DIAGNOSIS AND TREATMENT

The fecal flotation method is usually effective in making a diagnosis of the infection. Another method used is the direct smear technique. A diagnosis is confirmed when either the cysts or the trophozoites are viewed. The cysts present a smooth, thin-walled protective covering which protects the parasite contained inside. The trophozoite has a **piriform** (pear or teardrop) shape. The trophozoite has bilateral symmetry and a light green coloration. Giardia can be effectively treated with medication and proper follow-up medical care.

CANINE HOOKWORM

Ancylostoma caninum, canine hookworm, lives in the canine small intestine and causes significant disease. The hookworm fastens itself to the wall of the small intestine where it takes blood meals via intestinal wall penetration using its hook-like mouth.

In most cases, infection occurs when a dog ingests the eggs or larvae in contaminated food, soil, water, maternal milk, or an infected host. The canine may also become infected by larval penetration through the animal's skin. Vertical transmission to the fetus is also possible. The parasite can be detected 2-3 weeks after the initial infection.

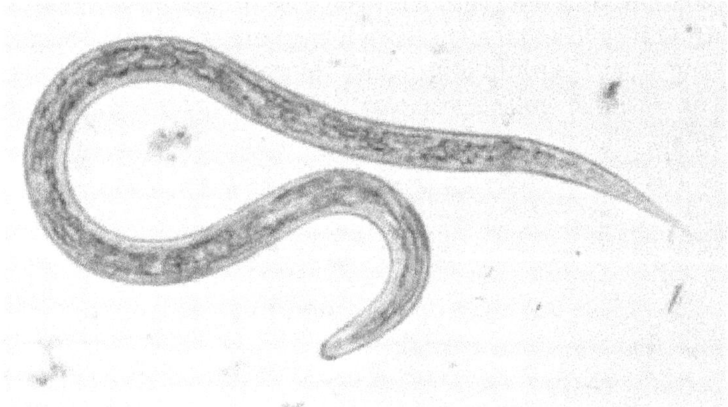

DIAGNOSIS AND TREATMENT

Ancylostoma caninum can have very detrimental effects on the host animal. Some of the more severe symptoms include anemia, weakness, and **melena**. Melena describes black, tarry, blood-bearing feces, indicating disease in the upper GI tract.

The canine **hookworm** parasite (*Ancylostoma caninum*) can be detected by fecal flotation testing. The parasite's eggs can be observed as clear, smooth, thin-walled eggs found in the feces. The worms are not usually seen by the naked eye due to their small size. The worms range in size from about 0.5-0.75 inches in length. Further, the mature hookworm is capable of fastening itself firmly to the wall or lining of the small intestine and thus is not normally dislodged.

Infected dogs can be treated with fenbendazole, moxidectin, milbemycin, and pyrantel. However, a preventive stance is recommended, reducing the animal's exposure to feces within its immediate surroundings by keeping the environment clean and removing fecal material.

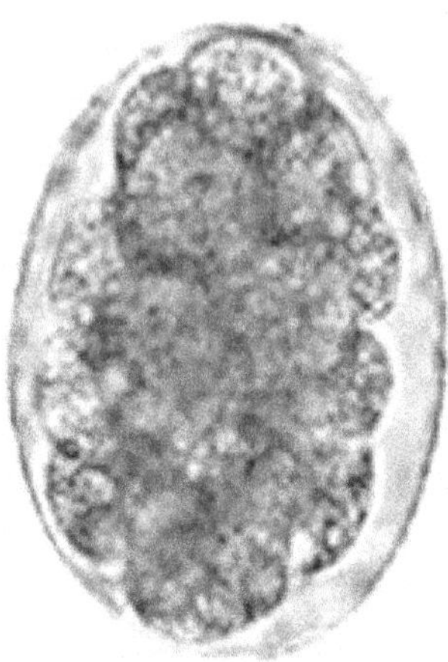

Dipylidium Caninum

The **common tapeworm**, *Dipylidium caninum*, resides in the small intestines of infected cats and dogs. The tapeworm itself presents with a long ribbon-shaped body. These worms have a head, neck, and segmented body parts. The segmented body parts are formed in the neck region of the worm.

The prepatent period (the time between the initial infection and reproductive maturation) for *Dipylidium caninum* is about 3 weeks. The older body segments (**gravid proglottids**) are found on the tip of the worm's body and are discarded at maturational intervals. The discarded proglottid segments are able to independently reproduce, as each contains both male and female reproductive organs. (Gravid means egg-bearing.) The proglottids stay active as long as host warmth is retained. They are passed in the feces, and the segment opens up to release the eggs that are inside. These eggs are eaten by an adult louse or flea larva, ultimately to infect or be ingested by another animal.

Cat owners may observe dehydrated or active tapeworms or artifacts; however, egg packets are not always present in a fecal flotation. Treatment includes a single dose of oral or subcutaneous anthelmintic, such as the broad spectrum praziquantel.

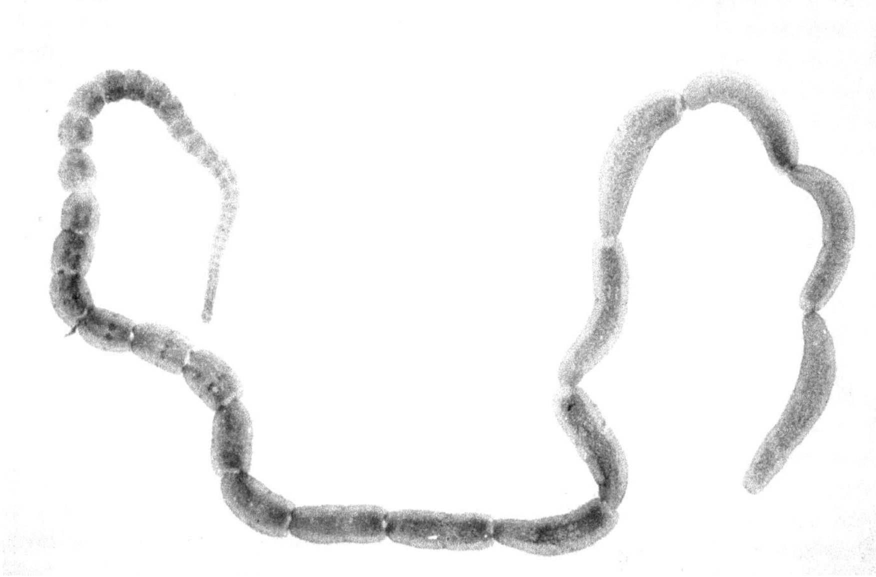

Ectoparasites: Skin Scrapes

Skin scrapes are used to examine integumentary problems in animals; a #10 scalpel blade is used in multiple places to scrape the skin. For deep skin scrapes, this occurs until blood oozes; for superficial skin scrapes, only gentle pressure is used. A drop of mineral oil is placed on a clean slide, the resulting sample is added, and a coverslip is placed on top. Under a low-power magnification, the slide is examined for parasites, which may include *Sarcoptes* and *Demodex* species. False negatives are possible.

Trichography involves plucking hair samples (including the hair bulb) with hemostats. Place a drop of mineral oil on a slide and pluck 10-20 hairs in a quick, smooth motion. Place them on the slide.

Skin Digestion Technique

The **skin digestion technique** is useful for the identification of external parasites. **Skin scraping** samples which have a significant amount of scurf (scales, epidermal shards) and skin debris are ideal for the skin digestion technique. The following is required for this technique: 15 mL conical centrifuge tube, 4% NaOH solution, hot plate, beaker, and centrifuge. A scalpel is used to place the sample in the centrifuge tube. Then, about 10 mL of NaOH solution is applied to the sample within the centrifuge tube. Next, the tube is positioned in a glass beaker water bath and boiled for 5-10 minutes.

The centrifuge tube is then placed in the centrifuge for 5 minutes at 1,000 rpm. Upon removal of the tube, the supernatant should be poured off from the top of the tube. Then, a drop of the sediment should be placed on a microscope slide and covered with a coverslip. Finally, the slide should be inspected for parasites using a microscope which has been set at 10x magnification.

Mange: Demodicosis

Demodex canis is a mite normally found in dog hair follicles and the sebaceous glands of the skin. Canine demodicosis (**demodectic mange**) is when a great deal of these arise due to the body's immune system becoming compromised due to illness. There are three types of demodectic mange: localized, juvenile-onset generalized, and adult-onset generalized. Localized demodectic mange usually affects dogs less than a year old and consists of up to five small lesions of alopecia, scaling, and redness found around the face and forelimbs. The localized form may develop into the juvenile-onset generalized form due to a hereditary immune system abnormality. Adult-onset generalized demodectic mange is the result of a compromised immune system due to an underlying disease that will need to be identified and managed in order to treat the demodectic mange. *Demodex canis* is diagnosed by performing a skin scraping to look for mites.

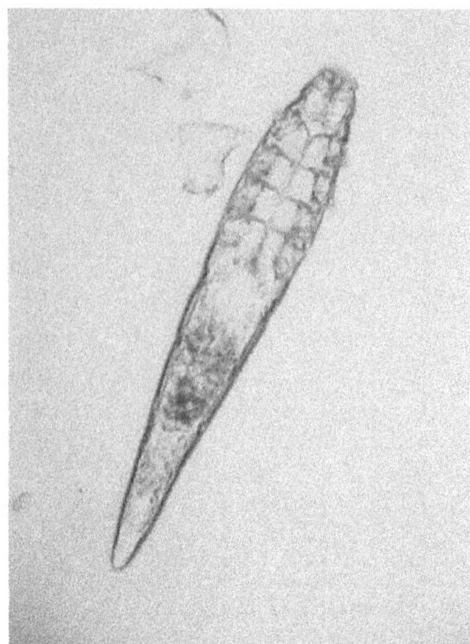

HEMOPARASITES: ELISA

Parasitic blood infestations will cause the body to develop antibodies to the presence of these foreign bodies. The **enzyme-linked immunosorbent assay** (ELISA) kits detect these antigens in the blood. While this test can reveal a host's antibody response to parasites, it cannot detect the microfilariae themselves. ELISA tests are particularly beneficial in the detection of occult heartworm (Dirofilaria immitis).

Commercial kits available for this use include Dirochek from Synbiotics, PetChek/Snap from Idexx, and Witness from Binax. The tests are performed on a tray with an indented surface. The kit supplies a membrane or wand that has parasite-specific monoclonal antibodies bound to its surface. Blood samples containing this particular antigen can thus become bound to the antibody. Next, an additional antibody is labeled with an enzyme and applied to the sample. This will also bind to the antigen. A color-producing agent is then applied.

If parasite-specific antibodies are present after the introduction of this agent, then an antibody-enzyme complex will be formed, producing a specific color. The specific color is an indicator that the antigen (i.e., the parasite) is present. If there is no parasite-specific antigen in the sample, the enzyme-labeled antibody will wash away without any color-change.

MITES: CHEYLETIELLOSIS

Cheyletiellosis has long been called "walking dandruff" for the mite's propensity to carry skin scales around with them as they move about. *Cheyletiella* **mites** can infest dogs, cats, and rabbits. Mites are creatures with 8 legs that extend beyond the margins of their bodies. The adult mite is oval in shape and can take up residence on the host's skin surface or on hair shafts or in hair follicles. The mite's stages of development require approximately 21-35 days for completion. The entire life cycle takes place on the host.

The adult mite is capable of living for 2-14 days off the body of the host. When off the host, mites have the ability to infect an animal through environmental contacts. Even so, mites normally infect an animal through more direct contact (i.e., moving among animals that come into physical contact with each other). Walking dandruff has the following symptoms: obvious scurf or dandruff scales, visible mites on the surface of the skin, pruritus (itching, resulting in scratching for relief), inflammation of the skin, crusts, and small swellings or spots.

Walking dandruff is detected by skin scrapings, the cellophane tape method, combings, or via microscopic study. Once diagnosed, walking dandruff can be treated with appropriate medications.

Superficial or Light Skin Scraping Method

Scraping the skin for external parasite identification requires a number 10 scalpel, mineral oil in a dropper bottle, microscope slides, and a microscope. The scalpel blade is first moistened on a slide laden with mineral oil. It is then ready to obtain a scraping. The blade of the scalpel should be held in a perpendicular position towards the skin to ensure that an incision in the skin is not accidentally made. Grasp the skin gently between the thumb and index finger of one hand. The other hand should be used to make contact with the skin as the scraping motion is performed. Some parasites require deeper scrapes than other parasites. Therefore, a tentative determination should be made to classify the presenting case according to potential types: Sarcoptes (burrowing mites), Demodex (hair follicle mites), Chorioptes, and Cheyletiella (both surface, non-burrowing skin mites). The burrowing mites require a deep scrape or rub to be collected.

Deep Skin Scraping Method

Non-burrowing mites such as Demodex, Chorioptes, and Cheyletiella require only superficial skin scraping or rubbing for specimen collection. This should be sufficient to dislodge the loose scales (flaky pieces of skin) and skin crusts in which they live. **Crusts** are dry, hardened outer layers of blood, pus, or other bodily secretion that form over a cut or sore on the skin.

Burrowing mites (Sarcoptes) are more difficult to collect. To ensure adequate material collection, the skin in an affected area should be taken down just deep enough to produce a slow leak of blood.

The material that is collected through either scraping method should be placed on a prepared slide laden with mineral oil. The slide should then be covered with a coverslip. The slide is scrutinized under a microscope at 10x magnification. At least 10 slides should be inspected to ensure accuracy in making the external parasite identification.

Fleas: Ctenocephalides spp.

There are 2 common species of *Ctenocephalides*: *Ctenocephalides felis* (the cat flea) and *Ctenocephalides canis* (the dog flea). Adult flea coloration is reddish-brown to black in appearance. The adults do not have wings but are able to jump great distances.

Adult fleas live 4-25 days, feeding by drinking the blood of the host. They lay eggs on the host's skin, which fall off in the surrounding environment (bedding, living areas, etc.). Upon hatching, (in 1-6 days) the larvae live on organic debris and adult flea feces. Upon larval maturation they spin a cocoon in which they reside, and, after 1-2 weeks, the pupa is a fully developed adult flea. However, the pupa will not leave the cocoon until adequate environmental stimuli indicate they are near a suitable host (e.g., heat, physical pressure, carbon dioxide, or movement). If no stimulus prompts emergence, the flea can remain in a quiescent cocoon state for up to 350 days.

Flea-infected animals may experience flea allergy **dermatitis**, inflammation that appears as redness, itching, or swelling of the skin, which may lead to excessive scratching. The animal should be closely observed in order to detect fleas or residual flea feces, which appears as small specks of dirt on the animal. Treatment includes medication and thorough cleaning of the animal's bedding and environment.

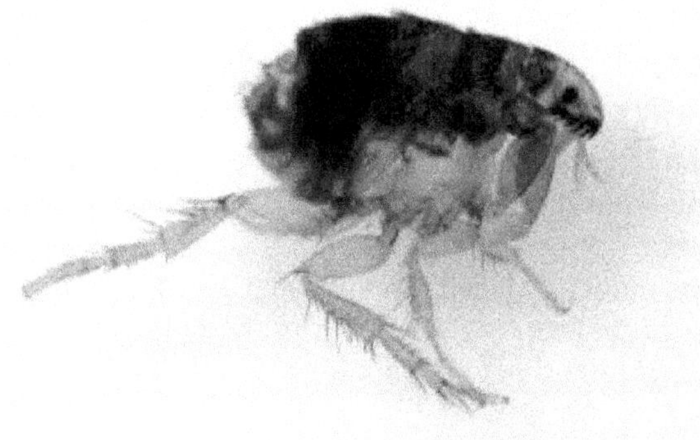

LICE: PHTHIRAPTERA

Lice lay eggs, which are known as **nits**. The nits are typically glued to the hair shaft so as not to fall from the host. Lice are also transferred from one host to another through physical contact. Lice have the ability to spend an entire life cycle on a single animal or host.

There are 2 kinds of parasitic lice (Phthiraptera): **sucking lice** (suborder Anoplura) and **chewing lice** (suborder Mallophaga). Anoplura species are wingless and flat-bodied and are parasites of various species of mammals:

- Haematopinus spp. will infect cattle, pigs, and horses.
- Linognathus spp. infects dogs, cattle, and sheep.
- Solenopotes spp. infects cattle.
- Pediculus spp. infects humans.

Likewise, different species of Mallophaga are parasites of both birds and mammals:

- *Damalinia spp*. infects horses, cattle, goats, and sheep.
- Felicola subrostratus infects felines.
- Trichodectes canis infects dogs.

DIAGNOSIS AND TREATMENT

Lice infestation is typically readily evident through close visual observation. The animal may exhibit excessive itchiness, accompanied by a scruffy, dry, or brittle hair or fur coat.

When infestation is evident, the animal should be deloused with medication to kill the lice. Medication should be applied to all the surfaces with which the animal has had contact. This includes the animal's bedding and surrounding living area. Failure to fully treat the animal and all the infective surfaces can readily result in a reinfestation of the lice. Reinfestation will likely require yet another thorough treatment to be applied to the animal and all surfaces involved.

RINGWORM: DERMATOPHYTOSIS

Diagnosing ringworm is done by using a dermatophyte test medium (DTM) culture. Dermatophytes metabolize protein in this culture medium and release alkaline metabolites that turn the medium a red color. Obtaining a sample from the patient's lesion can be done by using a new toothbrush to brush over the lesion or plucking some hair from the lesion with a pair of sterile hemostats and placing the sample into the medium. The DTM plate must be kept in a dark place with the lid closed loosely for up to two weeks. Examine the sample daily, and record if there is growth or color change. After two weeks, place a strip of clear tape over the sample in the

DTM to obtain a sample on the sticky side of the tape. Place a drop of new methylene blue stain on a slide, stick the tape on top of the stain, and then examine the slide under 40x magnification.

Microscopic examination of skin or hair samples without culturing may allow for quicker diagnosis.

Hemoparasites: Buffy Coat Method

The **buffy coat method** is used to examine a blood specimen for blood parasites. When blood is spun in a centrifuge, the 3 primary components of blood are separated from each other. The top layer is clear plasma; the bottom layer is red blood cells. In between is the buffy coat—a thin, creamy-yellowish (sometimes greenish) layer of white blood cells. If the buffy coat is placed on glass slides and examined under a microscope, the presence of parasites in the blood can often be revealed. The method requires the following: microhematocrit tubes and sealer, centrifuge, microscope slides and coverslips, saline solution, methylene blue stain, and a small file or glass cutter.

A microhematocrit tube is filled with blood. This tube of blood goes through the centrifuge process for 3 minutes, and the PCV is then read. Next, the tube is scored at the level of the buffy coat. Then the tube is cautiously snapped in half before lightly tapping the buffy coat onto a slide. One drop of saline solution and one drop of methylene blue stain are added to the slide, followed by a coverslip. The slide is then inspected for the presence of microfilariae.

Hemoparasites: Modified Knott's Technique

Modified Knott's technique is used to identify and quantify blood parasites. There are many kinds of blood-borne parasites (commonly classified as: rickettsial, protozoal, helminth, and viral).

The modified Knott's technique requires a 15 mL centrifuge tube and centrifuge, 2% formalin solution, methylene blue stain, Pasteur pipettes and bulbs, and microscope slides and coverslips. A centrifuge tube is used for the sample of EDTA (anticoagulant) blood (1 mL) and 2% formalin or water (9 mL). The solution causes hemolysis. This mixture is placed in the centrifuge at 1,000 rpm for 5 minutes. An alternative allows the solution to remain still for 1 hour. The supernatant or liquid on the surface is gently decanted off, so as not to disrupt the sediment. Next, 2 drops of methylene blue are applied to the undisturbed sediment. Aspirating gently with the pipette mixes the solution. A minuscule sample is positioned on a microscope slide and covered with a coverslip. The microscope is set at 10x magnification. This setting is used to examine the entire slide for microfilariae or larvae of an infesting parasite.

Dirofilaria Immitis: Canine Heartworm

Canine heartworms or *Dirofilaria immitis* occupy the heart and pulmonary artery of the host animal. Heartworms can infect dogs, cats, and other non-domestic animals through a mosquito vector or transplacental infection of microfilariae.

The **prepatent period** is the time between the initial infection and when the parasite reaches reproductive maturity, which is typically 6-8 months for *Dirofilaria immitis.*

Animals that have been infected by heartworms will exhibit symptoms of lethargy, exercise intolerance, and cough, which may be more noticeable when the animal is exercising. Chronic heartworm infection can cause severe weight loss, fainting, coughing up blood, and congestive heart failure. Animals that are more active can exhibit symptoms of heartworm infection earlier than less active animals. Likewise, animals that are heavily infected may also exhibit earlier symptoms of heartworm infection.

In the *D. immitis* life cycle, larval stages L1 through L4 represent the progressive stages of larval maturation.

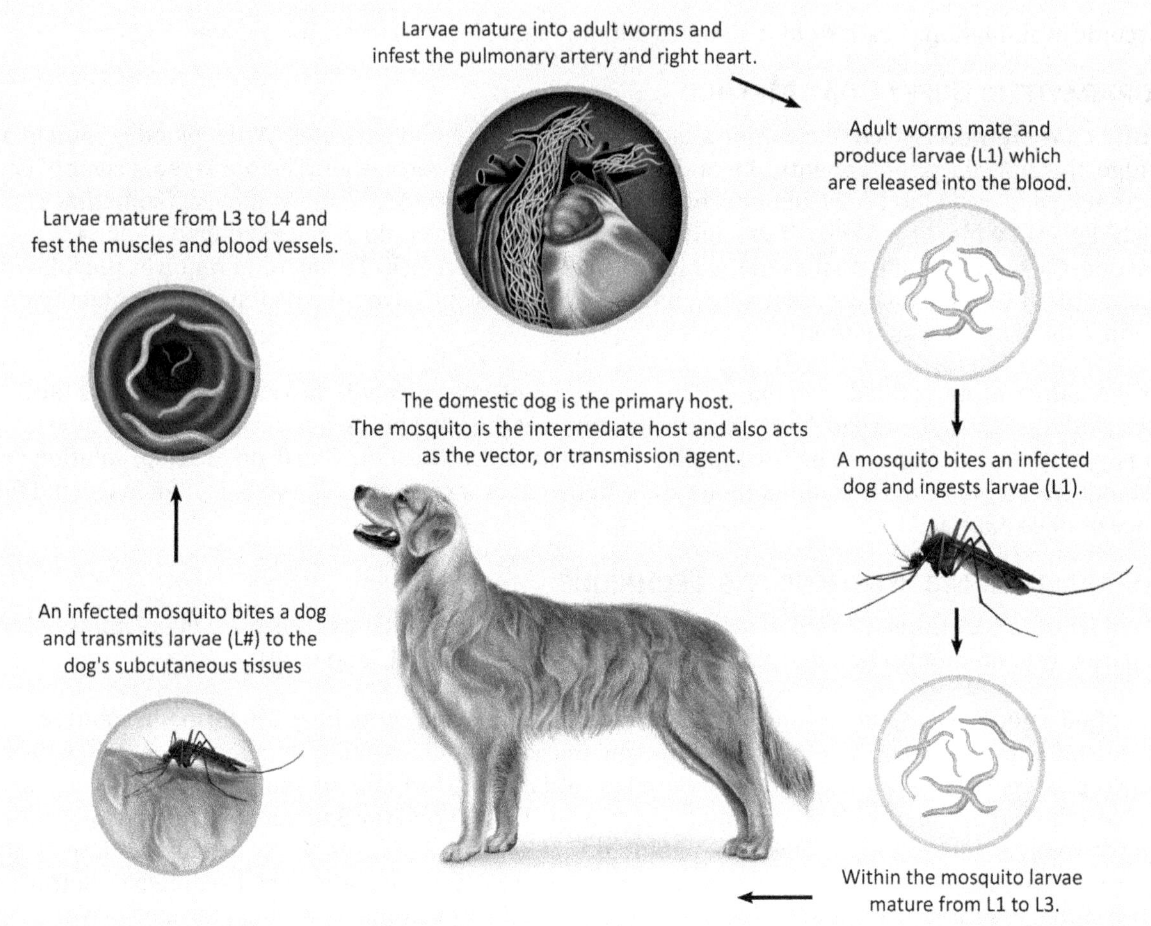

Dirofilaria Immitis Diagnosis

Testing for **microfilariae** (early larval stages of certain nematodes) is usually done using the modified Knott's test or wet or Giemsa-stained smears; these methods are not very sensitive, especially if the parasite load is low, and are considered supplemental.

The buffy coat method should be employed to increase the chance of an accurate diagnosis and identification of the heartworm.

Antibody testing is perhaps the most frequent method of diagnosis because it is more sensitive; immunologic assays such as SNAP tests are used to detect the antigens of gravid adult female heartworms. The SNAP test is performed with a drop of blood and a few drops of conjugate.

Dirofilaria immitis Treatment

If the dog tests positive for heartworms, radiographs of the chest will be taken to assess for any damage caused to the heart and lungs, as well as additional blood work to determine kidney and liver function. Dogs should be tested for heartworms before they start on heartworm prevention to be sure that they are negative. Also, dogs already on heartworm prevention should be tested annually. Puppies will start on heartworm prevention right away, because the prepatent period for heartworm disease is 6 months and puppies would not be tested until after that.

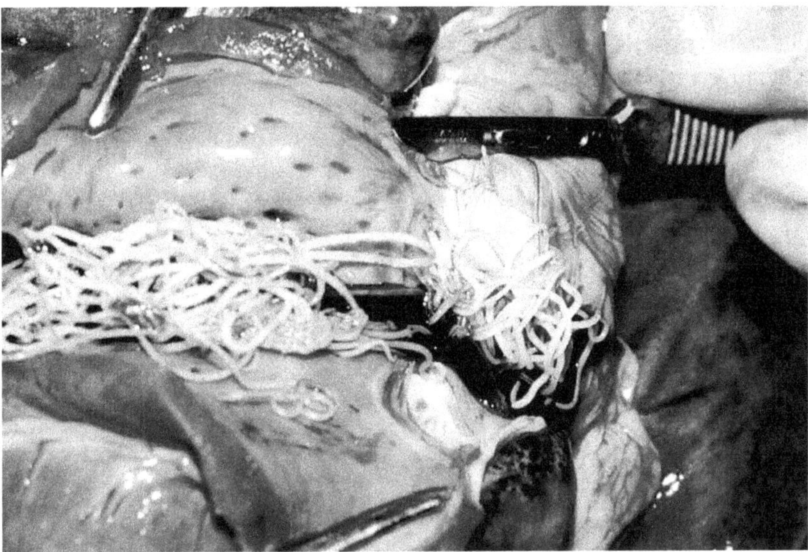

Babesia spp. and Anaplasma Marginale

Babesia spp. are blood-borne parasitic protozoa that cause **babesiosis**. Transmitted by ticks, it affects many domestic animals including cattle, horses, sheep, goats, pigs, and dogs. The particular type that is associated with the infection of dogs is known as *Babesia canis*, and the type found in horses is known as *Babesia caballi*.

These blood parasites can be found inside RBCs. The presence of a pairing of large, pear- or droplet-shaped blood cells can be observed in blood films from infected animals. The cells typically amass together under the buffy coat. Thus, the buffy coat (i.e., smears, etc.) may also be used for identification. *Babesia* spp. can be carried by the *Ixodes* tick, which can be detected through serology antibody testing.

Anaplasma marginale are blood parasites found within RBCs that cause **anaplasmosis**. These parasites look like tiny circles within the cell, and they turn a dark color when RBCs are stained. This dark stain occurs in the RBCs of cattle and wild ruminants. They may be mistaken for Howell-Jolly bodies, due to their similar appearance and roughly equivalent size.

Other Hemoparasites

Mycoplasma haemofelis (formerly called *Hemobartonella felis*; also called **feline infectious anemia**) is a flea-borne blood parasite that appears as cocci or rods. However, as a true mycoplasmic organism, it has no cell wall and cannot survive independently. It is easily stained with Wright's stain, which produces a dark purple color. These parasites are observed on the boundaries of feline RBCs and are routinely treated with tetracycline and transfusions.

Hemobartonella canis are blood parasites located on the surface of canine RBCs. These parasites look like extended chains of cocci or rods and may be stained a dark purple color with Wright's stain. This parasite is most commonly found in dogs that have had a splenectomy or that have compromised immune systems. This type of blood parasite is comparable to the *Eperythrozoon* spp. found in pigs, cattle, and llamas.

Cytauxzoon felis are tick-borne parasites that live within erythrocytes. The erythrocytes contain **piroplasms** that may appear as round or oval "signet rings," or in "safety pin" forms, tetrad forms, or as round dots. The dotted form may appear in linked cell chains. The nucleus stains dark red to purple with a light blue cytoplasm. These parasites are also located inside the feline's lymphocytes and macrophages. However, this type of blood parasite is not common.

Clinical Microbiology

Prokaryotic and Eukaryotic Cells

Prokaryotes are single-celled organisms without a nucleus (the structure that houses the majority of a eukaryotic cell's genetic material) or specialized organelles. Bacteria are the most common prokaryotes.

Eukaryotic cells have a nucleus contained in a nuclear envelope and specialized organelles. Most eukaryotes have 3 main parts. The first part is the outer **cell membrane** that allows oxygen and food particles to pass through and waste to be excreted. The second part is the inner **cytoplasm** that contains cytosol and organelles. In animal life, cytoplasm occupies over half of the cell's volume. Cytosol is the watery portion of the cytoplasm, excluding all structures and organelles. The third part of the eukaryotic cell, also found in the cytoplasm, is the **nucleus**. It contains the genetic material that controls cell growth and reproduction.

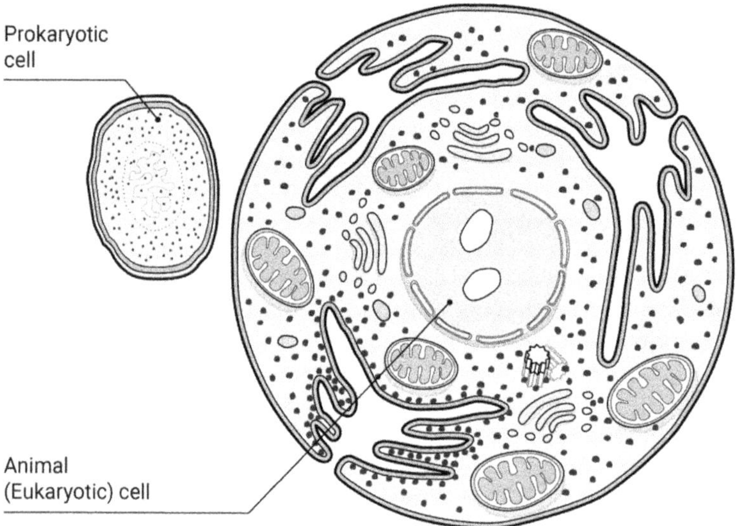

Organelles

Organelles found in **cellular cytoplasm** include:

- **Ribosomes** are cellular organelles that manufacture cellular proteins. They can be found freely floating in the cytoplasm, arranged in small clusters, or attached to endoplasmic reticula (intracellular tubular membranes which transport materials). Ribosomes manufacture essential proteins by reading the RNA produced by genetic DNA, and translating it into the kind of protein indicated.
- **Mitochondria** are specialized organelles that make up as much as 25% of the cytoplasm. Mitochondria transform organic substances from foods into ATP, a useable source of chemical energy.

- The **endoplasmic reticulum** is a network of tubes that alters and transports proteins, produces and stores macromolecules (i.e., glycogen and natural steroids), and sequesters calcium.
- **Golgi bodies** process cellular products, releasing them back into the cell or excreting them as needed.

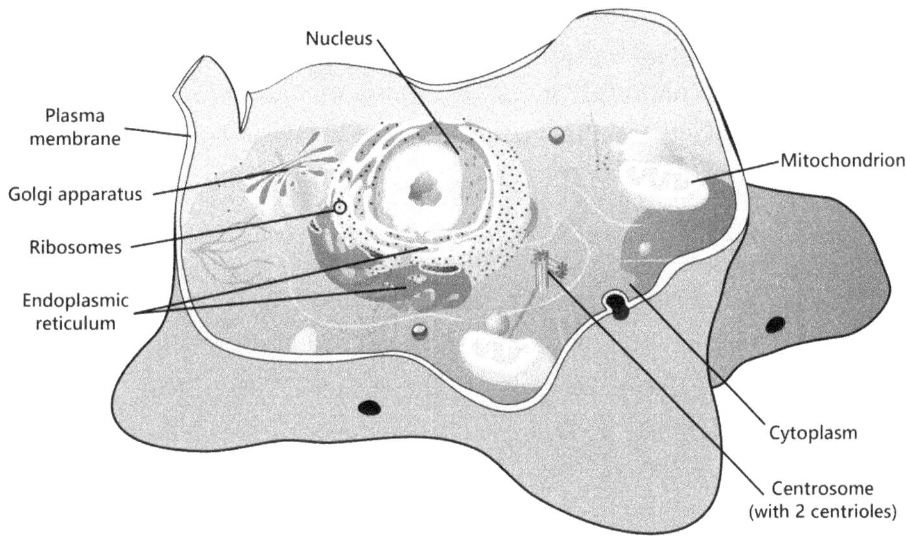

VIRAL REPLICATION

A **virion**, or complete virus particle, consists of genetic material (DNA or RNA) and a protein **capsid**.

Both RNA and DNA viruses require host cells for replication. Viral entry into the host organism can occur at the mucosal surfaces of the respiratory tract, the urogenital tracts, or the gastrointestinal tract. The virus will fasten itself to the cell membranes of those mucosal cells. The virus then invades the cell and uses the nucleic acid replication infrastructure of the cell to replicate its own genetic material and proteins. Virions are released from the cells by either **lysis**, which is **cytolytic**, meaning that the host cell dies, or **budding**, which is **cytopathic** and does not kill the host cell.

SIGNS OF VIRAL INFECTIONS

When noticeable disease symptoms are present, it is considered clinically identifiable. However, not all diseases have immediately noticeable symptoms. Some are described as silent, nonapparent, or subclinical infections. The danger in these infections lies in the ability of the host to infect others before it is noticeably ill.

A few models of apparent and nonapparent infections are found in rabies, FIV, and equine infectious anemia viruses. Some viral infections are most readily apparent when the infected cells stop functioning. A host can also have an impaired immune system due to an infection. This is true of horses infected with the equine infectious anemia virus (EIAV). Sometimes the detrimental impact to the immune system may actually produce conditions more problematic than those caused by the virus alone.

PREVENTING VIRAL DISEASES

Immunizations help prevent viral disease; viral infections can also be reduced when hands and surfaces are disinfected on a regular basis. In addition, the bodies of deceased animals must be properly and hygienically disposed of quickly and appropriately to prevent further infection.

General principles of health maintenance are also important in minimizing infectious disease: appropriate diet, access to fresh water, limiting stress and overcrowding, and a dry living environment.

Further, newly acquired animals should only be introduced to the herd after an appropriate period of quarantine. **Quarantine procedures** are recommended to maintain the health of the other animals. A quarantined animal should be fully isolated from all available people and animals. This isolation should prevent the spread of a viral or other infection and reduce all healthy animals' exposure to any diseases caused by infective processes. Quarantined animals should be prevented from having nose-to-nose contact with other animals, as through a fence or a cage.

Maintaining Microbiologic Samples

Certain tests available for microbiologic examination include bacterial cultures, fungal cultures, western blotting, virus isolation, and many others. Most of these tests rely on the growth of intact viable organisms or the detection of the nucleic acids and proteins of these pathogens. Most tests require that each tissue or fluid specimen be obtained aseptically and shipped in sterile, clearly labeled bags. Tissues and fluids for most assays can be kept frozen until shipment, but if the sample can be delivered within 24 hours, then keeping the sample chilled is preferred. Degradation of certain toxins such as *Clostridium perfringens* and *C. botulinum* can happen if not frozen right after collection.

Sterilizing and Heat-Fixing Microbiology Samples

A **Bunsen burner**, usually fueled from a wall gas outlet, is used to flame-sterilize the metal inoculating loop that is used to transport microorganisms from the specimen sample to a culture dish. The Bunsen burner is also employed to "heat fix" bacteria to a microscope slide. This is critical, as the bacteria might otherwise be washed away during the staining process.

An **electric heating element** can also be used to sterilize inoculation loops. The electric heating element is normally made from ceramic and operates electrically. Thus, natural gas is not required with this device. The electrical device gives a consistent burn to the applied surfaces, which is an advantage of an electrical device over a gas fueled Bunsen burner.

Another sterilization device is known as an **alcohol lamp**. This device is less expensive, but it does require more time to complete the sterilization process as the metal loops take longer to be sterilized using an alcohol lamp than a Bunsen burner. An alcohol lamp is fashioned from glass. A wick extends into the alcohol held in the base. The lamp is ignited with a match or other combustible source.

Sterile Specimen Collection

A sterile region in the body is defined as one that does not typically contain bacteria or fungi within its regions or hollow spaces. While not absolutely sterile, blood samples, urine samples, spinal fluid samples, joint fluid samples, solid organ samples, milk samples, and lower respiratory tract samples should not normally contain bacteria. These types of samples are frequently cultured to determine whether or not bacteria are present. Various non-sterile zones are found in the hair or fur regions, skin, sputum or saliva, intestinal tract, feces, ears, upper respiratory tract, nostrils and associated nasal regions, and the trachea. As non-sterile zones, these areas are expected to be full of resident bacteria and normal flora. By contrast, it is a potentially serious problem when disease-causing bacteria are found in areas expected to be sterile.

Collecting and Culturing Swab Specimens

A sterile cotton swab or a culturette can be used to collect a specimen from an animal. The swab will be used to swipe ears, nares, and abscesses. Fluid directly from the specimen may be squeezed directly onto the swab, if possible. There is a small measure of liquid or gel placed in the prepackaged swab containers. This gel can be used in conjunction with the sterile swabs to operate as a transport medium. This transport medium allows the organisms to remain in a state that can best be used for germination or further development when transported to another location. This viable state can last for a period of up to 48 hours, if the swabs are maintained in a proper environment in the interim.

A swab is typically used to inoculate a third of the surface region of the culture plate with microorganisms. The culture media potentially consist of BAP, CNA, and/or MAC. After the microorganisms have been introduced, then the swab is positioned in a THIO broth (a culture media for anaerobic and microaerophilic bacteria and sterility tests). The technician will either break or cut the end of the swab off, so it does not extend beyond the opening of the tube in which it is stored.

The inoculated plates are streaked to give the bacteria a linear growth pattern on the surface of the medium. This streaking is created when a contaminated needle, swab, or inoculation loop is drawn across the medium. The streak pattern also gives the bacteria needed isolation. Next, a flamed, sterile slide can be inoculated and stored for incubation over 24 hours. The incubation period allows the cells or microorganisms to develop under a controlled temperature. This steady development is necessary so that the microorganism can continue to grow and multiply within the medium.

Collecting and Culturing Solid and Urine Specimens

Solid specimens require alternate collection and culture techniques. These specimens can be defined as those collected from hard lumps, solid matter, and tissue samples. Tissue samples are derived from organs, skin, and scales. These samples must be cultured in order to allow the biological material to grow under special conditions. This is performed by placing the collected substance in a small volume of liquid base or broth over a period of 24 hours. The liquid base or broth is then **sub-cultured**, meaning the bacterial growth is transferred from another culture medium onto plated media. Aseptic techniques designed to prevent infection from pathogens are applied in the collection of tissue samples. Necrosis or tissue death is a grave concern that must be prevented from occurring.

Two methods used to collect urine samples are cystocentesis and catheterization. **Cystocentesis** (needle aspiration) is the technique used to collect the most optimum urine specimens for culture purposes because extraneous contaminants are nearly completely avoided. However, a sterile **catheterization** tube inserted through the urethra can also be applied with equal success, when due care is taken.

Collecting and Culturing Liquid Specimens

Specimens with a fluid base can be extracted with a syringe or sterile tube. These items are useful in aspiration of the following: abscesses, tracheal washes, bronchial washes, nasal discharges, joint fluid, or spinal fluid. The extracted fluid from the specimen is used in the inoculation of the culture plates. Typically, BAP, CNA, and MAC plates are employed in this task. Some extracted droplets from the sample are also cultured in a THIO broth. A third of the surface of the microscopic slide is inoculated using a pre-flamed, cooled inoculation loop. The inoculated plates are streaked to give the specimen a linear growth pattern on the surface of the medium. This streaking is created when a contaminated needle or inoculation loop is drawn across the medium. The streak also gives the bacteria needed isolation. Some of the remaining specimen collected from the syringe or tube is then used for a gram stain.

Growth Media

Trypticase soy agar (TSA) can be used to study bacterial hemolytic reactions; TSA plates enriched with blood or other specialized growth media are intended to propagate fastidious organisms (those with complex nutritional needs). A **blood agar plate** (BAP) is a similar medium which contains 5% sheep blood.

Trypticase soy broth (TSB) is a versatile medium that is able to culture most bacteria, even most fastidious bacteria. It is used for most blood cultures and sterility confirmation tests.

MacConkey II Agar (MAC) is for gram-negative organisms. It employs crystal violet and bile salts to hinder gram-positive bacterial growth. This medium also incorporates a neutral red indicator, which is able to change color (pink to purple, based on developing pH) in the presence of lactose fermentation. The altered coloration differentiates the lactose-fermenting bacteria (LFs) and non-lactose fermenters (NLFs). The medium inhibits the growth of *Proteus* spp.

Colistin is an antibiotic employed against intestinal infections that arise from a wide assortment of organisms. The medium that combines this antibiotic with nalidixic acid is known as **Columbia Colistin-Nalidixic Acid Agar (C-CNA)**. It is able to pick out gram-positive organisms, and it contains 5% sheep blood.

The **Salmonella-Shigella (SS) agar** culture medium is selective for specific pathogenic and gram-negative enterobacteria: *Salmonella* spp. and some *Shigella* spp. SS agar can employ lactose fermentation-generated color changes to allow various distinct colonies to be brought into view. This medium also employs ferric citrate to differentiate the bacteria that generate H_2S (hydrogen sulfide). The ferric citrate brings about a black coloration when H_2S-producing bacteria are active.

Campylobacter Agar with 5 Antimicrobics and 10% Sheep Blood (Campy BAP) is a particularly sensitive medium. This medium is used most often when developing *Campylobacter* spp. These organisms can be obtained from fecal specimens in a microaerophilic setting.

Culture Incubator

In clinical microbiology, the use of a **culture incubator** may be necessary to cultivate organisms outside a normal host environment. The incubator can maintain very exact temperatures to successfully support organism growth. These temperatures serve to duplicate the optimum growth conditions found in natural circumstances. One of the more commonly used temperature settings is 37 °C or 98.6 °F. In certain incubators, oxygen concentration and humidity can also be varied for optimum conditions. Veterinary cultures are usually derived from specimens grown at 37 °C, including specimens from reptile and amphibian cultures. This temperature allows a majority of the organisms to grow. However, the body temperatures of reptiles and amphibians can fluctuate with the temperature of the creature's environment. This form of fluctuation is referred to as poikilothermia. Most standardized tests require a temperature of 37 °C.

Gram Stains

The first step in a Gram stain is to retrieve the specimen to be tested by either taking a colony from a suspended plate positioned in water or placing a droplet of THIO broth (thioglycolate) onto a microscope slide and allowing the specimen to air dry. After heat-fixing, the slide will be inundated in Gram's iodine for a one-minute period, followed by a thorough rinsing with tap water. The slide is next inundated in a decolorizer for a period of 10 seconds, followed by another tap water rinse. However, if the slide remains overly dark-toned, then the procedure should be repeated.

The slide is then inundated in a safranin counterstain for 30-50 seconds, followed by a final tap water rinsing; it can then be air-dried.

Lastly, the slide should be viewed beneath an oil immersion (100x magnification) objective lens. Bacteria with a coloration ranging from purple to dark blue are gram-positive. Bacteria with a pink coloration are gram-negative. The bacteria are thus identified in accordance with Gram's classification methods. The result of completing the steps correctly gives the veterinarian the opportunity to make a diagnosis using the results of the gram stain process.

Maintaining Laboratory Equipment and Supplies

Light Microscope

One optical instrument used for specimen evaluation is known as the **light microscope**. This instrument has a number of eyepieces, a light source, a light condenser, a stage, objective lenses, and focus knobs. The term **monocular** is used to describe an instrument with one eyepiece. The term **binocular** is used to describe an instrument with 2 eyepieces. In a microscope, the eyepiece allows further magnification of the viewed field. The magnification or enlargement is normally set at 5, 10 or 15 times. This is written as the following: 5x, 10x, or 15x. The light source can be adjusted to provide the viewer with varying shades of concentrated luminosity. The instrument comes with a condenser that allows the light to be diminished or increased. Slides are placed on the stage or platform for inspection purposes. The stage or platform can be adjusted or moved horizontally or vertically by turning one of two knobs. The specimen on the slide is magnified or enlarged by using the objective lens. The microscope employed in clinical microbiology requires the following available settings: 10x, 40x, and 100x objectives. The focus is adjusted for coarse focus or fine focus by moving one of two knobs.

Microscope Maintenance

Some supplies needed for cleaning the **microscope** include cotton-tipped applicators, distilled water, suction bulb, Kimwipes, optical cleaning solutions, and a soft brush. After each slide, the ocular lens, objective lenses, stage, and stage clips should be cleaned, and the entire microscope should be cleaned daily. To clean an objective lens, a cotton-tipped applicator dampened with an adequate cleaning solution can be used, and then the lens is dried with a Kimwipe. Use distilled water to wipe away any debris from the lenses and the microscope body, then dry them with lens paper. Inspect the cord for frayed wires or any damage, and then lower the stage or raise the arm to gain access to the objectives for cleaning. A suction bulb can be used to remove tiny hairs that get stuck in the eyepieces; the eyepieces are then wiped with Kimwipes and 70% ethanol and dried. Kimwipes moistened with water should be used after fecal solution gets onto the stage to prevent pests and dust from adhering to it. Use a microfiber cloth and warm water to wipe down the microscope body, then dry it.

Ultrasonic Cleaner Maintenance

Ultrasonic cleaners use high-frequency sound waves to create high- and low-pressure waves inside the machine, creating tiny bubbles that will burst. When these bubbles burst, they create gentle scrubbing (cavitation) as they contact soiled instruments. To clean the ultrasonic cleaner, the appropriate cleaner is added to the distilled water filling the chamber and the machine is turned on so that once cavitation occurs it pushes the cleaner into the tiny, hard-to-reach areas of the machine. Cavitation erosion happens over time as a natural wearing process of the surface of the chamber, but it can happen faster if there are dirt particles on the bottom of the chamber that can wear the metal enough to cause leaks. Instruments must always be placed into the basket in the ultrasonic cleaner and should not be put onto the bottom of the chamber. The metal and other dirt particles from soiled instruments can create rust films in the tank, as can tap water if it is being used to fill the chamber instead of distilled water. Certain cleaning chemicals are available to remove rust films.

Centrifuge Maintenance

The **centrifuge** is used to spin a substance such as urine, feces, or blood and separate its components based on density. The inside of a centrifuge is normally made of ceramic, aluminum, or stainless steel and should be cleaned daily with the appropriate cleaner, which may vary depending on the interior material. To thoroughly clean the centrifuge, the rotor and sample tube holders should be removed and washed with warm water and liquid dishwasher soap, along with the inside of the centrifuge. Full-strength bleach and other caustic cleaners shouldn't be used because they can damage stainless steel. Steel wool and wire brushes can also damage the interior coating and create corrosion, so they should be avoided as well. Water should never be poured into the centrifuge because that can cause damage to the motor, gaskets, and sensors.

REFRACTOMETER MAINTENANCE

The **refractometer** is used to measure the urine specific gravity as well as the plasma total protein. The refractometer can be calibrated by placing a drop of distilled water on the prism, closing the lid, and reading it while holding it to the light and looking through the eyepiece; it should read 1.000 for distilled water. If the reading is off for calibration, then the instrument can be adjusted by turning the screw on the bottom counterclockwise, which moves the dividing line under 1.000, and then turning it clockwise until it reaches 1.000. The refractometer should be stored at 60-100 °F for accurate readings. After each use, the refractometer needs to be cleaned with a soft cloth moistened with a little water to wipe the prism and lid and then dried, or else the next reading will appear blurred.

Chapter Quiz

Ready to see how well you retained what you just read? Scan the QR code to go directly to the chapter quiz interface for this study guide. If you're using a computer, simply visit the online resources page at **mometrix.com/resources719/vtne** and click the Chapter Quizzes link.

Animal Care and Nursing

Transform passive reading into active learning! After immersing yourself in this chapter, put your comprehension to the test by taking a quiz. The insights you gained will stay with you longer this way. Scan the QR code to go directly to the chapter quiz interface for this study guide. If you're using a computer, simply visit the online resources page at **mometrix.com/resources719/vtne** and click the Chapter Quizzes link.

Animal Terminology

General Terminology

- **Breed**: Subgroups within a species with similar phenotypic characteristics, usually intentionally selected (e.g., Hampshire pig, Brahman cattle, golden retriever dog)
- **Dam**: Female parent
- **Intact**: Not castrated
- **Sire**: Male parent
- **Species**: Most familiar taxonomic unit used for identifying types of animals (e.g., dog, cat, horse)

Species-Specific Terminology

Poultry

- **Broilers and fryers**: Chickens less than 10 weeks old with tender meat
- **Roasters**: Chickens between 8 and 12 weeks old with tender meat, though slightly less tender than broilers and fryers
- **Drake**: Adult male duck
- **Gander**: Adult male goose
- **Hen**: Adult female turkey or chicken
- **Layers**: Chickens used for egg production
- **Poult**: Young turkey
- **Stew birds**: Older poultry used for meat, used for stews and soups
- **Tom**: Adult male turkey

Livestock

Species	**Equine (horses)**	**Bovine (cattle)**	**Caprine (goats)**	**Ovine (sheep)**	**Porcine (pigs)**
Group	Herd	Herd	Herd, flock	Flock	Passel, sounder
Intact, adult male	Stallion	Bull	Buck, billy	Ram	Boar
Adult female	Mare (>3 years old)	Cow (>3 years old)	Doe, nanny	Ewe (>1 year old)	Sow
Castrated male	Gelding	Steer	Wether	Wether	Barrow
Juvenile female (<3 years old or before giving birth)	Filly	Heifer			Gilt
Juvenile (before weaning)	Foal	Calf	Kid	Lamb	Piglet

- **Colt**: An intact male horse, younger than 3 years old
- **Jack**: Male donkey

- **Jenny**: Female donkey
- **Mule**: Offspring of a horse and a donkey

Animal Handling and Restraint

Handling and Restraining Small Animals

Though small animal veterinary practices most commonly encounter dogs and cats, they will also likely serve other small animal species, including birds, reptiles, and other small mammals. Proper handling and restraint of all of these species is important for the safety of the patients and practitioners. Positive pet and owner experiences at the animal clinic will lead to safer and less stressful future visits, which will decrease the amount of time spent managing fearful or aggressive animals. However, regardless of their size or species, all animals have the ability to harm themselves or their caregivers under the wrong circumstances, so great awareness and care are vital.

Animal clinics can be overwhelming to pets. When interacting with patients, it is safest to assume some level of excitement, ranging from mild overstimulation to fear and anxiety to outright aggression (towards people or other animals or both). The ability to assess the level of fear or aggression in an animal and anticipate changes that may occur rapidly will help protect the people and animals in the clinical setting.

Types of Displayed Aggression

Fearful aggression is often displayed when an animal feels threatened. Sometimes being on a leash or being confined in a cage will bring out fearful aggression if the animal is trying to escape but can't get away. Also, if an animal realizes that being aggressive helps to remove the threat, then they will continue that behavior. **Territorial aggression** is more common in dogs than in cats and occurs when the animal becomes aggressive toward someone or another animal coming onto its property but does not seem bothered by the same interaction outside of its territory. **Predatory aggression** is an attack with the intent to kill prey with no warning. **Food** or **possessive aggression** is displayed when the animal becomes aggressive if someone or another pet approaches when it is eating or has a possession such as a toy.

Large and Small Dogs

All dogs should be on a leash while they are in the veterinary practice, which will enable safe handling, restraint, and relocation of the animal. Dogs with bite warnings in their patient file should be muzzled, regardless of their size. New patients should be monitored with extra care for any signs of nipping or biting, and a muzzle should be used at the first sign of either. Small dogs will almost always be examined and treated on a table; large dogs may be examined or treated on a table or on the floor, depending on the size of the dog, the reason for their presentation, and how long their treatment will take. Working with a large dog on the floor is great for a quick nail trim or when expressing anal glands, but lengthy or detailed treatment is best on an elevated surface. Large dogs, especially if they are hyperactive, may require two people to restrain them. Geriatric large dogs on a table may also require additional assistance.

Standing Restraint

One commonly used restraint position for dogs is to have the dog stand and the holder face the dog's side, placing one arm underneath its abdomen and the other arm under the dog's neck and over its shoulders, holding the dog close to the handler's body. Properly holding a dog in this position will minimize their ability to bite the handler, but the technician should always be aware that a dog might still try. This restraint position is useful when expressing a dog's anal glands or trimming nails on the hind paws.

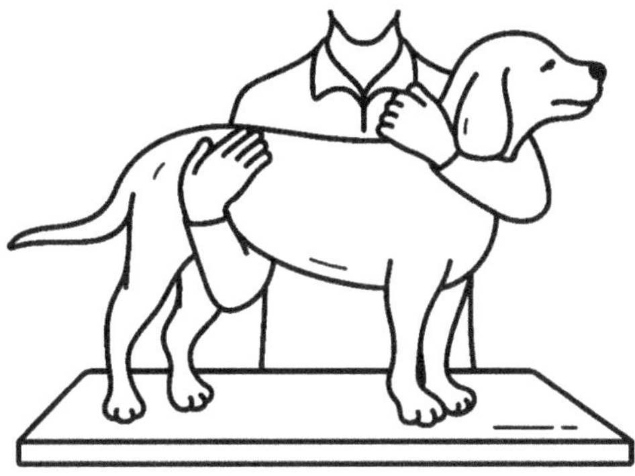

Seated Restraint

To restrain a seated dog, the holder places one arm around the hind end of the dog and the other arm underneath the neck, holding the dog close. This is helpful for a brachial or jugular blood draw or while trimming nails on the forepaws. Note that this position may allow the dog to slide, which may make them stressed. Brace the dog to prevent sliding or provide a slip-resistant surface for them to sit on.

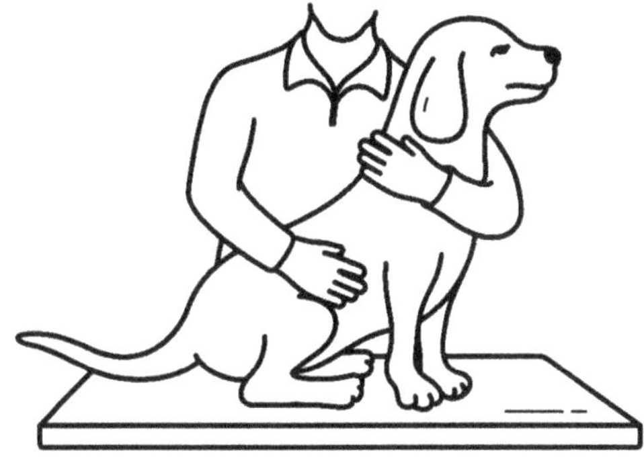

Recumbent Restraint

To hold a dog in **sternal recumbency**, have the dog lie squarely on its sternum and belly. The holder should hold the dog from the side with one arm in front of the neck and over the shoulders to secure the head, holding the dog's muzzle away from the holder's face and neck as much as possible. The holder's other arm should wrap over the dog's back and reach the opposite forelimb, allowing the holder to assist with cephalic venipuncture, if needed.

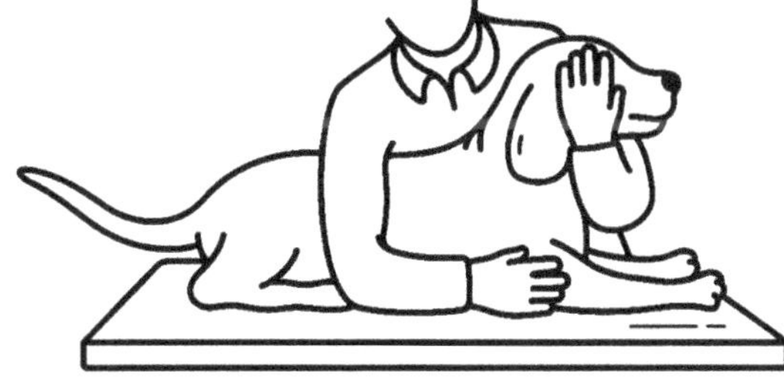

To hold a dog in **lateral recumbency**, the holder stands or sits along the dog's back while the dog is lying on its side. Hold the dog's head down by applying firm pressure with the arm over the neck, then hold the distal front limbs with that hand and a finger in between the two legs to secure the grasp. The holder's other arm will lie across the dog's caudal half in order to grasp the hind limbs in a similar manner.

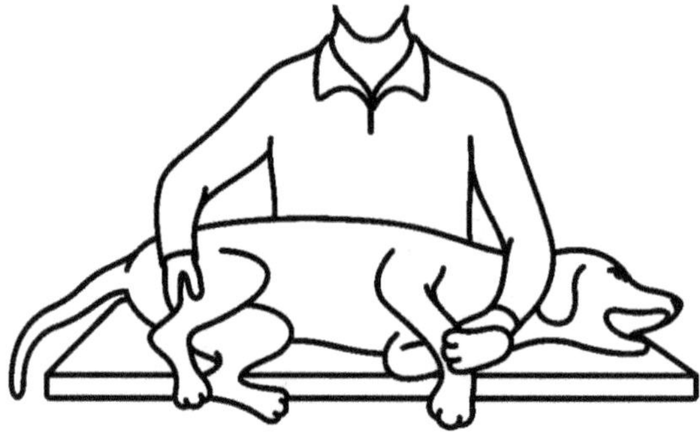

Cats

Towels are helpful when manipulating cats; they can be completely wrapped in the towel to immobilize the limbs while exposing the face and head, and the towel can also be rearranged to expose a single limb or area of the body requiring examination or treatment.

When drawing blood from the back leg of a cat, it is common to restrain the animal in lateral recumbency. To hold a cat in lateral recumbency, one hand will hold the cat by the scruff while stretching the cat on its side with its back against the holder's body. The back leg that is closest to the table is left down while the restrainer's other hand is holding the leg on top while occluding the vein of the leg on the table.

Sternal Recumbency and Seated Restraint

Sternal recumbency and seated restraint are both used for jugular blood draws on cats. These require similar techniques to the canine restraints, with a few differences. To hold a cat in sternal recumbency, the restrainer will stand on one side of the cat as it lies squarely on its sternum and belly. Wrap one arm over the cat's body to tilt the cat's head back by gently but firmly bracing the mandible so its nose is pointing up. The other hand should grasp the front paws and stretch them gently but firmly off of the table. This technique should only be performed on cats that will tolerate it.

Muzzles and Cat Bags

There are muzzles made just for cats, and they slip over the nose, cover the eyes, and Velcro behind the ears. There is a small hole where the nose and mouth are so the cat can breathe, but the eyes are covered, which helps to calm a feline patient. Sometimes a combination of a cat muzzle and wrapping the cat in a towel will help calm the cat even further by making them feel secure with the towel swaddled around them and calm because they cannot see what is happening around them. There are cat bags that the cat's body is placed in and the head is left out while the bag is zipped up along the cat's back. There is a hole in the front of the bag to extend a front leg through either to place an IV catheter or draw blood from if needed. Again, the cat bag and cat muzzle will work well together. If the cat is extremely aggressive or frightened, it may be necessary to use sedatives.

Birds and Other Small Animals

Avian species commonly treated in veterinary practices vary greatly in size and safety measures required for handling and treatment. Leather gloves should be worn with raptorial species (falcons, hawks, owls, vultures, and eagles) to protect against their sharp beak and talons. Ear protection may be necessary when working with parrot species, as their alarm cries can be quite loud. Towels are also helpful, but safe restraint requires close monitoring for respiratory distress. Birds lack diaphragms, so their respiration depends on the expansion of the thoracic wall to draw air into the lungs.

Towels are also helpful when restraining reptiles, but like birds, close monitoring of respiration is necessary. As a note, calcium and vitamin D deficiency is common in domesticated reptiles, making them prone to bone fractures.

When restraining small mammals, the use of appropriately sized towels is encouraged.

Species	Hand hold	Scruff	Notes
Rabbit	Use the football hold: support the sternum with one hand and the back end with the other.	Do not scruff without hindleg support.	Do not obstruct the nose. Support the back legs at all times.
Guinea pigs	Towels are helpful.	Not ideal.	Biting is common.
Chinchillas	Towels are helpful.	Not ideal.	Struggling and attempting to flee is common.
Ferrets		Scruff gently while supporting the hind limbs to induce relaxation.	Biting is common, especially in females. Use treats to distract.
Hamster	Towels are helpful.	Do not scruff.	Be sure cheek pouches are empty before gas sedation to prevent aspiration.
Mice		Scruff gently.	Gas sedation is helpful.
Hedgehog	Use leather gloves to protect from quills.		Use gas sedation after fasting to prevent vomiting.
Gerbil	Do not handle by the tail to prevent degloving.		Gas sedation is helpful.

Handling and Restraining Livestock

When handling and restraining livestock, several things need to be remembered. Mature horses and cows typically weigh between 800 and 1,400 pounds, depending on their breed and gender. Some of the larger horse and cattle breeds can reach weights of 2,000 pounds. Caution is required when working with animals of this size. Never wrap a lead rope around the hand or wrist, as animals startle easily, and the lead rope should be easy to release. The handler should never place body parts between an animal and an immovable object, such as the bars of stocks or a chute, to avoid being crushed.

Livestock Field of Vision

It is also important to keep in mind that because livestock species are animals of prey, their fields of vision differ from humans, dogs, and cats. Horses and cattle have less than half of the binocular field of vision that humans do: binocular vision allows for accurate depth perception, while monocular vision allows for a wider field of view. With roughly 280° of monocular vision, horses and cattle are very sensitive to movement, especially when it is unfamiliar. Slow, gentle movements are important, especially when working with a new animal. Never throw or wave objects near an animal, especially near its head. Additionally, no animal should be approached from behind or within their blind spot. Whether dealing with a horse, cow, cat, or dog, approaching an animal in their blind spot could startle an animal and cause them to fight or flee.

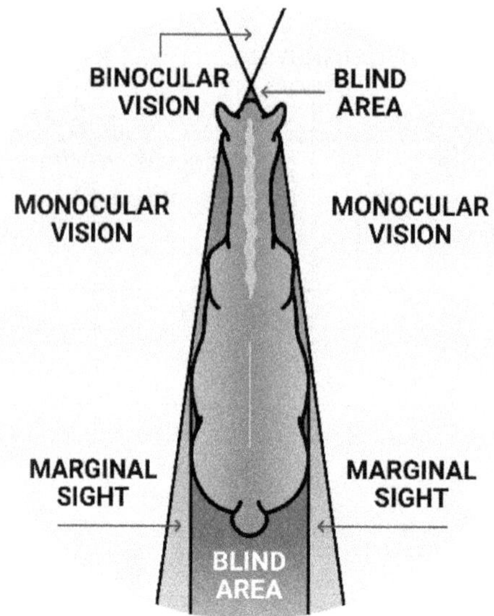

Working with Stressed Livestock

When under stress, common fight-or-flight responses should be remembered, and the safety of both patient and practitioner should be prioritized. Gates should always be closed, doors barred, and closed-chute systems used to prevent animals from escaping when they are being relocated or manipulated. However, if an animal gets loose, handlers should always have a way to escape or something to climb to get out of the way of a stressed animal. Though livestock species are animals of prey, when flight is prevented, they may react aggressively. Horses may reactively bite or kick, and cows may kick or charge in response to stress. Continuous observation of an animal's body language is critical to working safely with livestock.

Horses

When approaching a horse, especially in a stall, get the animal's attention (for example, by talking, making kissing sounds, or clicking the tongue) before opening the gate to avoid startling the animal and to encourage it to turn and face the gate. Nearly all domesticated horses will be manipulated using a halter and a lead rope. When approaching the horse with either, be sure no loose ends are dragging (which might resemble a snake) or waving. When putting on a halter, be sure that the lead rope is already attached to the ring that will be under the chin. Approach the horse's left shoulder from a slight angle and gently raise an arm to touch the animal. With the opposite arm, feed the loose end of the lead rope over the horse's neck so that it is loosely looped around the neck while the halter is put on. If the horse is already wearing a halter, slowly approach in the same manner, and after touching the horse's shoulder, slide the hand up the neck and clip the lead rope onto the halter ring located under the horse's chin.

Reasonably trained horses should be accustomed to this process and should be easily led by halter and lead rope.

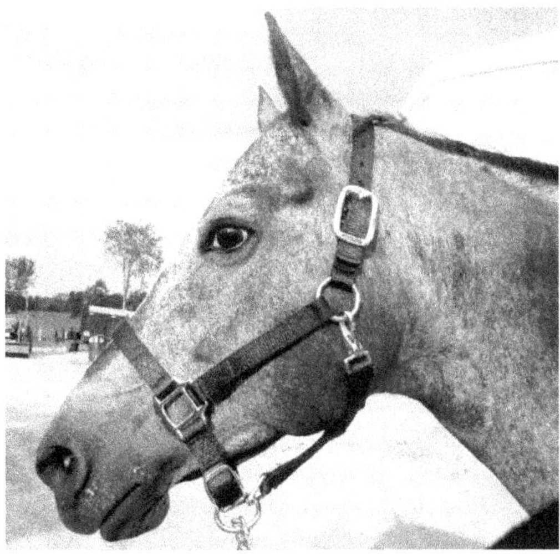

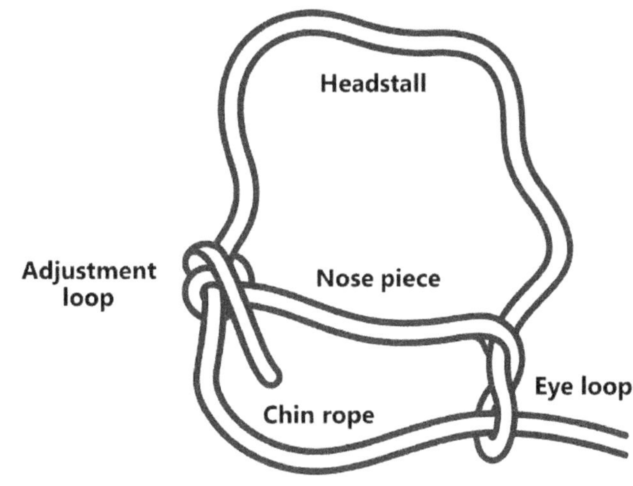

Skin Twitching and Chain Shank

Skin **twitching** is the process of squeezing and twisting loose skin on the horse's neck with the hand in order to calm or distract the animal. This manual twitch can also be applied to the ear, keeping in mind that the cartilage of the ear is sensitive, and this should never be done with a physical twitch. Mechanical twitches can be applied to a horse's upper lip.

A **chain shank** is another common restraint technique which uses a modified lead rope for additional control when handling a horse. The chain shank has a clip on one end, followed by roughly a foot of chain, attached to a length of rope. The chain can be fed through the chin ring on the horse's halter, through the left, square-shaped cheek ring of the halter, fed over the horse's nose, through the cheek ring on the right side, and clipped back onto itself under the horse's chin. The chain can also be fed over the horse's gums instead of over its nose, known as a **lip chain**. However, this should only be used by handlers with great skill as the chain can cause damage to the horse's mouth and gums.

Cattle

Cattle are not handled in the same way as horses. **Show cattle** will theoretically be halter-broken, **dairy cattle** tend to be more easily handled, but most **beef cattle** encountered in a large animal practice will be herd animals that will be examined and treated within a chute (pronounced *shoot*) system.

A **chute system** is a series of fences and gates designed for the subdividing and directing of groups of cattle so that they can be safely and systematically examined and treated. For example, if a whole herd is rounded up and directed into a corral, calves may be directed into one pen, cows into another pen, and bulls into another. This is done for efficiency (because equipment necessary for treatment varies between groups) and to prevent trampling (a small calf weighing 150 lb does not need to be in the same confined space as a cow or bull weighing 1,800 lb).

Using the Chute System for Cattle

From their pens, cattle can be directed up the main hallway-like chute single-file toward the squeeze chute for examination and treatment, also known as **working**. A **squeeze chute** is designed with a headgate, tailgate, and sides that are adjustable in order to change the width of the chute. As the cow moves its head through the **headgate**, a handler will close the headgate around the cow's neck while the second handler puts in the **tailgate bar** and slowly squeezes the cow with the sides of the chute to prevent it from jumping, twisting, or falling and injuring itself. Applying enough pressure in the squeeze chute allows the cow to stand up and balance while also effectively calming the animal. Once the cow is properly in the chute, a halter can be used to restrain the head to the side if the head (particularly the horns, mouth, or eyes) needs to be examined.

The use of electric cattle prods when working with cattle is discouraged.

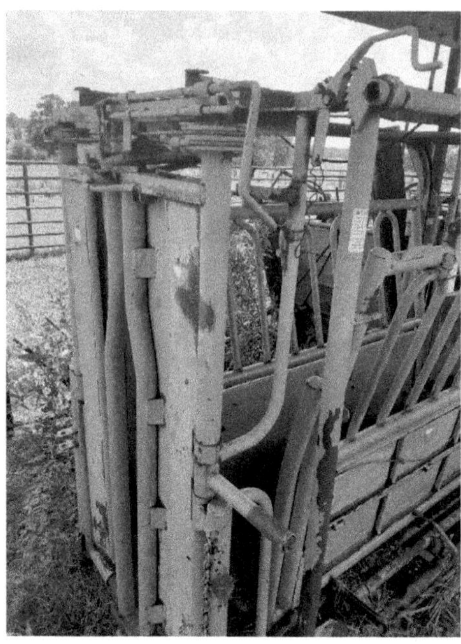

Goats and Sheep

Some goats and sheep may be easily restrained with a rope halter but not always. Sheep can be restrained by **flipping** or **setting up**, where they are maneuvered to a seated position with their back against the handler's legs as the handler holds the forearms. Goats will not tolerate this position, and they can instead be backed into a corner, where the handler straddles the goat and elevates its jaw with one hand while the handler squeezes its sides with their legs.

Pigs

Pig sorting panels are boards (usually wooden or plastic) with handle-holes cut out that are used to help move pigs through a chute or in a pen. They are roughly 2.5 feet tall, 2.5 feet wide, and an inch or two thick, and prevent pigs from slipping around handlers as they are relocated.

Hog snares can be used for greater control of an animal when they are being worked, but care and expertise are needed. The loop of the snare can be adjusted and slipped into the mouth and over the snout of a pig and tightened; however, pigs should not be moved around with a snare, and the snare should be held by a handler, not tied off to something, in order to prevent injury.

Note: pig squeals are incredibly loud, and wearing ear protection when working with them is advised.

Information and Evaluation

Basic Physical Examinations

A thorough physical exam is vital in obtaining information about the chief complaint and current health status of a patient. The technician should adhere to a preset, standard routine regarding the physical examination. This will help ensure a more complete and uniform examination. The routine also prompts the technician to adhere to important portions of the exam which may easily be overlooked when a less consistent routine is used. Each body system requires a thorough perusal in a comprehensive examination.

BODY CONDITION SCORE

A **body condition score (BCS)** scale is designed to evaluate the patient's body fat. Two systems are used, depending on veterinarian preference: a 1-9 scale and a 1-5 scale.

Score on 9-point scale	Description	Score on 5-point scale	Description
1/9	Emaciated	1/5	Very thin: ribs and pelvic bones are easily distinguishable, and the patient has very little body fat or muscle mass.
2/9	Very thin		
3/9	Thin	2/5	Underweight: the ribs can be felt easily, and there is no obvious waistline or abdominal tuck to the patient.
4/9	Underweight		
5/9	Ideal weight	3/5	Ideal weight: the ribs can be felt with no obvious amount of fat covering, and the abdomen is tucked nicely.
6/9	Overweight	4/5	Overweight: the ribs are palpable with difficulty, the waist is absent or barely visible, and an abdominal tuck may be present.
7/9	Heavy		
8/9	Obese	5/5	Obese: large fat deposits over its chest and back, and the abdomen appears distended.
9/9	Severely obese		

This score chart is important because it is a visual to show the owner where the pet's weight should be and what they should look like. After they recognize that their pet may be overweight, a feeding plan can be set, and regular weigh-ins can be scheduled to monitor progress.

WEIGHT AND TPR

One of the first sets of measurements the veterinary technician is charged with collecting on each animal is weight and TPR (temperature, pulse, and respiration). When weighing an animal, it is important to be sure that the scale has been tared before putting the animal on it, whether weighing a small kitten or a rodeo bull. Most animal temperatures are taken rectally. Pulse rate can be calculated by palpating the jugular vein or auscultating or palpating over the heart. Count the number of beats per 10 seconds, 15 seconds, 20 seconds, 30 seconds, or 60 seconds, and multiply by 6, 4, 3, 2, or 1, respectively, to get the beats per minute. Respiration is calculated in much the same way; count the number of times the chest rises and falls in a 15-second period and multiply by 4 (or any combination of the time frames and values above). Note that the normal, healthy values for each species vary; young animals tend to have higher TPR measurements than their adult counterparts; measurements should be taken on reasonably calm, still animals.

Species & Age	Temperature (± 1 °F)	Pulse (bpm)	Respiration (breaths per minute)
Puppy	100	200+	15-35
Adult dog	100-102.5	60-120 (depending on the breed size)	15-25
Kitten	100	220-260	15-35
Adult cat	100-102.5	150-200	20-30
Calf	101.5-103	100-140	30-60
Adult cow	100.4-103.1	50-60	20-25
Foal	99.5-102.2	45-60	60-80
Adult horse	99.5-101.3	38-45	8-12

MENTATION

Mentation refers to the mental activity or level of consciousness of the patient. Mentation status should be documented for each patient and can be labeled as normal, dull, obtunded, stuporous, and unresponsive.

Normal means the patient is bright, alert, and responsive to stimuli and its surroundings. **Dull** means that the patient is interactive by nudging or walking up and seeming interested in people but seems depressed. **Obtunded** means the patient is reacting to stimuli but not necessarily interested and is slower moving and more depressed. **Stuporous** means the patient is disconnected and only responds to painful stimuli, whereas **unresponsive** means the patient is disconnected and does not respond to any sort of stimuli.

HEART AND LUNG SOUNDS

Part of the physical examination is to examine the **chest cavity** of the patient. The veterinary technician or veterinarian will locate the heart by placing the stethoscope over the side of the chest between the fifth and sixth intercostal space. Once the heartbeat is heard with the stethoscope, you can record the heart rate and listen for any murmurs or abnormalities. Also, while listening to the heart, you will listen to lung sounds to make sure they sound clear with no crackling. The anatomy of the thoracic cavity begins with the diaphragm, which separates the abdominal cavity from the thoracic cavity. The heart is located in the thoracic cavity and is responsible for pumping and carrying blood rich with oxygen and nutrients to the rest of the body, providing the cells with energy. The lungs are located in the thoracic cavity as well and are a main part of the respiratory system. They have the important function of delivering oxygen to the blood and removing carbon dioxide from the blood through an exchange that occurs in the alveoli.

NORMAL CARDIAC RHYTHM

A thorough examination should be completed and all of the following cardiac performance indices and measures should be recorded: heart rate, rhythm, intensity, any deficiency or absence of standard sounds, and any unusual sounds—all of which can be classified as cardiac arrhythmias (sometimes referred to as dysrhythmias). Two of the more common and prominent abnormal rhythms in the heart are tachycardia and bradycardia. **Tachycardia** is a sustained overly-rapid heart rate. **Bradycardia** is an unusually slow heart rate. Irregular beats, skipped beats, and incomplete beats are often associated with both of these forms of **arrhythmias**. The condition known as hypocalcemia can result in bradycardia. **Hypocalcemia** is a condition where the animal has an extremely low level of calcium present in the blood.

ATRIOVENTRICULAR BLOCKS

The term **atrioventricular block** is abbreviated as AV block. This condition occurs when the atrial depolarization is not relayed to the ventricles, or when there is an unduly prolonged delay between atrial depolarization and ventricular depolarization. There are 3 recognized degrees of AV block. First-degree AV block is characterized by a lengthened PR interval, arising from dysfunction of the AV node. There are few symptoms or problems associated with this degree of AV block. In second-degree AV block, one or more (but not all) of the atrial impulses fail to communicate on to the ventricles. While few patients show symptoms, those who do may experience fainting and dizziness. In third-degree AV block (sometimes referred to as "complete" heart block), no atrial impulses (sometimes called supraventricular impulses) are relayed to the ventricles. This leaves the ventricles to generate a rhythm from alternate conduction sites (often septally derived). In an electrocardiograph, the P wave and the QRS complex can be seen to function independently from each other. These factors will be used to establish the presence of a complete heart block. Some animals with second-degree heart block may be in poor health. However, an animal with second-degree heart block may or may not be diagnosed with a heart disease.

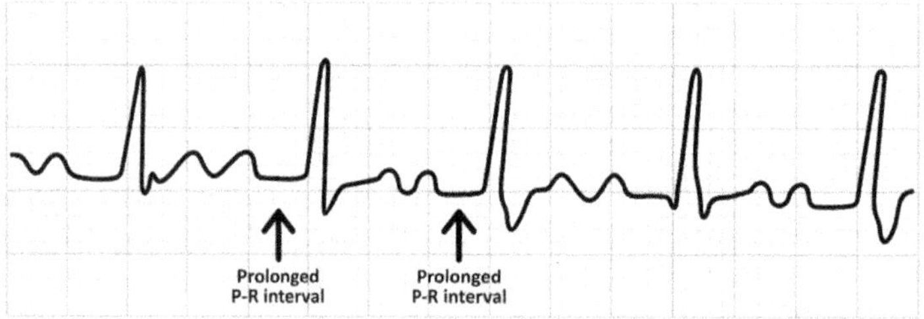

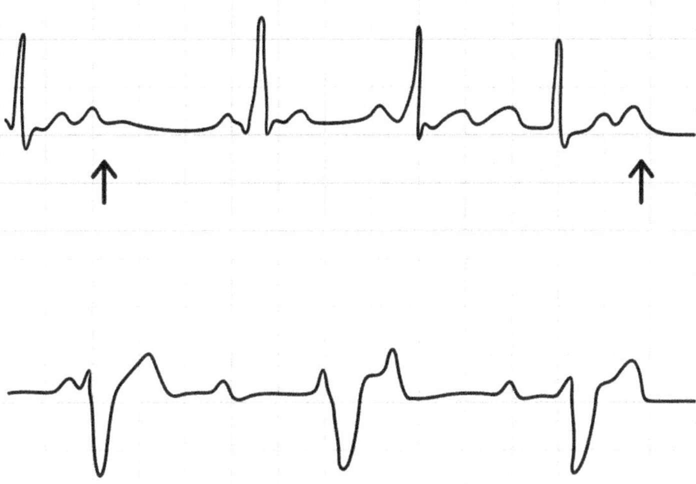

Normal Respiration

The normal respiration rhythm has a consistent pattern: 1) a **pause**, 2) followed by **inspiration** or breathing inwards, and 3) **expiration** or breathing out. Animals that are in an excited condition can exhibit deeper inspiratory breaths than expiratory breaths (i.e., gasping, etc.). This can be seen in an abnormal respiration rhythm. Further, strenuous exercise may bring on the following: coughing, nasal discharge, epistaxis (nose bleeds), hyperpnea (abnormally deep or rapid breathing), and dyspnea (difficult or labored breathing). These symptoms can indicate that the animal has a respiratory condition. An endoscopy will be beneficial in helping the veterinarian to determine the condition of the pharynx and trachea.

Skin and Coat Condition

There are a number of potential issues associated with the condition of an animal's skin and coat. Therefore, the technician should be careful to note whether or not the animal's skin or coat has a healthy shine to it. A dull coat may indicate that the skin is dry and may ultimately contribute to a condition known as alopecia. **Alopecia** is the loss of hair or the persistent absence of hair from the body. In some animals, this can be aggravated by excessive scratching and ultimate injury to itchy, dry skin.

The skin's **elasticity** or **turgor** (hydrated plumpness) should also be examined. This evaluation can help detect problems associated with dehydration. Skin that is poorly hydrated usually does not exhibit proper flexibility, and thus will not snap back into place when pulled outward. Instead, the skin is slow to go back into place. The skin at the thoracolumbar region in particular should be pulled upon to determine if the skin can be described as properly or poorly turgid or pliable. However, turgor must be evaluated in relation to the degree of dehydration. Thus, specific documentation may describe skin turgor as: good or normal, decreased, poor, or doughy. Briskly responsive, pliable skin is diagnosed as normal.

Palpation

A complete physical examination should also include the detection of any fleas, lice, mites, ticks, or lesions. The technician should examine the animal by **palpation**, a gentle pressure applied by the fingers over the animal's body. This should be useful in detecting lumps, swellings, and in producing reactions to painful points that the patient may be experiencing. Any unusual masses or changes in organ size, or other tissue enlargements, should be recorded. These observations will be used to further determine the patient's overall health. Indeed, all available information should be used to diagnose and treat the patient fully and properly.

Eyes, Ears, and Nares

The animal should also be examined for proper reflexes and appropriate responses to visual stimuli. This is essential in determining problems associated with the eyes. Likewise, the technician should record any leakage or matter that is released from the eyes. The color of this leakage may be clear or purulent. **Purulent** describes an exudate that contains pus or a similar yellowish or greenish fluid. This may indicate an infection in the animal.

The examination should note any irregularities in the cornea. Likewise, the clarity of the conjunctiva (the membrane covering the eye's surface) and the color of the sclera (the whites of the eyes) are both noted. The technician will manipulate the ear in checking its health. The technician will note any auditory stimuli response, abnormal or disproportionate odor, and the presence or absence of matter in the ear canal.

The technician will note the quality of any movements involving the patient's head. Any favoring of one side, disequilibrium, poor coordination, etc., should be recorded. The technician will check the nares or nostrils. The color and consistency of mucus released in the nasal region should be noted. This includes any sneezing or congestion observed. The nostrils should also be checked for any obstructions that may be causing a congested response.

The Respiratory System

The technician will need to listen to the patient's internal organs with a **stethoscope**. This is referred to as **auscultation**. For **pulmonary auscultation** the stethoscope should be placed on the back or the side of the thorax. The **thorax** is located between the neck and the abdomen. Moving the stethoscope to various points throughout the thoracic area can aid in obtaining a complete evaluation of the upper and lower lobes of the lungs and the trachea. This may be particularly important with larger animals. The technician should listen closely for any sounds that are irregular. This can involve crackling, wheezing, stridor, rhonchi, or rales. **Stridor** refers to a severe, struggling, high-pitched gasping for air, arising from an obstructed or highly constricted airway. **Rhonchi** are wet, mucus-laden wheezing or snoring sounds. **Rales** refer to a crackling, bubbling sound that emanates from the chest region. Some sounds may present only at the time of inspiration or expiration, but others present during both inspiration and expiration.

Sounds coming from the animal's upper airway and trachea should be checked further, particularly if an obstruction appears to be involved. Likewise, any problematic breathing should be noted. The animal's respiratory pattern, rate, and depth, and any changes noted with exertion may be important. The animal may exhibit hyperventilation or hypoventilation, panting or shallow breathing, and dyspnea.

Hyperventilation refers to a deep, quick-paced breathing that may be induced by anxiety or by an organic disease process. In particular, the disease of an organ may contribute to problems associated with carbon dioxide levels in the blood. The animal may then experience dizziness or weakness.

Hypoventilation refers to a shallow breathing that allows carbon dioxide to build up in the bloodstream. **Dyspnea** refers to difficult or labored breathing, often associated with heart disease coupled with overexertion. These problematic symptoms should be recorded. Felines that exhibit quick, shallow breaths or open-mouth breathing may be in physiological distress. This observation should be carefully noted to further promote the proper diagnosis of the animal.

The Gastrointestinal System

The technician will appraise the gastrointestinal system by checking the animal's mouth, teeth, and gums. The technician should make a note of all fractured, missing, or discolored teeth found in the animal's mouth. The animal's gums should be inspected for periodontal disease. Likewise, the presence of **halitosis** (bad breath) should be recorded. The technician will also make notes regarding any signs of malocclusion or unusual alignment of the teeth. The technician will seek to determine the age of the animal as related to dental status and overall health.

The animal's tonsils should be examined for any growth or excess size. In addition, the technician should document any disproportionate salivation or problems associated with swallowing. The technician should record any greenish- or yellowish-colored mucus. The mucous membranes must be pale pink in color to be considered normal. Any irregularities should be recorded. The gingival tissue should be checked for capillary refill time (abbreviated as CRT). This can be examined by applying gentle pressure on the gums and then quickly releasing in order to determine how long the gum tissue takes to return to a normal color. The refill process should be brisk and uniform in its re-saturation.

Abdominal Organs

The stomach breaks down food, and gastric acid in the stomach helps digest the food. The digested food leaves the stomach and enters the small intestine, which is a tube-shaped organ extending from the stomach to the large intestine. The small intestine has three parts: The first is the **duodenum**, the **jejunum** is the middle, and the **ileum** is the smallest part that connects to the large intestine. The gallbladder and the pancreas attach to the duodenum. Enzymes and other secretions important for digestion are produced by the liver and pancreas and pass through the pancreas to mix with food in the duodenum. The jejunum contains tiny fingerlike projections (villi) that absorb nutrients. The large intestine connects the small intestine to the anus and absorbs water to maintain hydration, as well as stores waste for defecation. The large intestine is divided into three parts: the ascending colon, the transverse colon, and the descending colon where fecal matter exits the anus.

Palpating the Abdomen

When examining a patient, the abdomen must be examined for signs of **distension** (swelling due to internal pressure) or any lesions or bruising. The abdomen must also be palpated beginning at the spine, moving around and down toward the belly. Palpate with one or both hands to feel for any masses, fluid, or even fetuses if pregnancy is suspected. By palpating the abdomen, the veterinarian may find an enlarged organ, a mass, an obstruction in the small intestine, or even an extremely full bladder, which could indicate obstruction. The patient may show pain upon palpation, which may need to be investigated further. The stomach, liver, spleen, and pancreas lie in the cranial abdomen; the kidneys and part of the spleen are located in the middle of the abdomen; and the bladder, prostate, uterus, and colon are in the caudal part of the abdomen. The small intestine is found throughout the entire abdomen.

Common Clinical Signs of Equine Gastrointestinal Ailments

Gastrointestinal ailments in horses can be attributed to a number of possible problems. These problems include overfeeding, parasites, twisted intestines, defective feed, an irregular feeding schedule, and sudden changes in feed. An animal exhibiting the following clinical signs could be suffering from a gastrointestinal ailment: restlessness, getting up and down frequently, agitation, hoof pawing, persistently pacing the stall or confinement area, rolling, biting at, or persistently watching their flank, and kicking at the abdominal region. Other bodily symptoms include: a distended abdomen, sweating, grinding teeth, increased heart and respiration rates, increased CRT (capillary refill time, usually in the gingival area), and diminished appetite. The animal's mucous membranes and gums should be checked. The gums can have a visible red or blue toxic line located right above the horse's teeth. The mucous membranes can change to a pale, bright brick red or bluish color. **Cyanosis** is indicated by a bluish color and means there is not enough oxygen in the horse's bloodstream. The following conditions may also be present: hypermotility, hypomotility, or the entire absence of gastrointestinal motility. The horse may even sit in a stance like a dog or with its legs extended out in a sawhorse-like posture.

Evaluating Hydration

The body is designed to balance fluids and other biochemistries between intracellular and extracellular components within the body. Metabolic functions and the restoration of lost fluids through drinking both play a part in how that fluid is allocated, maintained, and utilized. Some metabolic functions include losing fluids through respiration, excretion, and episodic routines such as sweating and milk production.

Fluid can be lost by atypical adverse conditions. These adverse conditions may include the following: vomiting, diarrhea, or abnormally excessive urination. Some diseases induce **polyuria** (excessive urination). Available fluids may also be reduced due to the patient's state of health. For example, chronic disease or severe injury can negatively impact the patient's ability to take in fluids. Ill dogs that have rapid respiration or excessive panting may also suffer from further fluid loss.

Tests can be given to determine the degree of dehydration present. A dehydration test measures the packed cell volume or PCV, total plasma protein or TPP levels, urine-specific gravity, and a lower rate of urine production.

Evaluating Hydration Status

A patient's **hydration status** can be evaluated through physical examination in a few different ways. The **skin tent test** will check the amount of moisture in the skin by pulling the skin over the thorax or lumbar region away from the back. If the patient is well hydrated, the skin will return immediately to its normal position, but if the skin stays standing, that means the patient is dehydrated. If there is a slight loss of the **skin's elasticity** from the skin tent test, that indicates a 5-6% dehydration. An increased capillary refill time, sunken eyes, and a more obvious delay in the skin returning to its normal position during the skin tent test indicate a 7-10% dehydration level. Dry mucous membranes, sunken and dull eyes, tachycardia, rapid and weak pulses, along with no return of the skin to its natural position during the skin tent test indicate a 10-12% dehydration level. A 12-15% dehydration level can lead to death.

Dehydration

The following factors should be considered in determining degree of dehydration: weight (especially recent rapid changes likely due to fluid loss), **skin turgor**, moistness of mucous membranes, heart rate, and **CRT** (capillary refill time). These factors must be evaluated through a physical inspection of the animal. The presence of poor or doughy skin turgor should produce a closer examination for other signs of dehydration. Ideally, the degree of dehydration should be determined. Dehydration is classified as follows: mild (6-8% fluid loss), moderate (10-12% fluid loss), and severe (12-15% fluid loss). Regions of the body that have an excessive amount of skin, such as the neck, are not good candidates to test for turgor.

Mild or Moderate Dehydration

Animals with a rate of dehydration under 5% of total normal fluid status do not typically show obvious signs or symptoms. However, animals with rates of 5-6% dehydration will usually exhibit a mild decrease of skin turgor evidenced by a lack of pliability to the skin. Animals with 8% dehydration will exhibit a more moderate reduction of skin turgor, a minor rise in CRT, and some dryness in the mucous membranes. The CRT can be examined by applying gentle pressure on the gums and then quickly releasing in order to determine how long the gum tissue takes to return to a normal color. The refill process should normally be brisk and uniform in its re-saturation of the gum tissue.

Severe Dehydration

Animals with dehydration rates of 10-12% total body fluid loss will exhibit moderate to severe loss of skin turgor, hollow-looking eyes, a marked rise in CRT (capillary refill time), dry mucous membranes, rapid heart and respiratory rates, cold limbs, and perhaps signs of shock. The CRT can be examined by applying gentle pressure on the gums and then quickly releasing in order to determine how long the gum tissue takes to return to a normal color. The refill process should normally be brisk and uniform in its re-saturation of the gum tissue.

The animal exhibiting 12-15% dehydration will be extremely metabolically depressed. In addition, the animal will likely already be in shock. This animal is in danger of dying from the severe level of dehydration and shock.

Common Conditions and Treatment

Respiratory Diseases

Common clinical signs of respiratory diseases include nasal discharge, which can be unilateral (occurring on one side) or bilateral (occurring on both sides) and can be characterized as:

- **Serous**: Clear liquid
- **Mucoid**: Opaque and sticky
- **Mucopurulent**: Green-yellow and mucoid
- **Hemorrhagic**: Bloody

Other possible signs include sneezing, facial swelling, **dyspnea** (respiratory distress), and sometimes anorexia. Common disease conditions include rhinitis or sinusitis, bronchitis, pneumonia, pyothorax, and pneumothorax.

Tracheobronchitis (Kennel Cough)

Kennel cough is caused by *Bordetella bronchiseptica*, a strain of bacteria associated with respiratory disease in canines, but it may also affect cats, rabbits, and very rarely humans. *Bordetella* is very contagious and is transmitted through direct contact or through the air. In young puppies or older dogs with a compromised immune system, *Bordetella* can cause major illness and even death. Mostly, in healthy adult canines, *Bordetella* causes mild illness. The *Bordetella* vaccine is a noncore vaccine; therefore, it is not administered to all dogs or cats and is typically used for those likely to come in contact with the bacterial organism in kennel situations, such as at the groomer or boarding facility. Puppies may receive the intranasal *Bordetella* vaccine as early as 3–4 weeks of age, and they can receive the injectable vaccine at around 6–8 weeks of age, with a booster between 10 and 12 weeks of age. Dogs should then receive a booster *Bordetella* vaccine every 6–12 months.

Feline Herpesvirus Type 1

Feline herpesvirus type 1 (FHV-1) causes feline viral tracheitis, a highly contagious feline disease involving upper respiratory infection including sneezing, discharge from the eyes and nose, and fever. The virus can survive in the environment for up to 24 hours and is commonly spread through direct contact. Latent infections do occur; a cat previously infected with FHV-1 will experience disease symptoms (including shedding) again after a stressful experience. FHV-1 is ubiquitous globally and affects both domestic and wild cats of all ages.

Feline Calicivirus (FCV)

One of the most common causes of feline upper respiratory infection and oral ulceration is **feline calicivirus (FCV)**. There are more than 40 different strains of calicivirus, and the severity varies greatly between strains.

The virus can be shed by an infected cat's oral, nasal, and conjunctival secretions, as well as through the urine and feces, for up to 21 days. After recovering, many cats develop a carrier state in which they continue to shed viral particles occasionally or consistently. The carrier state can last a few months or even a lifetime; therefore, those cats are contagious. The virus can survive in the environment for up to a week, allowing fomites to indirectly spread FCV. Like FHV-1, FCV is ubiquitous globally and infects both domestic and wild cats of all ages.

Clinical signs include ulcers found on the tongue, gums, hard palate, nose, or lips.

Cardiovascular Diseases

Heart Disease

Heart disease affects the heart's **myocardium** (muscle of the heart), valves, rhythm conduction, or **pericardium** (membrane around the heart). It may be hard to detect in animals because the heart can compensate in order to protect the body; however, over time, heart disease can lead to heart failure. Heart failure can present with the following signs: exercise intolerance, **syncope** (fainting due to hypotension), weakness, **tachypnea** (rapid breathing), increased capillary refill time, cough, anorexia, or depression.

Congestive heart failure (CHF) describes the resulting symptoms when heart disease causes poor cardiac output and resulting poor venous return to the heart. **Left-sided congestive heart failure** will lead to pulmonary edema, dyspnea, tachypnea, resulting in abnormal respiratory sounds, and sometimes cough. **Right-sided congestive heart failure** will cause edema in the thoracic and abdominal cavities and jugular distention.

Sinus Bradycardia

A particularly slow but regular ventricular heart rate can be described as **sinus bradycardia**. This term is generally used when the heart rate is less than 70 beats per minute for dogs that weigh under 20 kg or 45 lb. This rate is also given for dogs that have a heart rate of less than 60 beats per minute when weighing over 20 kg or 45 lb. Heart rates measured at 100 beats per minute or less are indicative of sinus bradycardia in cats. Animals experiencing profound bradycardia can exhibit symptoms such as weakness, hypotension, and syncope. Both excessive and reduced parasympathetic tone may result in sinus bradycardia. Sinus bradycardia can sometimes also be attributed to respiratory disease. The disease can cause the animal to experience a number of problems, including struggling to draw in air, gastric irritation, increased cerebrospinal fluid pressure, hypothyroidism, hypothermia, hyperkalemia, and hypoglycemia. Certain drug therapies may also induce the condition.

Sinus Arrhythmia as Related to Respiratory Rate

Sinus arrhythmia (also called respiratory sinus arrhythmia or RSA) refers to a normal variation in heartbeat as influenced by respiratory patterns. Both inspiratory and expiratory respirations can alter the heart's sinus rhythm. Typically, the heart rate increases during inspiration and decreases during expiration. Theorists suggest that this maximizes cardiac output during more effective ventilatory periods. Variations are more pronounced in younger animals and moderate with age. The "sinus" term refers to the sinus node (or the sinoatrial node), which is the heart's natural pacemaker. It is important to know about respiratory sinus arrhythmia, as these changes will be apparent during an EKG. Neurologically induced cardiac variations (as seen in altered vagal tone and parasympathetic system responses, including emotions) can also contribute to the magnitude of sinus arrhythmia experienced. Finally, any respiratory disease in an animal may also bring about an altered sinus arrhythmia.

Heartworm Disease

Heartworm disease is spread by mosquitoes, and both dogs and cats are susceptible to it. Clinical signs differ between the species. Cats can present with coughing, vomiting, lethargy, anorexia/weight loss, and dyspnea; dogs can present with coughing, right-sided congestive heart failure, syncope, exercise intolerance, dyspnea, and **hemoptysis** (coughing up blood). There is no effective treatment protocol in cats, and treating dogs can be prolonged, risky, and involved (possibly including surgery and with the risk of pulmonary thromboembolism), so monthly heartworm prevention should be strongly recommended for pet owners.

Heartworm Prevention

Heartworm preventatives, including ivermectin, moxidectin, milbemycin oxime, and selamectin, are effective against heartworm disease. Heartworm preventatives work by killing the infective larvae that have infected the patient within the previous month. **Ivermectin** (Heartgard, Iverhart Plus, and Tri-Heart) is an antiparasitic drug that is administered as a chewable oral tablet monthly at a very low dose as a heartworm preventative. Medications include **pyrantel pamoate**, which also will kill hookworms and roundworms (Heartgard Plus). **Milbemycin oxime** (Trifexis and Sentinel) is an antiparasitic drug given as a monthly oral tablet that will also kill roundworms, hookworms, and whipworms. **Selamectin** (Revolution) is a topical monthly application that is an antiparasitic drug that kills heartworm infective larvae as well as fleas, hookworms, roundworms, and ear mites. **Moxidectin** (ProHeart 6 and Advantage Multi) is an antiparasitic drug that kills heartworm infective larvae and hookworms. Advantage Multi is a topical drug applied once monthly, and ProHeart 6 is an injectable given SQ once every 6 months.

Gastrointestinal and Hepatobiliary Diseases

Signs commonly associated with upper gastrointestinal diseases include: regurgitation, **dysphagia** (difficulty eating), vomiting, hypersalivation (a common precursor to vomiting and a sign of nausea), gagging, and dehydration (if vomiting has been occurring a while). Signs of lower GI disease possibly include: diarrhea, presence of blood or mucus in the stool, constipation, and **tenesmus** (straining on urination or defecation). Blood in the stool can be described in two ways: **melena**, when the blood is partially digested, indicating possible disease in the small intestine, and **hematochezia**, when the blood is undigested and present on the outside of the stool, indicating possible disease in the colon or rectum.

Gastrointestinal Obstruction

Gastrointestinal obstruction is common, especially due to foreign bodies in dogs when they swallow a chew toy or household object. It can also be the result of neoplasia (a growth) or intussusception (when a section of bowel "telescopes" on itself). If the foreign object is stuck in the esophagus, it could result in vomiting or regurgitation. If the foreign object is stuck in the bowel, it could result in abdominal pain, sepsis, diarrhea, or shock. Patient history, radiography, and ultrasound are used to determine the presence and location of a foreign object or other cause of a gastrointestinal obstruction.

Pancreatitis

Pancreatitis is the inflammation of the pancreas, a glandular organ in the abdomen that produces digestive enzymes and regulatory hormones (insulin, glucagon). This occurs when trypsin (a protease) is activated early in the pancreas—rather than in the duodenum where it is supposed to be activated—causing damage to the pancreas. The disease can be acute (more common in dogs) or chronic (more common in cats). Predisposing and contributing factors include: a high fat diet, genetics, dietary indiscretion or abrupt dietary changes, trauma, drug or medication toxicity, or hormonal disease.

Acute clinical signs include anorexia, fever, vomiting, and diarrhea, which may later develop into hypotension, renal failure, disseminated intravascular coagulation (DIC, also colloquially "dead in cage"), and multiple organ failure. Chronic clinical signs include anorexia, lethargy, weight loss, and hiding (especially in cats). It can be hard to detect and can lead to diabetes mellitus and exocrine pancreatic insufficiency (EPI, a disorder of the pancreatic digestive enzymes).

Treatment involves hydration therapy in response to the vomiting and diarrhea (V/D) and nausea, as well as pain management.

Canine Parvoviral Enteritis (PVE)

Canine parvoviral enteritis (PVE) is common and highly contagious to all dogs; however, young (6 weeks to 6 months), unvaccinated, and not fully vaccinated dogs have the highest risk of infection with CPV. The virus spreads via direct fecal-oral contact, as well as indirectly via fomites; it can survive in the environment for weeks, months, or years, depending on the conditions, and is resistant to many disinfectants. Fecal viral shedding occurs just days after infection, often before the presentation of clinical signs, which occur acutely and include: V/D (often hemorrhagic), dehydration, nausea, anorexia, depression, lethargy, abdominal pain, fever, leukopenia (reduction of white blood cell count), and neurological signs. Viral shedding can continue for 10 days after disease recovery.

Diagnosis is confirmed through fecal antigen testing in conjunction with patient history and clinical signs. However, large volume diarrhea can dilute fecal antigens and give a false negative early in the course of the disease. Treatment is supportive: hydration therapy, antiemetics, antibiotics, and nutritional support.

Preventing the Spread of Canine Parvovirus

To prevent environmental contamination and the spread of canine parvovirus (CPV) to other dogs, infected patients must be kept in an isolation ward in the hospital away from other patients. When personnel handle dogs with CPV, they must be wearing gloves and a gown (specified for that infected patient), and they must also step through a diluted bleach foot bath with their shoes before entering or leaving the isolation room. Every surface should be cleaned with a diluted bleach or an accelerated hydrogen peroxide disinfectant.

Vaccinations for canine parvovirus should be administered to puppies at 8 weeks, 12 weeks, and 16 weeks of age; there is a booster a year later and then every 3 years to prevent and control this deadly virus. Modified live vaccines protect against all strains of canine parvovirus. CPV can remain viable in the environment for long periods of time; therefore, in kennels, shelters, and hospitals, every surface needs to be cleaned, disinfected, and dried twice before reuse.

Feline Panleukopenia Virus (FPV)

Feline panleukopenia virus, also known as feline distemper and feline parvovirus (FPV), is a highly contagious and often fatal disease in kittens. The virus can persist in the environment for up to one year under the right conditions. Virions are shed by feces, urine, blood, and secretions for up to 6 weeks after recovery. Vertical transmission, direct oronasal infection (including breastmilk), and indirect infection via fomites spread FPV. Stray cats are usually exposed to FPV before they reach 1 year of age, and those that survive an acute FPV infection will build a strong immune response. FPV infects and kills the rapidly dividing cells of the bone marrow, intestines, and lymph nodes. Usually if kittens are infected transplacentally, they will be stillborn, but if they become infected immediately after birth from nursing, it could cause cerebellar hypoplasia as a result of the virus damaging the part of the brain responsible for muscle activity.

Like CPV, FPV is treated supportively with hydration therapy, antiemetics, antimicrobials, nutritional support, and sometimes immunotherapy.

Urinary Diseases

Dysfunction of the urinary tract can cause a range of symptoms associated with specific terminology, including:

- **Anuria**: Failure of kidneys to produce urine
- **Azotemia**: Elevations of creatinine and blood urea nitrogen (BUN) in the blood
- **Bacteriuria**: Presence of bacteria in the urine
- **Dysuria**: Discomfort, pain, or burning on urination
- **Glucosuria**: Glucose in the urine
- **Hematuria**: Blood in the urine
- **Oliguria**: Production of only small amounts of urine
- **Polydipsia**: Excessive thirst
- **Polyuria**: Excessive urination
- **Pollakiuria**: Frequent urination
- **Proteinuria**: Increased protein levels in the urine
- **PU/PD**: Presence of both polyuria and polydipsia
- **Pyuria**: Presence of white blood cells in the urine
- **Stranguria**: Straining to urinate
- **Uremia**: High levels of waste products in the blood
- **V/D**: Notation indicating the presence of both vomiting and diarrhea

Chronic Kidney Disease

The **kidneys** (paired, bean-shaped organs located within the abdominal cavity on either side of the spine) filter waste and excess fluid from the blood. Glomeruli (singular: **glomerulus**) are the filters of the kidneys; their function is estimated as GFR: **glomerular filtration rate**.

Chronic kidney disease (CKD) involves a progressive loss of renal function due to tissue damage. It is most common in geriatric animals. Symptoms of CKD may include: azotemia, hypertension, proteinuria, PU/PD, V/D, lethargy, anorexia, dehydration, oral ulceration, and uremia.

CKD is classified into 4 stages:

- Stage 1: Subclinical, usually undetected
- Stage 2: Glomerular filtration rate (GFR) <25% of normal, azotemia present, possible decreased ability to concentrate urine (leading to PU/PD)
- Stage 3: GFR decline, azotemia present, clinical signs present, re-evaluate every 3-6 months
- Stage 4: GFR decline, severe azotemia, clinical signs present, re-evaluate every 1-3 months

Because CKD is often a result of another disease process, treatment involves identifying and treating the primary disease. Treating the possible complications of CKD (including hypertension, metabolic acidosis, and urinary tract infection [UTI]) is also important.

ACUTE KIDNEY INJURY

Acute kidney injury, formerly known as acute renal failure, can be caused by toxins, ischemia, and infection and may present with the following clinical signs: V/D, anorexia, depression, oliguria, and oral ulceration. AKI is graded (I-V) based on serum creatinine:

- Grade I: Less than 1.6 mg/dL
- Grade II: 1.7-2.5 mg/dL
- Grade III: 2.6-5 mg/dL
- Grade IV: 5.1-10 mg/dL
- Grade V: More than 10 mg/dL

Severe AKI is serious and has a 50% survival rate. Treatments include hydration therapy and attempts to increase urine output. For animals with severe anorexia, a parenteral feeding tube is advised. Dialysis (peritoneally or hemodialysis) may also be necessary.

UROLITHIASIS

A **urolith** or **calculus** is a mineral-salt stone found in the urinary tract; they are named based on where they are found: nephrolith (nephron), urocystolith (bladder), ureterolith (ureter), or urethrolith (urethra). Depending on the location of the stone, urolithiasis may be accompanied by vomiting, abdominal pain, depression, anorexia, stranguria, and polyuria.

Treatment may involve surgical removal of stones, catheter removal of stones (if they are small enough), lithotripsy (the use of shock waves to break down stones so they are small enough to pass), or dissolution via urinary acidification. Prevention of recurrence of urinary calculi includes owner education, dietary changes, and monitoring of urine by the owner.

UTI

Urinary tract infections can be secondary to other disease processes, including diabetes mellitus, hyperadrenocorticism, and CKD. They may also be the result of infection due to a catheter or a urolith. UTIs can present with dysuria, hematuria, and polyuria, which can cause a pet to urinate in inappropriate places even if potty trained. Urine samples may contain red and white blood cells, as well as bacteria, the most common of which is *E. coli*. Treatment with antibiotics should include owner education about the importance of administering the complete round of medication as prescribed.

FLUTD

FLUTD stands for **feline lower urinary tract disease**, also called feline urologic syndrome. Conditions of the syndrome include: urolithiasis, neoplasia, trauma, feline interstitial or idiopathic (sterile) cystitis (FIC), and urinary tract infection. The lower urinary tract consists of the bladder, ureters, and urethra. The most common clinical signs are polyuria, hematuria, and stranguria. FLUTD occurs most commonly in cats 2-6 years old. Obstructive FLUTD, in which the urethra is obstructed, is a medical emergency; it is seen most commonly in male cats.

Endocrine Diseases

Hyperthyroidism

Hyperthyroidism occurs when the **thyroid gland**, which is wrapped around the front of the trachea just below the larynx, is overactive and produces too much thyroxine (T_4) and triiodothyronine (T_3), leading to an increased metabolic rate. It is most common in middle-aged and geriatric cats, and it is uncommon in other species.

Presentation to the clinic usually occurs when a pet owner notices weight loss, increased appetite, increased excitability or activity, PU/PD, V/D. Professional examination could reveal the following: elevated serum T_4 levels, **tachycardia** (elevated heart rate), heart murmur, hypertension, enlarged thyroid gland or presence of a thyroid tumor, **dyspnea** (shortness of breath or difficulty breathing), or congestive heart failure.

Apathetic hyperthyroidism is less common and involves vomiting, depression, and anorexia.

Treatment options include thyroidectomy or hemithyroidectomy, radioactive iodine medication, antithyroid drugs, and adhering to a low iodine diet for the pet.

Hypothyroidism

Hypothyroidism occurs when there is a deficiency of thyroid hormones leading to a decreased metabolic rate. It is most common in dogs and usually occurs because of damage to the thyroid gland caused by lymphocytic thyroiditis or idiopathic thyroid atrophy. Lymphocytic thyroiditis can be immune-mediated and occurs when lymphocytes, plasma cells, and macrophages invade and destroy the thyroid gland, decreasing its functionality. Idiopathic (spontaneous or of unknown cause) thyroid atrophy describes the idiopathic replacement of thyroid tissue with adipose tissue.

Clinical signs of hypothyroidism include lethargy, depression, dullness, exercise intolerance, weight gain (with no corresponding appetite increase), obesity, low T_4 and T_3 hormone serum concentration, **nonpruritic** (pruritic means itchy) **alopecia** (patchy hair loss), and hypothermia or heat-seeking behaviors.

Treatment consists of daily oral hormone replacement medication.

Diabetes Mellitus (DM)

Diabetes mellitus (DM) is a disease process resulting from insulin deficiency. **Insulin** is produced and secreted by the pancreas and facilitates the cellular uptake of glucose, which maintains normal blood glucose levels. Type 1 DM, also called insulin-dependent DM, describes insufficient insulin production and is more common in dogs, especially middle-aged canines. Type 2 DM, also called non-insulin-dependent DM, is the result of endogenous insulin resistance and is more common in cats. Remission of diabetes mellitus in cats is likely with prompt, attentive treatment; however, with dogs, remission does not occur.

Clinical signs of diabetes mellitus include **polyphagia** (excessive eating), weight loss (usually from a previously obese state), and PU/PD. Diagnosis can be confirmed by the presence of hyperglycemia and glycosuria; in cats, it is important to check for elevated fructosamine levels in order to rule out stress-induced hyperglycemia, which is common.

Diabetes mellitus can be challenging to manage; dogs require insulin injections once or twice per day. Dietary changes, attempts at weight reduction, and constant monitoring of insulin levels and changing of insulin doses are required. Untreated, diabetes mellitus progresses to diabetic ketoacidosis (DKA).

Diabetic Ketoacidosis (DKA)

Diabetic ketoacidosis (DKA) occurs when diabetes mellitus goes untreated. Due to prolonged insulin deficiency (whether absolute [type 1 DM] or relative [type 2 DM]), the body must use an alternative carbohydrate metabolism pathway. This produces toxic ketones, which are excreted in the urine (**ketonuria**) and may cause the breath to smell fruity.

DKA usually presents as an emergency with a history of anorexia, PU/PD, vomiting, weight loss, abnormal temperature (hypothermia or hyperthermia), neurological signs (ranging from depression to a comatose state), and signs of abdominal pain. Emergency treatment usually involves responding to the dehydration, metabolic acidosis, and decreased serum potassium, phosphorus, and sodium levels.

Hyperadrenocorticism (HAC)

Cushing syndrome describes the condition resulting from elevated circulating cortisol levels, which has several potential causes. It is hard to diagnose and is progressive.

Clinical signs are the result of hypercortisolemia and include: PU/PD, increased appetite and weight gain, lethargy, alopecia, muscle atrophy, enlarged pot-belly abdomen, and commonly secondary UTIs.

Cushing disease, also called pituitary-dependent hyperadrenocorticism (PDH), causes 80-85% of Cushing syndrome cases; most cases occur in dogs, and it is rare in cats. PDH is caused by an ACTH-secreting pituitary tumor. In dogs, it is commonly diagnosed using the low-dose dexamethasone suppression test. Pharmacological treatment occurs in response to the symptoms caused by hypercortisolemia.

Adrenal-dependent hyperadrenocorticism is much less common and is caused by one or more adrenal tumors, which may be unilateral or bilateral, that secrete cortisol. Treatment involves the removal of the adrenal tumor.

Hypoadrenocorticism

Hypoadrenocorticism or **Addison's disease** is the disease process caused by a deficiency of adrenal hormones, especially cortisol and aldosterone. It most commonly affects dogs, though it sometimes occurs in horses. It may cause anorexia, V/D, PU/PD, weight loss, bradycardia, weakness, collapse, anemia, hypoglycemia, **hyperkalemia** (increased serum potassium levels), and **hyponatremia** (decreased serum sodium levels), and it can present acutely as an emergency. It is difficult to diagnose and requires continuous treatment to manage. Adrenal function testing, including the ACTH stimulation test, can be used in diagnosis.

Immune-Mediated Diseases

IMHA

Immune-mediated hemolytic anemia is the most common cause of hemolytic anemia. **Hemolysis** is the rupturing of red blood cells. In dogs, IMHA is usually considered primary; the immune system **idiopathically** (of unknown cause) develops autoantibodies that react with self-antigens of circulating red blood cells. In cats, IMHA is commonly secondary to a blood parasite.

IMHA may cause lethargy, exercise intolerance, **icterus** (jaundice), tachycardia, heart murmur, **splenomegaly** (enlarged spleen), and **hepatomegaly** (enlarged liver). Pulmonary thromboembolism is a resultant additional risk in dogs.

Diagnosis involves checking for evidence of autoimmune disease, such as **autoagglutination**, which is the clumping of **erythrocytes** (red blood cells) due to autoantibodies. IMHA can be treated with immunosuppressants, blood transfusions, hydration therapy, and anticoagulants. It has a 20-75% mortality rate.

Myasthenia Gravis (MG)

Myasthenia gravis is a neuromuscular disease that causes generalized muscle weakness. In its congenital form, there is an inherited deficiency in the acetylcholine (ACH) receptors of the post-synaptic membrane. In its acquired and immune-mediated form, there are autoantibodies against the ACH receptors in the synapse. As a review, a **synapse** is the junction between two neurons, across which neurotransmitters, such as ACH, are passed.

MG presents with generalized muscle weakness, exercise intolerance—though rest helps—and possibly regurgitation due to megaesophagus. Administering IV edrophonium chloride will usually quickly resolve exercise-induced stiffness, weakness, or tremors, indicating the presence of MG, which can be confirmed by the presence of serum ACH-receptor autoantibodies.

Drug therapies include the administration of anticholinesterase (cholinesterase is the enzyme that breaks down ACH) and immunosuppressive drugs.

Infectious & Parasitic Diseases

Zoonosis

Zoonosis is any disease that can be transmitted from animals to humans, or any disease that normally is in an animal but can infect humans. There are three routes of transmission including contact, aerosol, and vector-borne. Contact may be direct (e.g., ingestion or puncture wounds) or indirect (e.g., exposure to fomites by handling the dirty laundry, dishes, or housing of an animal). There are certain zoonotic parasites such as hookworms that can be transmitted from dogs and cats to humans through the feces. Roundworms are also zoonotic parasites that can be transmitted to humans through feces, and they can cause visceral and ocular larva migrans (where larvae settle in the eye). Rabies, which is fatal, is also a zoonotic disease transmitted through saliva, bites, or scratches from infected animals.

Methods of Transmission

When encountering a pet in the clinic, it is important to know the methods of transmission of suspected diseases in order to protect the animals and people who come into contact with the infected animal. The various methods of disease transmission are direct transmission, indirect transmission, and vertical transmission. Vertical transmission involves the spread of disease from mother to offspring, before or after parturition (the process of giving birth), either transplacentally or through breastmilk.

Direct Transmission

The direct contact of mucous membranes or broken skin with infected excretions (urine, feces) or secretions (tears, sweat, saliva, mucus, semen) is defined as **direct transmission** of disease. This can include nose-to-nose transmission, fecal-oral transmission, and the spread of disease via respiratory droplets. The spread of disease by direct contact can be slowed or stopped in a herd or between pets by isolating sick animals and quarantining animals suspected to be infected or newly introduced to a herd.

Indirect Transmission

Indirect transmission of disease does not require direct contact with an infected animal, making stopping the spread of disease much more difficult. Pathogens may spread by way of:

- **Airborne transmission**—involves the suspension of pathogens in the air for up to several hours, allowing it to be inhaled long after an infected animal has left
- **Vectors**—living organisms that play host to the pathogen by either transporting it or supporting its life cycle, such as fleas, ticks, or mosquitoes
- **Vehicles**—inanimate objects that transport or support the life cycle of a pathogen; includes fomites, food, water, biologic products, and medical supplies, such as shoes or gloves, causing iatrogenic spread

Tick-Borne Illnesses

Ticks carry bacteria capable of causing disease in animals and humans. Travel history and exposure to tick habitats should be considered when an animal presents with signs of disease, especially acutely. Owners should be counseled to save ticks if one is discovered on a pet.

Dogs and cats can acquire **anaplasmosis**, with clinical signs including joint pain leading to lameness, fever, vomiting, and diarrhea. Clinical signs of **ehrlichiosis** in dogs and cats include depression, anorexia, fever, joint pain, and bruising. **Rocky Mountain Spotted Fever (RMSF)** can infect dogs and cats, but the tick must be attached for at least 5 hours to transmit RMSF. Signs of RMSF are anorexia, joint pain, fever, vomiting, diarrhea, pneumonia, kidney and liver failure, and neurological signs. Clinical signs for **Lyme disease** include fever, swollen lymph nodes, and anorexia; in more severe cases, kidney disease and heart conditions may develop. There is a vaccine given for Lyme disease for dogs. All of these diseases are commonly treated with a course of antibiotics.

Clinically Significant Ticks of North America

Scientific name	Common name(s)	Adult Female	Adult Male	Diseases carried
Amblyomma americanum	Lone star tick			• Granulocytic ehrlichiosis • Heartwater • Rickettsiosis • Tick paralysis • Tularemia
Dermacentor variabilis	American dog tick			• Canine tick paralysis • Rickettsiosis • Rocky Mountain Spotted Fever (RMSF) • Tularemia
Ixodes scapularis	Eastern blacklegged tick Deer tick Blacklegged deer tick	Adult female Male and female nymphs also carry disease.		• Babesiosis • Canine anaplasmosis (Anaplasma phagocytophilum, A. platys) • Ehrlichiosis • Lyme disease (Borrelia burgdorferi) • Rickettsiosis • Tick paralysis

Feline Leukemia Virus (FeLV)

Feline leukemia virus (FeLV) is a retrovirus that is spread through saliva, nasal secretions, feces, and urine, as well as through nursing mothers to their kittens. Retroviruses invade cells and insert a copy of genetic material with the help of the reverse transcriptase enzyme. Cats that live primarily outdoors are at a higher risk of contracting FeLV, but exposure does not always mean that the cat will become infected because the virus may not replicate. There are three specific groups of FeLV, including FeLV-A, FeLV-B, and FeLV-C. FeLV-A affects all cats infected with FeLV and causes severe immunosuppression, is easily transmitted, and is the group used in making the FeLV vaccines. FeLV-B occurs in about half of cats infected with FeLV and causes neoplastic disease. FeLV-C affects less than 1% of infected cats and causes severe anemia. There is no treatment for FeLV, so vaccinating is crucial.

Canine Distemper Combination Vaccine

The **canine distemper vaccine** is a combination vaccine that protects against more than just the distemper virus. The canine distemper vaccine protects against **distemper**, **canine adenovirus-2** and **canine adenovirus-1 infection** (hepatitis and respiratory), **parvovirus**, and **parainfluenza**. The abbreviated vaccines are labeled DA2PP or DA2PPV. The D is for canine distemper, which is a virus that affects the respiratory system, digestive system, and the brain and nervous system of canines. The distemper virus is highly contagious and can be fatal. A2 refers to the canine adenovirus-2, which can cause respiratory disease. P stands for parvovirus, which is an incredibly contagious and potentially fatal disease that attacks the immune and digestive systems, causing diarrhea and vomiting. PV refers to parainfluenza virus, which is a viral respiratory disease in dogs.

Leptospirosis

Leptospirosis is caused by the *Leptospira* bacteria that are found in water and soil, and there are numerous strains that can cause disease. Leptospirosis is zoonotic, where infection in humans can cause flu symptoms and could cause kidney and liver disease. Leptospirosis is very common in dogs but is rare in cats. Dogs are exposed to the *Leptospira* bacteria by drinking out of contaminated rivers, ponds, streams, or from living in areas where infected wildlife mammals may be present. If the dog's mucous membranes or open wounds come in contact with the infected urine of wildlife mammals, the dog can become infected. Dogs may also become infected if they eat an infected animal or get bitten by an infected animal. *Leptospira* bacteria can be transmitted through the placenta to puppies as well.

Neurologic Diseases

Rabies Virus

Rabies is acute viral encephalomyelitis caused by *Rabies lyssavirus,* a *rhabdovirus* that damages the central nervous system. Rabies is mainly transmitted through infected saliva by the bite of an infected animal that results in an open wound, and it may also be contracted through saliva coming into contact with mucous membranes. After an animal or person is bitten by an infected animal, the virus migrates through the peripheral nerves to the spinal cord and up to the brain. It then travels through the peripheral nerves to the salivary glands and is shed intermittently. Once clinical signs appear, the virus is considered contagious, but in cats and dogs, the virus is contagious a few days prior to noticeable clinical signs. After the virus replicates in the central nervous system, every organ will become affected.

Rabies: Clinical Signs and Safety Considerations

While aggression is stereotypically associated with rabies, any behavioral changes—including depression—accompanied by neurological signs could be a sign of rabies, and caution should be taken when examining the animal.

Veterinary professionals should be very cautious when working with suspected rabies cases, even if the suspected infected animal is already dead. Gloves, gowns, and goggles should be worn, and pre-exposure prophylaxis for veterinary professionals is recommended. Since rabies can only be positively identified through a postmortem examination, it becomes necessary to also euthanize animals that are suspected of having rabies.

TETANUS

The bacteria known as *Clostridium tetani* can be found in some soils. This bacterium is responsible for the infection known as **tetanus**. The bacterium typically enters the body through a puncture wound. The neurotoxins created by the clostridium tetani are able to severely impact the nervous system. Animals can present with the following symptoms: muscle stiffness as evidenced by a sawhorse stance; a decrease in water and feed consumption; hypersensitivity to light and noise; and muscle fasciculations. The tetanus antitoxin booster binds the circulating tetanus toxins to the antitoxin in the vaccine. The puncture wound requires cleansing, and in addition, any excess fluids around the site should be drained off. Topical penicillin is rubbed onto the injury. The animal should be given an IV infusion with penicillin and other fluids. It is recommended that horses receive an annual tetanus vaccination; however, dogs and cats are not very susceptible to tetanus.

DERMATOLOGIC DISEASES

RINGWORM

Ringworm (dermatophytosis) is a fungal disease that infects the skin, hair, and claws of patients. The ringworm fungus feeds on the keratin found in the layers of these areas. Most ringworm is caused by the *Microsporum canis* species in dogs, although some cases are caused by the *M. gypseum* or *Trichophyton mentagrophytes* species. Once infected, dogs will develop lesions of alopecia and crusts, as well as bumps on the skin (mainly on the face, ears, tail, and feet). Ringworm is zoonotic and is spread very easily by contact with contaminated objects or infected animals; however, some humans and animals can be asymptomatic carriers, which means that they have ringworm but show no symptoms. Coming in contact with an infected animal does not necessarily mean that it will cause infection; it depends on the species of fungus and the age, health condition, and other factors of the host.

CTENOCEPHALIDES FELIS

Ctenocephalides felis is a common cat flea. The fleas lay their eggs in the fur of the host (dog or cat), and the eggs will fall onto the carpet or outside onto the dirt where they hatch about 1–6 days later. The flea larvae that just hatched will feed on organic debris in the environment and the feces of adult fleas. In order for the larvae to develop, the environment must be warm, shaded, and moist. Fleas inside of a house will dig deep into carpet fibers or floor cracks and damp basements. Mature larvae produce a cocoon where it pupates, and once the pupa is mature, it emerges from the cocoon when stimulated by physical pressure or heat. If not stimulated, the adult flea may remain in the cocoon for a few weeks or up to a year if conditions allow. Adult fleas normally do not leave their host unless forced off, and they begin feeding immediately once on the host. Fleas mate in a couple of days after feeding and can produce up to 50 eggs a day, and they continue producing eggs for up to 100 days.

NEOPLASTIC DISEASES

Neoplasms, or growths, may be described as either **benign** (non-cancerous) or **malignant** (cancerous). Cancer is often defined in terms of the tumor site, the severity, and the type of tissue in which the growth is located. Other terms often used to describe a growth include mass, lump, lesion, neoplasm, tumor, and malignancy. Normally, the primary danger associated with a benign tumor is derived from the place it occupies inside the body. A tumor can prevent the body from functioning normally and thus can be dangerous or even life-threatening. More serious tumors are those described as both cancerous and metastatic. These types of tumors are invasive and malignant. These cancer cells often break free and move into a secondary region of the body. The regions frequently involved include the lymph nodes, bones, lungs, and other internal organs. This spreading of cells from the primary site to the secondary position is known as **metastasis**. These locations need not have any relative connection. The terms primary and secondary are used only to designate the original tumor as opposed to any that later emerge if the cancer spreads.

TYPES OF THERAPY TO TREAT TUMORS

Localized tumors have not spread to other parts of the body and are often fairly simple to remove if they are also encapsulated (i.e., a lump with clear margins) but may be more difficult if they are diffuse (fuzzy, or tentacle-like). It is important to note that malignant tumors should be removed along with approximately 2-3 cm or 1-2 inches of healthy tissue bordering the tumor.

- **Cryosurgery** is done by freezing tiny external epithelial lesions with liquid nitrogen or N_2O. The cancerous tissue is thereby frozen, following which it dies and can be sloughed off, debrided, or otherwise removed.
- **Chemotherapy** applies cytotoxic agents to the cancerous regions. Chemotherapy cannot be described as a cure-all for cancer, as it is toxic not only to cancer cells but to healthy cells as well. However, chemotherapy has been able to create a state of remission in some patients. The types of cancers which best respond to this type of treatment are known as systemic and metastatic cancers.
- **Radiotherapy** applies a dose of ionizing radiation to the cancerous region. It interrupts the cell's DNA replication, which results in its death.
- **Cauterization** uses various methods to burn away tiny epithelial tumors.

Sarcoma

Sarcomas are classified as a malignancy that grows in muscle, tendon, bone, fat, or cartilage, along with various other soft tissues. Sarcomas originate in mesenchymal connective tissues or the embryonic mesodermal tissues found in muscle, bone, fat, or cartilage.

The formation of the term has specific meaning. The prefix (sarco-) comes from the Greek word *sarkos*, meaning "flesh." The suffix *-oma* also comes from the Greek and means "swelling" or "tumor." The suffix *-oma* is typically used to refer to a tumor, benign or malignant. Thus, the term fibroma refers to a tumor that has its starting point in the fibers of muscle or nerves. This type of tumor is benign. Chondrosarcoma refers to a malignant tumor that originates in the cartilage, and sarcoma refers more generally to any cancer of connective tissue. Other malignant tumors ending in the suffix *-oma* include melanoma, insulinoma, seminoma, and thymoma.

Melanoma

Melanoma is a malignant tumor or cancer that may or may not be accompanied by dark pigmentation (if pigmented, it is usually black). This type of cancer is more commonly found in dogs than in cats. Melanoma can be unrelenting, and it often grows quickly. The tumor can **metastasize** or spread within the body quite rapidly. The spreading of this cancer occurs when the original tumor is transported by the lymphatic system to the lymph nodes or via the vascular system in blood cells. Dogs have a 1 in 20 chance of having any tumor diagnosed as malignant melanoma. The most common sites for development of melanoma are on the skin, on the animal's digits, and in the mouth (more particularly found on the face, trunk, feet, and scrotum). Animals with malignant melanoma are generally older, frequently 9-12 years of age. The tumor may have produced ulcers or bleeding. This form of cancer responds best to early detection and treatments. The chances for metastatic spread are increased with late detection of the cancer. Often, late detection will have given the cancer time to spread to various bodily organs.

Late-Stage Melanoma and Squamous Cell Carcinoma

The late diagnosis of malignant melanoma may preclude successful treatment. Certainly the prognosis is never as good as it could have been with earlier detection. **Late-stage melanoma** is not treatable with chemotherapy or radiation. The animal can be expected to survive for 2-3 months when the cancer reaches its most advanced stages.

Both cats and dogs can be diagnosed with **squamous cell carcinoma**. This is the most common type of malignant tumor that can develop in the epithelial layer of the skin, but it can also develop in the mucous membranes. This type of cancer is primarily found in cats, but it can also occur in dogs. It attacks the adjacent tissue and can spread to destroy bone in the animal's skeletal structure. The tumor appears grayish white or pink and has an abnormally shaped mass. It is most often located in the gingiva, tonsils, and nose. Ulceration is associated with this cancer. Squamous cell carcinoma is aggressive but treatable. The veterinarian may apply surgery, radiation, or hyperthermia in the removal of the tumor.

Epulis and Gingival Hyperplasia

Epulis is a non-malignant cancer that begins along the periodontal ligament. It will attack the adjacent tissue and spread to the bone. There are 3 kinds of epulides: fibromatous, ossifying, and acanthomatous. **Fibromatous epulides** are fashioned from a resilient tissue fiber. **Ossifying epulides** are fashioned from bone cells and fibrous tissue. The ossifying tumor can develop into cancer.

Acanthomatous epulides are detrimental to the bone structure. They are extensively intrusive and will infiltrate (grow into) normal bone. Once it has engulfed the bone it will destroy it. The animal may exhibit drooling, loss of appetite, difficulty eating, and bad breath. The tumor may also be of such a size and located in such a way as to cause the animal difficulty in breathing.

Gingival hyperplasia is a condition which occurs in animals that produces an excessive growth of gum tissue. This can be a genetically inherited condition, or it can be drug induced.

Complications of Chemotherapy

Cytotoxic agents are capable of destroying neoplastic cells, primarily by disrupting nucleic acid and protein synthesis. Cytotoxic agents (often referred to as chemotherapy medications) are toxic to all cells, but tend to be taken up faster by cells that are rapidly dividing—a characteristic common to cancer cells. Because bone marrow cells also divide rapidly, patients often become immunosuppressed when cytotoxic agents delay the production of crucial blood and immunological cells.

Common side effects of chemotherapy include alopecia, cardiotoxicity, vomiting, diarrhea, pancreatitis, hepatosis, neutropenia, thrombocytopenia, anemia, neurotoxicity, and renal toxicity.

Staff should wear protective garments to reduce harmful side effects induced by even incidental contact with powerful cytotoxic agents. Recommended garments include latex gloves, long-sleeved lab coats or long-sleeved surgical gowns, and safety goggles. The sleeves on the garments should have close-fitting cuffs. In addition, the waste products must be discarded according to specific biomedical waste guidelines. This waste includes syringes, IV administration sets, gauze, and gloves. The waste should be discarded in a plastic bag that has been securely closed.

Nutritional Diseases

Obesity

Obesity can cause irreversible damage to the pet's organs, bones, and joints. Obese pets are more prone to diabetes because the extra fat leads to insulin resistance in cats. Obese cats also run the risk of developing hepatic lipidosis, which can result if the cat becomes stressed and stops eating and the body starts metabolizing body fat for calories. The liver in a cat is not meant to process large amounts of fat, so it becomes overwhelmed and eventually fails, which can be life threatening. Pets can develop arthritis because there is an excess of weight being put on the joints leading to pain and discomfort caused by the degeneration of the joints. Obesity, especially in brachycephalic breeds, can cause trouble breathing because of the extra fat constricting the chest, making it harder for the pet to take deep breaths, and also causing the pet to cough because the lungs cannot inflate fully. To maintain a healthy weight for a pet, be sure to use an actual measuring cup to measure the amount of food per serving, limit treats, and only give healthy table food such as fruits and veggies (be sure that whatever food is given is not toxic to the animal). Give the pet daily exercise in some form, whether it is walking a dog or using a laser pointer for a cat to chase. There may be an underlying medical issue contributing to the pet's obesity such as Cushing syndrome or hypothyroidism, and testing should be done to rule out suspected disease.

Musculoskeletal Diseases

Osteoarthritis in Small Animals

Osteoarthritis results when the cartilage in the joints degenerates over the course of the patient's lifetime, causing pain and inflammation. The degeneration of joints could be caused by numerous things, such as infection or trauma. Joint and cartilage destruction and inflammation often result from degenerative joint disease, and after enough damage has taken place on the joints, grinding sounds may be heard during movement. Diagnosing osteoarthritis commonly involves the patient's overall disposition, pain upon palpation of the joints, and the owner's evaluation of their pet's movement and painful signs at home. Signs of osteoarthritis are lameness, muscle wasting, and inability to get up or down stairs or jump onto the bed. The pet may also have trouble getting up after laying down. Radiographs can show soft-tissue swelling around the joint, an increase in joint fluid, and a narrow joint space.

Reproductive Management

Female Reproductive System

The female reproductive system consists of many interrelated organs and anatomical features. The ovaries are a pair of organs necessary for female reproduction. The oval-shaped ovaries are located in the female's abdomen. **Ovaries** are responsible for the production of ova and hormones. The ova are female reproductive cells. **Ova** is the Latin word for "eggs," and the words may be used interchangeably. In most species, the ova will pass from the ovaries to the uterine horn or uterus, down to the uterine tubes (or Fallopian tubes or oviduct). The **uterus** has the following parts: uterine horns, body, and cervix, leading to the opening of the uterus. **Uterine horns** are the projections from the uterus that extend toward the uterine or fallopian tubes. Some animals do not have uterine horns.

Some animals are **polytocous** or **multiparous** (which means that the animal is able to have more than one baby at a given time), and will typically have longer uterine horns in order to carry several offspring. Species that typically have only one baby at a time are known as **monotocous** or **uniparous**. Their fetuses will grow and develop in the uterus itself. There are three layers within the uterus and uterine horns: **endometrium**, **myometrium**, and **perimetrium**. During the birthing process, the fetus will pass out of the uterus to the exterior environment. The vehicle for this passage is known as the vagina or **birth canal**. The **vulva** is the name given to the external female genitalia, which consists of the labia and opening to the urethra and internal sex organs.

Estrous Cycle: Proestrus

The duration of time that a female mammal can exhibit signs of sexual receptivity that may attract a mate is known as the **estrous cycle**. During this period of time the female has reoccurring physiological changes that can be attributed to the effects of reproductive hormones. There are 4 estrous phases: proestrus, estrus, diestrus, and anestrus. Some schema include a fifth phase called metestrus, which is very brief (1-5 days) immediately following the estrus phase.

Proestrus is the time period designed to prepare the uterus to receive an embryo. **Follicle stimulating hormone** or FSH induces ovarian follicles to develop and give off estrogen. **Estrogen** is a steroid hormone produced by the ovaries, which builds up in the uterus and uterine horns. During proestrus, estrogen induces endothelium to grow and form an inner layer in the uterus. This inside layer develops in preparation for a potentially fertilized egg to implant.

Estrous Cycle: Estrus, Metestrus, Diestrus, Anestrus

With the onset of **estrus**, the female is able to function in the reproductive process and ovulation occurs. The female's uterus and uterine horns are fully prepared to accept an embryo. Canines also experience a surge in **luteinizing hormone** (LH), which comes from the pituitary gland. The luteinizing hormone is responsible for ovulation, and indicates that the egg or eggs from the ovaries are ready for fertilization. Ovulation in cats and rabbits occurs through the breeding process, as they are nonspontaneous or induced ovulators.

A third phase called **metestrus** begins as luteinizing hormone levels begin to drop. In this post-ovulatory phase, each egg-containing follicle changes, bursts, and grows into a corpus luteum. A corpus luteum is a yellow mass that produces progesterone to continue thickening the lining of the uterus. The corpus luteum is needed to begin and to maintain a pregnancy, and functions to produce hormones during **diestrus**, the next phase of the estrus cycle. Finally, all sexual hormonal activity ceases during the concluding phase called **anestrus** (the resting phase).

PREGNANCY

Pregnancy is the term used to describe when a female animal carries an unborn offspring inside her body. A healthy pregnancy lasts from the time of fertilization to the birthing process. During the estrus cycle, the corpus luteum will work to consistently produce essential pregnancy-related hormones throughout most or all of a pregnancy. The duration of the production of hormones will vary in accordance with the type of species. Some types of animals will require the hormones to be produced throughout the entire period of the pregnancy. Other types of animals will only require the hormones until the placenta is formed.

The **placenta** is a transient organ inside the uterus that pregnant female mammals produce to supply oxygen and food to a fetus. Nutrition, oxygen, and other substances are delivered to the fetus through the umbilical cord. The **umbilical cord** is a flexible tube that links the abdomen of the fetus to the mother's placenta. This tube is also used to expel waste. The intrauterine **corpus luteum** will break down or decompose if a pregnancy does not actualize (i.e., if a fertilized egg does not implant there).

Different species have different average lengths of gestation.

- Dogs: 61 days (2 months)
- Cats: 64 days (2 months)
- Cows: 292 days (9 months)
- Horses: 336 days (11 months)
- Pigs: 114 days (3 months, 3 weeks, 3 days)

SPAYING AND NEUTERING

Spaying or **neutering** a pet is important for the pet's health. Spaying a female animal eliminates the potential to develop uterine or ovarian cancer, and it also eliminates the risk of pyometra (infection of the uterus). Spaying a female also lowers the risk of mammary cancer. Neutering a male animal eliminates the risk of testicular cancer and greatly reduces the risk of prostate and perianal cancer. Spaying and neutering pets also helps prevent overpopulation. Humane societies and shelters are constantly overpopulated with dogs and cats, and there are not enough staff members or funds to provide help to all of the stray or abandoned animals, which results in many animals being euthanized. Neutering a pet will also benefit the owner because the females will not go into heat, and it significantly lowers aggression, urine marking, mounting, and their desire to seek out a female in heat. This decreases the urge to roam away from the home, subsequently decreasing the risk of getting hit by a car or fighting with other animals.

COMMON HEALTH ISSUES IN HORSES

COLIC

Colic in horses causes considerable pain in the abdominal region and is the number one cause of premature equine fatality. This common problem can be a result of the following:

- Poor feed quality or feeding and hydration patterns
- Intestinal tears, displacements, torsions, or hernias
- Disproportionate gas
- Sporadic cramps
- **Ileus** (gastrointestinal atony)
- Parasitic infections

- **Volvulus** (bowel obstruction resulting from intestinal torsion)
- Intussusception
- Impactions
- Obstructions
- Displacement
- Inguinal hernias
- Ulcers

The colic's degree of severity may not be readily evident depending upon the disposition of the horse. Therefore, careful observation is recommended. In addition, the horse can be placed on a treatment regimen involving the following: fluid therapy, anti-inflammatory drugs, mineral oil, anti-flatulence medication, and anti-ulcer medication. Intestinal injuries (tears, torsions, hernias, etc.) typically require corrective surgery. The horse will need the following checked: vital signs, motility, and fecal output. The horse's state of hydration may be observed when a nasogastric tube is passed and gastrointestinal reflux is achieved. The horse will require regular moderate exercise, typically by being walked. The animal should be reintroduced to food slowly and gradually to reduce risk to the animal's digestive system.

Colitis

The exact cause of **acute colitis** in horses has yet to be fully understood. However, it appears to be linked to the following: dietary changes, excessive consumption of carbohydrates, *Clostridium perfringens* or colitis X, *Clostridioides difficile*, Potomac horse fever, antibiotic therapy, and the overuse of NSAIDs. Acute colitis presents in a horse with the following signs: inappetence, listlessness, depression, abdominal pain, hyper- or hypomotile gastric motility, increased heart and respiration rates, discolored mucous membranes, increased CRT (capillary refill time), diarrhea, dehydration, hypoproteinemia, imbalance of electrolytes, metabolic acidosis, and shock. Shock, in this situation, can often be attributed to endotoxemia (caused by endotoxin molecules released during the rapid growth or death of gram-negative bacteria).

Mucous membranes that have a brick or dark red color, or else a muddy, bluish, or cyanotic coloration, can be associated with acute colitis.

Fluid Therapy Management of Colitis

A horse with **colitis** should be treated with **fluid therapy**, consisting of a balanced electrolyte solution. This should reduce the inflammation and spasms experienced by the horse in the colon and abdominal region. Sometimes adequate amounts of potassium, chloride, and calcium are missing from the animal's diet, which can be supplemented during fluid therapy. Fluid therapy can also be used for the correction of **metabolic acidosis**. Metabolic acidosis is caused by an increase in the acidity of the blood. The result is a low blood pH level. The correction is made by adding sodium bicarbonate or anti-inflammatory drugs to the fluid therapy administered to the animal. However, a plasma transfusion is required when the total protein is low.

A **vasodilator** is an agent that opens and expands the blood vessels. This agent can be effective in combating the natural tendency toward vasoconstriction found in the equine medial and lateral digital arteries (located between the hoof wall and the distal phalanx). One commonly used vasodilator is known as nitroglycerin.

Salmonellosis

Many horses with diarrhea are diagnosed with **salmonellosis**. Salmonellosis is the number one cause of infectious diarrhea in horses for at least 2 reasons. First, salmonella is a **zoonotic** organism (can be passed between animals and humans) that is essentially ubiquitous in the equine environment (up to 20% of all horses may "shed" the organism, as it is present in their natural intestinal flora). Second, it is extremely contagious to other equines. Therefore, this contagious disease must be managed very carefully.

Salmonellosis can also be triggered by stress in the animal. Significant stress can be caused by the following: transportation by trailer (especially in the heat), sudden changes in feeding, use of antibiotics, sickness, surgery, or immunosuppression. It is important for signs of the disease not to be mistaken for similar signs displayed in animals with colitis. The animal can also have an acute case of diarrhea. Notably, the consistency and categorization of the diarrhea is profuse, watery, and foul-smelling. The animal may have **pyrexia** (a fever) and may also show signs of anorexia.

Management of Salmonellosis and Intestinal Clostridial Infections

In the event infectious salmonellosis is discovered, the animal should be isolated and only one handler should treat the animal to reduce cross-contamination risks. The handler should wear a gown, gloves, and protective boot covers. Thorough hand washing with a bactericidal solution is essential. Boots worn in the isolated horse's stall must be washed in a foot bath. Fluid therapy is given using a balanced electrolyte solution to reduce chances of dehydration and electrolyte disorders. Animals with hypoproteinemia may need a plasma transfusion. The animal's vital signs must be taken at regular intervals to ensure that the body is functioning adequately. The horse can be fed as often as its appetite allows. However, grain should not be included in the diet during this time.

Intestinal clostridial infections cause severe inflammation of the intestines. Colitis X, a widespread form of this disease, is usually discovered only after the death of the animal (during a postmortem examination) and is similar to colitis. Diarrhea is not observed in its early stages. Chronic pain is generated in the abdominal region within hours of contracting the disease. Hypermotility is typically seen. It is treated with an oral dose of antibiotics such as bacitracin. This disease should be treated in largely the same manner as that of colitis or salmonellosis.

Anterior Enteritis

Anterior enteritis can be linked to *Clostridium spp* (i.e., including multiple subspecies). However, this disease is normally thought of as **idiopathic**, with no apparent or known source. Clinical symptoms of this disease involve the following: severe colic, higher heart and respiration rates, and a probability of **pyrexia** (fever).

Horses are unable to expel excess stomach contents by way of **emesis** (vomiting). Thus, the treatment of anterior enteritis involves insertion of a **nasogastric tube** (NG tube). This tube is used to collect any gastric reflux fluids and to relieve gastric and intestinal fluid distension. Without placement of this tube, outright gastric rupture may occur from fluid overload. If the patient exhibits a lessening in symptoms after the NG tube is placed, then it is highly probable that the patient does not have an intestinal obstruction, and it is more likely that the patient has anterior enteritis. A rectal exam is needed for verification purposes and to make a more conclusive (albeit not always definitive) diagnosis.

Anterior Enteritis Treatment

Fluid therapy provides replacement of essential fluids, as oral fluid intake is trapped by the enteritis. A jugular vein access is usually needed, as the animal may require as much as 60-100 liters (16-26 gallons) of replacement fluids daily. The horse requires the monitoring of these vital signs: temperature, color of mucous membranes, CRT (capillary refill time) in the gingival area, and digital pulses. Toxemia can occur as a result of the bacterial toxins present in the horse's bloodstream. This poisonous condition can be a direct result of the severe intestinal upset that accompanies anterior enteritis.

Potomac Horse Fever (PHF)

Potomac horse fever (PHF) is also known as **monocytic ehrlichiosis** and **equine ehrlichial colitis**. Common vectors implicated in spreading the infective organism, *Ehrlichia risticii*, include flukes, ticks, helminths (parasitic worms), and aquatic insects. In the northeastern United States, a peak season exists for the spreading of this disease, largely between the months of June through August. Signs of the disease include depression, anorexia, and pyrexia; a decrease in gut sounds; abdominal pain; and watery diarrhea. Treatments involve the following:

- Isolation of the animal
- Oxytetracycline
- Fluid therapy consisting of a balanced electrolytic solution
- Frequent monitoring of vital signs

Laminitis is a serious concern. Vaccines preventing PHF have a high rate of effectiveness but are not 100% effective.

Hyperkalemic Periodic Paralysis (HYPP)

Some American Quarter Horse sires have a particular genetic mutation that brings about the disease known as **hyperkalemic periodic paralysis (HYPP)**, which can present with the following clinical symptoms: muscle fasciculations; incidences of colic, sweating, respiratory distress, and a prolapsed nictitating membrane ("third" eyelid); loose feces; and **ataxia** (unsteady gait). A blood test can be used to reveal if the horse is a homozygous affected animal, with 2 identical genes, or a heterozygous carrier. Ideally, however, the test will reveal that the horse has a normal genetic makeup. Breeding is not recommended for horses that have a positive blood test. In addition, horses that have HYPP should not be ridden, as gait and balance issues can present a danger to both the animal and the rider. The horse should be given a low potassium diet, and lots of fresh water. It is best not to give the horse alfalfa hay, feeding grass, or oat hay. In addition, stress should be reduced as much as possible.

Strangles

The bacteria *Streptococcus equi equi* can produce **strangles** in horses, which causes problems with breathing and swallowing. It is highly contagious, requires the animal to be placed in isolation, and has a low survival rate.

S. equi equi organisms can survive more than 4 weeks outside of the host if kept from heat and out of sunlight. Transmission of strangles occurs mainly through direct contact or shared items between horses such as feeding bins or anywhere a draining abscess has touched because they are infective. Strangles can also be transmitted by a handler's clothes or tools that have been exposed to the bacteria. Some horses may be carriers, which means they look otherwise healthy but carry the bacteria. They can randomly shed the bacteria for years, therefore always risking infecting other horses.

Symptoms and Treatment

The horse suffering from strangles will have significant abscesses on the lymph nodes, particularly those located underneath the mandible, the guttural pouches, and in the throat. Over time, the lymph nodes develop into empyema abscesses (pus-filled lesions), which require hot packs to facilitate the abscesses opening and draining. The abscesses may also require lancing to allow the fluid to drain. During this time the infected horse may experience **dysphagia**, finding it difficult to swallow. If this happens, the horse should be given additional fluids. The infected horse should also be fed slurries, which are a liquified mixture of water and feed.

Treatment requires constant access to fresh water. The infected horse should be kept warm and dry. The horse should also be given antipyretics and antibiotics. All materials that come into contact with the sick animal should be disposed of by fire or disinfected thoroughly. Though there is no cure, there is an intranasal vaccine that can reduce the seriousness of the symptoms.

Equine Herpes Virus 1 (EHV-1)

Equine Herpes Virus 1 (EHV-1) is a viral pathogen that primarily infects the respiratory tract and lymph nodes, as well as endothelial tissue in the nose, lungs, adrenal glands, thyroid, and central nervous system. Thus, neurological problems and spontaneous abortions in gravid horses may also occur. Typical infective symptoms include: fever, depression, inappetence, nasal discharge, and a cough. However, if neurologically afflicted, the horse can exhibit the following symptoms: ungainly movements, incontinence, posterior ataxia (lack of muscle control in the hind limbs), and an absence of tail tone. The horse may be found sitting as a dog or in a recumbent position. This is attributed to the paralytic state of the animal's hind legs.

To reduce fetal risks, the animal should be given a vaccination in the 5th, 7th, and 9th month of the pregnancy. The vaccine is Pneumabort K+1b. Abortion does not necessarily have to occur if the animal is infected during later gestational periods. Harm to the foal in utero is evident when a foal is delivered stillborn. A live foal may also die shortly after delivery. The horse may be given antibiotics, anti-inflammatory drugs, or corticosteroids. It is recommended that horses receive a preventive vaccination. However, abortions or neurological diseases can still occur if the vaccination does not provide enough protection.

Equine Herpes Virus 4 (EHV-4)

Equine Herpes Virus 4 (EHV-4) produces rhinopneumonitis and is common worldwide. However, its infection patterns differ significantly from those common to EHV-1. EHV-4 infections are largely localized to the respiratory tract and associated lymph glands, without the neurological and pregnancy issues.

EHV-4 is spread through close contact or through aerosolized body fluids (i.e., droplets scattered when sneezing, etc.). This viral disease targets the horse's upper respiratory tract and causes increased respiratory symptoms such as wheezing, rhonchi, rales, and stridor. In addition, the lymph nodes will swell from the infection. It is highly recommended that the horse be placed in isolation. The horse's environment should be protected against undue cold but should be well ventilated. The horse should be placed in a stall that is quiet and should not be placed under stress. The animal will require brief periods of exercise, as this is beneficial to blood circulation and lymph systems. This disease cannot be totally prevented by preemptive vaccination, but post-infection vaccination is thought to reduce the seriousness of the associated symptoms.

Equine Infectious Anemia (EIA)

Equine Infectious Anemia virus (EIA), also called **Swamp Fever**, can be spread by blood-feeding insects (mechanically; EIA does not replicate in insect vectors), and all body fluids and tissues of diseased animals can be potentially infectious. Because it can penetrate the placental barrier, EIA can also infect foals in utero. Iatrogenic spread by way of contaminated needles and medical supplies is a significant source of infection in horses.

Infection is for life, with recurring periods of remission and exacerbation, and asymptomatic spread is possible, though not common. Infected horses will have the following symptoms: pyrexia (fever), depression, weight loss, anorexia, and anemia. Infected animals are usually euthanized. In each state or province, local, state, provincial, and federal regulations should be consulted regarding the laws concerning euthanasia. Horses that are not put to sleep should be placed in isolation to prevent further contamination of other animals. This isolation must last the length of the horse's lifespan, as there is no known cure for EIA. Total isolation (including insect-free isolation) is the only way to keep other horses from contracting the disease.

Laminitis

Laminitis, most common in the front feet, is the irritation and inflammation of the epidermal (insensitive) and dermal (sensitive) laminae, the layers that hold the distal phalanx within the hoof wall. This can cause an irregular gait or severe lameness and can cause the hoof wall to detach.

Laminitis can result from many things, including: high fever, endotoxemia, sepsis, equine metabolic syndrome (from overconsumption of grain or sudden exposure to lush pasture), and road founder (trauma to the feet). Horses with laminitis may present with lameness, depression, lethargy, apprehension, pyrexia, anorexia, hoof sensitivity, and an increased digital pulse and temperature.

Radiographs can detect the extent of the laminitis. Treatment includes anti-inflammatory drugs, acepromazine, fluids such as LRS (lactated Ringer's solution), and trimming the hoof in a restorative fashion.

Vasodilators such as isoxsuprine hydrochloride and nitroglycerine can be applied to the horse's medial and lateral digital arteries. The horse should be given grass and hay to eat; it should not have access to grain. Veterinarians and farriers should work together on corrective measures.

Navicular Disease

Navicular disease is not fully understood; however, it is chronic, degenerative, and produces lameness and specific deterioration of the navicular bone (a small bone in a horse's foot). It may present with: stumbling, shorter strides, intermittent lameness, and possible evidence of hoof pain. Diagnosis should be confirmed with flexion tests, nerve blocking, and radiographs.

The horse can be treated with the following: anti-inflammatory medication, vasodilators, and corrective foot trimming and shoeing. One vasodilator often used for this condition is isoxsuprine hydrochloride. Some horses require a **surgical neurectomy**. This procedure is conducted along the nerve to the foot. The nerve is cut above the fetlock. However, this procedure should only be used when all other alternatives have been exhausted.

Vaccinations Given to Horses in the United States

There are routine sets of vaccinations that should be administered to horses based upon geographic location. The prevalence of a particular disease can relate directly to the region in which the animal resides. All horses in the United States should be given the following vaccinations:

- Rabies
- Tetanus
- West Nile virus
- Eastern and Western equine encephalomyelitis

Vaccinations that are available based on risk factors, primarily location, include the following:

- Anthrax
- Botulism
- Equine herpesvirus (rhinopneumonitis)
- Equine influenza
- Equine viral arteritis
- Leptospirosis
- Potomac horse fever
- Rotaviral diarrhea
- Snake bite
- Strangles
- Venezuelan equine encephalomyelitis (VEE)

Nursing and Rehabilitation

Patient Nursing Procedures

Layers of the Skin

Skin is composed of three layers: the epidermis, dermis, and hypodermis. The **epidermis** is the outer layer, which provides protection from sources of infection. The basement membrane is the protective layer connecting the epidermis to the dermis. The **dermis** contains the protein collagen, elastic tissue, and fibers that give skin its strength and support. The dermis contains sensory nerves that respond to painful stimuli, touch, and hot or cold temperatures. Finally, beneath the dermis is the **hypodermis**, which attaches the skin to the muscle and consists of connective tissue, providing insulation and protection to the body.

Placing an IV Catheter

Depending on the size of the patient, **IV catheters** vary in size: a 24 gauge is smaller and used in critical, smaller patients; a 20 gauge is larger and used in large-breed dogs. In surgery or emergency treatment, it is best to use a larger catheter in the patient, if possible, to allow a larger port of access to the vein. First, shave the area where the catheter will be placed, vacuum excess hair, and scrub the area rotating between chlorhexidine solution and alcohol approximately three times. The person restraining the pet will hold off the vein, and the person placing the catheter will locate the vein. Start low on the vein in case the catheter does not advance and you need to try again; that way, you can try again higher on the same vein. Insert the needle/catheter into the vein, and blood should flash into the hub of the end of the needle you are holding. Once blood is flowing back and the catheter is in the vein, swiftly advance the catheter over the needle into the vein as you are pulling the needle out of the vein. Place an injection plug into the end of the catheter to stop blood from flowing out. Last, tape the catheter in place so it is secure to the leg.

Wound Management

Appropriate wound treatment involves protective measures, evaluation, and treatment. The initial protective measure requires that the wound be covered with a dressing and/or a splint of some sort. The second step involves an evaluation of the wound's degree of severity. The most severe cases are those that require control of hemorrhaging. Once any hemorrhaging is under control, the wound should be checked to lessen further contamination and infection risks. Hair or other debris should be cleaned and clipped away from the area. The border surrounding the wound should be thoroughly cleansed with an antimicrobial/detergent scrub. This step also involves a sterile flush of any hollow body parts or organs. Getting rid of necrotic tissue is the step known as debridement. In addition, it may be necessary to place a drainage tube to allow excess air and fluid to exit the wound site.

Types of Open and Closed Wounds

Open wound refers to an injury that has an external break in the tissue.

- An **abrasion** is an open wound that involves a loss of the epidermis plus some of the dermis layer.
- An **avulsion** is an open wound that is a result of the tissues being torn from their attachments.
- An **incision** is an open wound caused by a sharp tool (surgery).
- A **laceration** is an open wound caused by tearing, which creates superficial and deeper tissue damage.
- A **puncture** is an open wound created by a sharp object (e.g., tooth) that could cause severe tissue damage and is at a high risk for infection.

Closed wounds are the result of damage beneath the skin's surface. Closed wounds consist of contusions defined as: **blunt force trauma**, which does not break the skin but does damage to it and the tissues underneath, and **crushing injuries**, which are closed wounds caused by excess force placed upon an area of the body over a length of time.

4 Phases of Wound Healing

There are 4 phases associated with wound healing: inflammatory, debridement, repair, and maturation.

- The **inflammatory phase** is the initial phase that follows an injury. This phase is associated with the appearance of scabs. Scabs are a crust over the injured area formed from blood, serum, and pus. This crust protects the wound so that healing can begin.
- The **debridement phase** commences about 6 hours after the injury takes place. Neutrophils and monocytes work to remove foreign material, bacteria, and necrotic tissue from the wound. Both neutrophils and monocytes can be described as white blood cells.
- In most cases, the **repair phase** starts approximately 3-5 days after the initial wound. However, the time associated with this phase is contingent upon foreign substances being adequately extracted from the infected area.

- The final phase is known as **maturation**, which can extend for a number of years and includes the process of scar lightening. Refashioning the collagen fibers and other fibrous tissue promotes complete wound recovery. Multiple phases may sometimes operate simultaneously, accomplished by a series of overlapping actions.

BANDAGING

The 3 principal layers of bandages are the non-adhesive primary layer, the secondary layer, and the tertiary layer. The **non-adhesive primary layer** is used without anything in between it and the wound. The type of tissue that forms over a wound, known as granulation tissue, should be treated with a non-adhesive primary layer. This bandage layer prevents further trauma to the injury site.

Exuded substances are soaked up by the cushioned, secondary layer. Common name brands include Kling or Sof-Kling.

Finally, the exterior layer, or tertiary layer, gives the 2 bottom layers more reinforcement. This reinforcement is due to the type of bandage used, including adhesive tapes, elastic bandages, Vet Wrap (3M), and conforming stretch gauze. The adhesive tape gives the bandage the ability to bond to the other layers. The elastic bandage and stretch gauze are expandable and flexible over the layers covering the wound.

TYPES OF DRESSINGS USED IN A BANDAGE APPLICATION

There are 3 types of bandages used on a wound: dry-to-dry bandages, wet-to-dry bandages, and wet-to-wet bandages.

Loose necrotic tissue should be addressed with a **dry-to-dry bandage**. The dry gauze stays in place with the follow-up application of a dry, absorbent wrap. The patient will experience pain whenever the bandage is removed, but dead and dying tissue is naturally debrided and removed with it.

It is best to use a **wet-to-dry bandage** on any infected or open wounds. If an exuded substance is present then the wound may require a wet, saline-moistened or medicated bandage placed inside and dry bandage coverings outside. This type of bandage is advantageous as it is able to treat infection and still absorb exudates that emanate from the wound. This type of bandage can also reduce pain associated with the removal of exuded substances attached to the binding. The bandages soak up excess fluid from the wound. The bindings are not taken off of the patient when wet. **Wet-to-wet dressings** can sometimes be useful for chronic wounds or for larger, ulcerated wounds that require internal tissue regrowth before epidermal tissue can grow and provide protective coverage. Deep pressure sores are one possible example. This form of bandage is removed while still wet.

REASONS AND PRECAUTIONS FOR BANDAGING THE LIMBS

A patient's limbs may require bandaging for a variety of reasons. These reasons include: to reduce or stop movement (i.e., in bone fractures), to prevent infection or contamination, and to stabilize a limb for purposes of fluid therapy (i.e., a subcutaneous infusion or IV line).

The best bandage application provides an even distribution of pressure throughout the bandaged area of the limb. Equally distributed pressure ensures reasonably unimpeded circulation in the limb. Using adequate padding and overlapping the bandage wrap by 50% will help ensure proper tightness when bandaging. In addition, the entire limb distal to an injury requires a bandage whenever the proximal appendage requires a bandage.

Whenever a limb bandage has been placed, it is necessary to carefully ensure adequate circulation. Toes and nails should be completely covered in order to prevent trauma, though the pad and third and fourth nail should be visible and accessible from the end of the bandage.

Bandages should not start at a joint, rather proximal or distal to it, in order to prevent skin injury caused by the bandage itself.

Reasons and Precautions for Bandaging the Head and Neck

The patient's head and neck may require a protective bandage after certain surgeries. The following surgeries are associated with this need: postocular surgery, aural hematoma repair, and ear surgery. In addition, a bandage of this type may be needed to firmly secure a jugular catheter or a nasogastric or pharyngostomy tube into place.

Wound edema is a condition in which serous fluid builds up in excessive amounts in the patient. In the head and neck area, this condition can endanger the patient's life. Therefore, the condition of the wound and surrounding swelling should be checked often. This may require removal of the bandage to allow an inspection of the site. The patient's respiration, skin color, and involved mucous membranes should be carefully checked. The bandage should be slack enough to allow the insertion of 2 fingers underneath the bindings. Patients with respiratory concerns should have their bindings loosened. It may be necessary to reapply a different bandage. Animals that are opposed to wearing a head or neck bandage may need to be given an Elizabethan collar. The Elizabethan collar is used to prevent the animal's access to the bandaging material.

Reasons and Precautions for Bandaging a Tail

There may be occasions when an animal's tail may also require a bandage. This bandage should incorporate and be able to cover the animal's wound. An animal that has had a tumor removed or a partial tail amputation will also benefit from the application of a bandage.

An animal experiencing a period of persistent diarrhea may also benefit from the application of a tail bandage. This bandage can bundle up both the appendage and any associated hair, and thereby better help in securing and maintaining the cleanliness of the animal.

An amputation can involve persistent bleeding. This bleeding can be induced, exacerbated, or perpetuated by excessive tail wagging or by bringing the intact portion of the tail in contact with a hard object. Tail wagging movements can be reduced by sedating the animal. However, this is only a temporizing intervention and one of last resort, due to the negative effects of such medication. An optional way to lessen tail movement is to slide a tube-shaped item over the bottom of the remaining portion of the tail. This should reduce the momentum of the tail wagging, and provide some additional protection to the animal's tail. Analgesics or painkillers can also be given to the patient to reduce the animal's distress and painful symptoms.

Managing Hospitalized Patients

Cleaning a Kennel

The first step to cleaning a kennel is to remove the animal and any bedding, bowls, and toys. Next, wipe away any feces, urine, or vomit from the kennel. Use a bristle brush to scrub the kennel with the disinfectant starting at the top with the ceiling of the kennel, all sides, the door, and the floor of the kennel. All hinges and latches need to be scrubbed as well. The disinfectant solution must sit for 5–10 minutes to be effective, and then it should be rinsed with water. All dishes should be soaked in the dilute disinfectant after being cleaned with soap and water. All blankets should be washed.

Maintaining an IV Catheter for a Patient

An intravenous (IV) catheter may be in place for up to 72 hours in a hospitalized patient. During hospitalization, the IV catheter must be monitored to make sure that proper placement is maintained and that the catheter is still **patent** or unobstructed. The patient may move around and twist the IV line or even pull on the IV catheter, which could pull it out of the vein. The patient could also attempt to bite or pull at the catheter with its teeth to try to remove it. To make sure the catheter is patent, a syringe of flush (lactated Ringer's or sodium chloride) can be administered through the catheter to feel if it is moving through the vein or pull back on the plunger to see if blood pulls into the syringe from the vein. The patient must be monitored to ensure that the foot doesn't get swollen if the tape for the catheter becomes too tight.

Getting a Hospitalized Patient to Eat

If the patient has not been eating enough food to meet its resting energy requirement (RER), then a feeding plan must be put in place to provide nutrients. In order to create a feeding plan, the patient's ability to eat should be evaluated. Enticing the patient to eat by placing a small amount of canned food in the mouth may be just enough to get the patient to eat. **Syringe feeding** is another method that is done with a liquid mixture of canned food and water in a feeding syringe. To syringe feed a dog, the tip of the syringe is placed inside of the cheek, emptying small amounts at a time while waiting for the dog to swallow. Another method is to place a **feeding tube** and administer either a liquid or blended food product through the tube. While in the hospital, the patient should be fed on a schedule according to their caloric requirements. To calculate the patient's RER (resting energy requirements), use the formula of 15 kcal/lb for the dog and 20 kcal/lb for the cat. The feeding schedule will be decided by how well the patient tolerates being fed, and feeding the amount close to the patient's RER is recommended.

Maintaining a Hospitalization Form for a Hospitalized Patient

If a patient is presenting with an illness that requires hospitalization, then routine monitoring of the patient must be recorded. Hospitals will commonly have a hospitalization form on the patient's kennel for the duration of the stay. The form will have the patient's name, client's name, signalment (species, breed, age, and sex), weight, date, and the illness or injury. Any medications given or that will need to be given will be recorded on the form including the strength, dose, and how many times per day it is to be administered. If IV fluids are being administered, that will be recorded on the form as well, along with the rate and type of fluids. Routine temperature, pulse, and respiration (TPR) measurements will be recorded on the hospitalization form throughout the day. The attending veterinarian will record how often the patient should be examined and if certain tests need to be run, such as a CBC, on the form. Once the requested treatments and exams are done, the person should initial the form so other staff members will know what has been done. Hospitalization forms are an effective form of communication.

Administering Medications

Oral Administration

The **oral route** of drug administration is used for tablets, capsules, solutions, and suspensions. Oral dosing is generally used for systemic effects after drug absorption from the GI tract; however, the disadvantage of the oral administration route is the slow onset of action for the drug as well as irregular absorption. Contraindications for oral medications include vomiting, injury in the oral cavity or esophagus, or problematic swallowing.

The patient should be given medication by mouth in an oral dosage that is liquid, semisolid, or in a pill or capsule form. **Liquid medication** can be injected into the pocket of the cheek via a dropper or syringe. Pills or capsules should be positioned toward the back of the animal's tongue. This is accomplished with one hand, while the other hand works to keep the animal's mouth open. Once the pill has been positioned, the animal's mouth is held closed until the animal has swallowed noticeably. Gently stroking the animal's throat downward while holding the mouth closed with the nose upward can help trigger a swallowing response.

Methods for Oral Administration to Dogs and Cats

A **pill popper device** is a long plastic handle with a rubber end with a slit to hold the pill. Once the popper is placed in the dog's mouth, the plunger is pushed from the opposite end forcing the pill out and into the dog's throat. Tablets and capsules can also be hidden inside of soft treats or canned food and be fed to the dog. In order to administer a tablet or capsule to a cat orally, pill poppers can also be utilized, though pill administration to felines is difficult. When possible, the medications should be administered in liquid or long-acting injectable form. If pills are the only option and pill poppers are not available, someone should hold the cat while the other person quickly lifts up the top jaw and places the pill at the back of the cat's tongue so that it is swallowed.

Topical Administration

Topical medications can be placed on or rubbed into the skin after sanitizing and clipping any hair in any region to be used for medication application.

However, it is perfectly acceptable to place appropriate topical medications directly on any lesions or wounds. The directions accompanying each medication will provide specific information regarding the amounts recommended to be applied at any given time. In addition, the directions should note the time it takes for the medication to be absorbed. The technician that applies the medication should wear gloves to prevent accidental absorption into their skin.

The topical route of administration is used for parasitic control, local skin treatments, and therapeutic agents. Drugs applied to the skin (topical) for a local effect include antifungals, anti-inflammatory agents, and antiseptics. Topical drugs come in different forms, including powders, creams, liquids, and sprays.

Parenteral Administration

Parenteral routes of administration include intravenous (IV), intramuscular (IM), and subcutaneous (SQ) injections. Medications by injection typically take effect much more quickly, will not be regurgitated or expectorated, and are more completely absorbed into the system than drugs administered orally. IV administration has a quick onset of action, usually within seconds, and the onset of action for the IM and SQ routes is within minutes.

When injecting animals raised for human consumption, it is important to document the medication, dosage, site of injection, and withdrawal period of the injection. IM injections should not be administered in the leg or the loin because the muscles in those areas are fabricated into valuable cuts of meat after slaughter. Instead, SQ and IM injections should be administered in the neck in the triangle of space between the spinal column, shoulder, and nuchal ligament.

Different species and injection methods require different needle sizes and injection sites:

	SQ			IM		
Species (All ages)	**Injection Site**	**Needle gauge**	**Needle length**	**Injection Site**	**Needle gauge**	**Needle length**
Dogs & Cats	Loose skin over shoulders and neck	20-18	1.0-1.5 inch	Quadriceps muscles (avoiding the sciatic nerve), also the caudal thigh muscles in dogs	23-21	1.0-1.5 inch
Horses	Neck triangle	20-18	1.0 inch	Neck triangle, semitendinosus, pectoral muscles, rump	20-18	1.0-1.5 inch
Cows	In the neck in the triangle of space between the spinal column, shoulder, and nuchal ligament	18-14	0.5-0.75 inch	In the neck in the triangle of space between the spinal column, shoulder, and nuchal ligament (2 inches smaller cranially than the SQ triangle)	20-16	0.75-1.0 inch
Goats & Sheep	Loose skin behind the elbow, on the side of the neck, in the flank area	22-18	0.5 inch	In the neck, in the loose skin behind the elbow	22-18	0.5-1.0 inch
Pigs	Juveniles: loose skin of flank and elbows Adults: behind the ear	20-14	0.5-1.0 inch	In the neck, behind and below the ear	20-14	0.5-1.0 inch

SQ Injection Technique

Certain medications such as antibiotic or pain control injections and even vaccines will need to be administered **subcutaneously** (SQ, or under the skin). To administer an injection SQ, first find the appropriate area of clean, dry, loose skin and gently pinch the loose skin between your thumb and forefinger. Pull the skin up to create a tent. The area pinched between your fingers creates a small indentation. Take the cap off of the needle, and insert the sterile needle into the skin tent indentation parallel to the skin's surface. Once inserted, pull back on the syringe plunger to be sure no blood is drawn back, and ensure that you are in the SQ layer. If no blood is seen, push the plunger and medication forward into the skin. Remove the needle once the syringe is empty.

Large quantities of injections should be distributed across multiple injection sites.

IM Injection

The animal receiving an **intramuscular (IM) injection** should have the injection site cleansed by using a cotton ball doused in alcohol. Some likely places for an intramuscular injection are in the muscles of the neck, the semitendinosus muscle (in the thigh), the gluteus muscle (in the flank), and the pectoralis descendens (a chest muscle). The medical staff should be careful to avoid injections near joints, blood vessels, or large fat deposits. The effectiveness (in duration) of some drugs can be extended with the application of an IM injection.

Some drugs require administration through intramuscular injections alone. For instance, an injection of procaine penicillin directly into the bloodstream will result in a harmful reaction in the patient. The medical staff should be on the alert for the following reactions after injection: restlessness, agitation, head tossing, snorting, eye rolling, violent thrashing, or a state of collapse.

IV Injections

The animal receiving an **intravenous injection** should have the injection site cleansed with a cotton ball doused in alcohol and firm swabbing of the injection site.

IV administrations can be given in the cephalic, femoral, saphenous, or jugular veins. The IV is the quickest route to produce the desired effect. This also is an ideal method when a large dose of medication or fluid must be given. The cephalic region refers to the area within or on the head. The femoral region refers to the area of the thigh or the femur. The saphenous vein is found in the leg and refers to 2 major veins which travel from the foot to the thigh. The jugular vein refers to one of the 4 main pairs of veins found in the neck.

Other Parenteral Administration Routes

There are additional distinctions which may be involved, including intradermal, intraperitoneal, intracardiac, intratracheal, intramedullary or intraosseous, intranasal, intrathecal, and intra-arterial. **Intradermal** (between skin layers) is abbreviated as ID. **Intraperitoneal** (into the abdominal cavity) is abbreviated as IP. **Intracardiac** (into the heart) is abbreviated as IC. Intratracheal (into the trachea) is abbreviated as IT. **Intramedullary** or intraosseous (into a bone) is abbreviated as IO. Intranasal (into the nose) is abbreviated as IN. **Intrathecal** (into the space around the spinal cord) is also abbreviated as IT, and thus is context specific. Intra-arterial (into an artery) is abbreviated as IA.

Otic and Optic Administration

Otic or aural administration refers to the application of medication to the ear. Medication should be applied to clean, dry ears dropwise without touching the dropper to the ear itself. Once applied, the ear should be gently massaged, allowing the medication to distribute properly; if the animal has otitis media or another ear infection, manipulation of the ear may be painful.

Optic administration of medication refers to the application of a drug directly to the eye. Medication is administered dropwise or as an ointment. To apply drops, tilt the animal's head back and gently lower the lower eyelid, dropping medication into the inner corner of the eye; hold the head back and steady until the animal has blinked a few times. To apply ointment, tilt the animal's head back and gently lower the lower eyelid, squeezing a line of ointment on the inside of the lower lid. Gently massage the lid while closed to distribute the medication. Observe the animal while the vision remains blurry.

Owners should be educated on how to administer otic or optic medications if prescribed.

Fluid Therapy

Contraindications

There are times when an animal's immediate condition may make it inadvisable to pursue rapid fluid replacement. For example, **pulmonary edema**, an excess of fluid accumulating in the lungs, is a concern that requires regular and frequent observations until all troubling fluid dynamics can be adequately addressed and resolved. Other problems that may make rapid fluid replacement therapy inadvisable include: pulmonary contusions, brain injury, severe ascites, cerebral edema from any cause, and congestive heart failure. If the animal shows signs of over-hydration, then fluid therapy must be halted. **Over-hydration symptoms** include: restlessness, an elevated respiratory rate, wheezing or other sounds of respiratory compromise emanating from the lungs, an abnormal rise in blood pressure, chemosis, and pitting edema. **Chemosis** is an enlargement or swelling of the eye whites. **Pitting edema** is a sign of fluid overload in the extremities, seen when the tissues are firmly pressed and do not rebound (leaving a "pit" or dent where previously pressed).

At the conclusion of fluid replacement therapy, the animal is again evaluated. The weight of the animal should be taken. The specific gravity and amount of any recent urine voiding should also be noted.

Routes

Fluids can be given to a patient in a number of ways. Fluids can be given through oral, subcutaneous, percutaneous, intravenous, or intramedullary routes into the body. A syringe or a feeding tube is often used in the administration of fluids by oral means. However, an oral administration route is not advisable in animals displaying certain adverse conditions. These include: vomiting, esophageal injury, and/or pancreatitis.

A subcutaneous fluid replacement route is often used in cases that exhibit symptoms of mild dehydration. However, the subcutaneous fluid route cannot be applied if the patient is in shock or in cases of severe dehydration. This is due to the relatively slow rate of absorption associated with poor peripheral circulation, which is a symptom of shock. Therefore, it is best to administer intravenous fluids to patients in shock accompanied by moderate to severe dehydration. Younger animals, or those that are very small, should be given fluids by intramedullary infusion. This method allows the fluid to be absorbed quickly, since it is delivered directly into the highly vascularized bone marrow.

Calculating the Fluid Replacement Volume

Fluid levels must be promptly replaced in patients that are suffering from hypovolemic shock or severely dehydrated conditions. These patients should receive 60-90 mL/kg/hr of fluids to replace the lost volume. The replacement fluids should be given to the patient over a 12- to 24-hour time frame in order to avoid inducing other problems. The total fluid amount needing to be replaced can be calculated by determining the daily fluid requirements. The calculation for the amount of replacement fluids required is the percent dehydration (as a decimal point figure) multiplied by the animal's body weight in kg, multiplied by 1,000 to obtain the replacement amount in milliliters.

The quantity of maintenance fluid needed is approximately 40-60 mL/kg/day. A measurement must be taken to determine the volume of urine excreted on a daily basis. In addition, diarrhea, vomitus, and other concurrently lost fluids should be measured. This includes any fluid that drains from an injury. This provides an estimated amount of the total fluid needed to provide rehydration, maintenance, and replacement fluid for that which is continuously excreted in one form or another.

Replacement solutions include Normosol R and lactated Ringer's solution or LRS. Maintenance solutions are known as: Normosol M and normal saline with KCl.

Importance of Understanding if Other Medications Have Been Taken

It is important to ask owners if their pet is taking any medications or supplements, or if they have treated the illness or injury the pet is presenting for. Certain medications should not be administered to dogs. Aspirin and ibuprofen, for example, are human NSAIDs, but they can be dangerous if given to dogs even if it is the correct dose due to sensitivity. They can also cause stomach ulcers and kidney failure. If an owner gives their dog Tylenol (acetaminophen) at the incorrect dose, this can cause liver and kidney damage, and it converts hemoglobin to methemoglobin, which results in decreased oxygen delivery to the tissues. If the owner has been giving their pet NSAIDs, then the veterinarian cannot prescribe an NSAID designed for dogs because they cannot be taken together. Any of these medications should be avoided at all costs in cats because even one dose of Tylenol given to a cat could cause death.

Monitoring Giving Lifelong Medications

If a patient is on a lifelong medication such as a thyroid medication, it is necessary to recheck the pet's thyroid level regularly to ensure that they are on the right dosage and determine that the patient's health status is normal while on the medication. If an animal is diabetic, then you will want to be sure that the client is administering the correct dose of insulin to the patient, because there can be serious complications if the pet is given an incorrect dosage, such as hypoglycemia if the pet is given too much insulin. If the patient is taking phenobarbital to help control seizure activity, it is crucial to ask the owners if the pet has had any seizures while on the medication and how they are doing in case the dosage needs to be adjusted. Also, if the patient is taking phenobarbital regularly, a phenobarbital level blood test will need to be run once a year to make sure that the dosage is accurate.

Physical Rehabilitation

Cryotherapy

Cold therapy or cryotherapy can be helpful in veterinary physical rehabilitation in the first 72 hours after surgery or acute injury. It can be applied locally via ice or cold packs. Towels soaked in ice water can also be used, but they should be changed frequently so that they are cold enough to be therapeutically useful. Localized cryotherapy promotes vasoconstriction, helps manage pain, and reduces cellular metabolism locally, which can prevent edema, muscle spasms, and an immune response near the injury or incision. Cryotherapy is especially helpful after injuries to tendons, ligaments, or bone and in managing osteoarthritis.

Heat Therapy

Heat therapy is most useful in veterinary physical rehabilitation starting 72 hours after surgery or injury, and it can be continued for the next five to seven days via hot packs, heat wraps, towels in hot water, or submersion in warm water. Beginning heat therapy too early will interfere with the healing process as it promotes vasodilation and impulse conduction in the tissues. It is also useful in pain management. Heat therapy is helpful after 72 hours in cases of chronic inflammation; muscle tension; pain; injury to tendons, ligaments, or bones; osteoarthritis; and IVDD (intervertebral disk disease).

Passive Range of Motion

Physical rehabilitation through passive range of motion activities helps promote blood and lymph flow through tissues, as well as promoting synovial fluid production in the joints. These non-weight-bearing movements help prevent stiffness and pain, although they do not prevent muscle atrophy caused by long-term lack of use. Passive range of motion activities are helpful after injury to or surgery on extremities or in cases of paralysis. Animals can be in lateral recumbency or standing (if they can safely tolerate it), while the therapist gently and fully flexes and extends one joint at a time on the limb. Alternating, slow, gentle adduction and abduction of the limb can also be helpful, as well as bicycling the limb to reach all joints and tissues with one set of motions.

Underwater Treadmill

The **underwater treadmill** works to improve the dog's range of motion, increase muscle strength, and increase endurance. The underwater treadmill also helps patients with soft-tissue injuries, weak muscles, and postsurgical care such as an amputation or orthopedic surgery. The temperature of the water is kept at around 95 °F, which helps with flexibility and allows for an improved range of motion for affected joints. Depending on the patient's size and progress, the level of the water and the speed of the treadmill are adjusted accordingly. A water level right above the feet is helpful to patients with reduced flexion in the carpus and hock. A water level at the elbows is great for athletic dogs to improve their endurance because there is a lot of resistance and not a lot of buoyancy. Water levels at the shoulder benefit patients with osteoarthritis or surgical recovery because this provides the most buoyancy with little weight on the joints.

Disposal of Hazardous Materials

Used sharps need to be disposed of into a sharps container directly after use. Items categorized as **sharps** include items with rigid corners or edges that could cut an individual, such as needles, blades, broken glass, and slides. After using a syringe, the needle should not be removed or bent in any way and you should not recap the needle. **Sharps containers** are sealed and made of a material that is resistant to punctures. After the container is full, the lid is closed, and it is nearly impossible to open again. Once sealed, sharps containers are water resistant. The sharps container should be labeled as a biohazard. A medical waste disposal company will pick up and dispose of the sharps.

Clinical Diagnostic Procedures

Running Quality Controls on Laboratory Instruments

Running **quality controls** on lab equipment should ideally be done at each shift. There should be a log book in which the results of the controls are logged and tracked to look for trends. Each quality control should be assessed for accuracy according to the reference ranges before patient samples are run. Quality control results are accurate when they fall into the average reference ranges. Differences in quality control results must be evaluated; for example, if one day the reading is at the high end of the reference range and the very next day it reads at the low end of the reference range, then something may be wrong with the instrument because this could reflect the difference between a normal and an abnormal value in a patient. Proper handling and storage techniques must be used with quality control material. Some may need to be refrigerated, and some may need to be reconstituted with distilled water (not tap water). Certain products have a short shelf life after being opened, so carefully reading instructions is vital.

Blood Pressure

Systolic arterial pressure (SAP) is created when the left ventricle contracts and blood is pushed into the aorta. Then, that left ventricle empties and relaxes, and it begins to fill again while the aortic pressure decreases, giving the **diastolic arterial pressure (DAP)**. The **mean arterial pressure (MAP)** is measured through a calculation from both the systolic and diastolic values. The actual calculation is $MAP = DAP + \frac{1}{3}(SAP - DAP)$. **Blood pressure** can be monitored directly using an arterial catheter (a catheter inserted into an artery) giving continuous monitoring or indirectly by use of a Doppler or an automated blood pressure cuff to detect the arterial blood flow in a peripheral artery.

Normal blood pressure values for a dog's SAP range from 90-140 mmHg, and MAP in dogs ranges from 60-100 mmHg. Normal systolic values for cats range from 80-140 mmHg, and normal mean pressures in cats range from 60-100 mmHg.

Review Video: Diastolic vs Systolic
Visit mometrix.com/academy and enter code: 898934

Doppler BP Measurement

The **Doppler measurement of BP** uses a crystal instead of a stethoscope to detect blood flow. The equipment needed to perform a Doppler BP reading includes a tape measure, a sphygmomanometer, ultrasound gel, inflatable cuff, and the Doppler unit. An appropriately sized cuff is chosen and placed on the patient's front limb (just below the elbow) or the hind limb, and then the cuff tubing is connected to the sphygmomanometer. A small area is shaved distal to the cuff over the artery (if it is the front limb, shave between the carpal and metacarpal pads). Apply ultrasound gel to the Doppler crystal, and then place the crystal on the shaved area to find an audible pulse. Inflate the cuff using the sphygmomanometer until you cannot hear the pulse anymore, and then slowly release the pressure while listening for the pulse to return. Record the number that the sphygmomanometer reads when the pulse is heard again. The reading mostly relates to the systolic BP in dogs, whereas in cats it is more closely related to the mean arterial pressure.

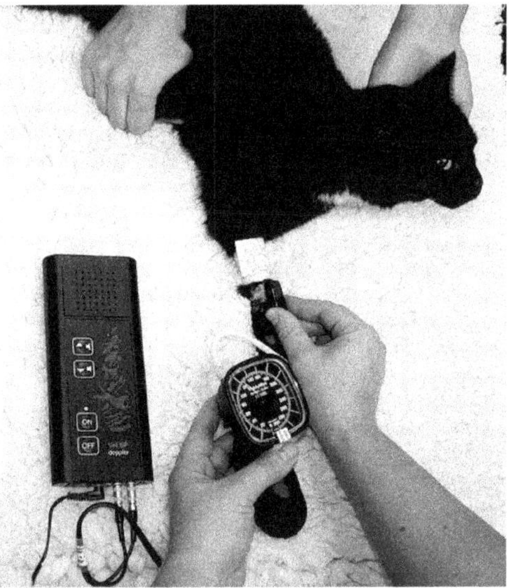

Oscillometric BP Measurement

To perform an indirect **oscillometric blood pressure (BP) reading**, the cuff size needs to be accurate for the patient. An appropriate cuff size will have a width measurement that is 40% of the limb circumference in dogs and 30% in cats. The cuff can be measured by laying it lengthwise along the limb, making sure that the edges measure 25-50% of the circumference of the limb. The limb chosen should be level with the heart. Common placements are the midradius on the front leg, midtarsus on the rear leg, or the tail base. The tubing from the cuff should run along the artery at the chosen limb and lead toward the BP monitor, not the patient. The cuff should be placed around the limb securely but not too tightly, and it should never be taped in place because this would result in inaccurate readings. This BP monitoring is done with a machine that will inflate and deflate the cuff and display the systolic, diastolic, and mean arterial pressure on a screen.

Electrocardiography

Non-invasive **electrocardiography** can be accomplished through the use of bioelectrical leads placed in such a way as to externally sense the heart's electrical conduction activity. The device is used in making a profile of the electrical impulses that govern and regulate the function of the heart. Each impulse is given immediately prior to various areas of the heart experiencing muscle contraction or movement. The abbreviation for electrocardiogram is EKG. EKG tracings are visible when drawn by a heated stylus on heat-sensitive graph paper, or as transiently displayed on a monitor screen.

The Cardiac Cycle

The **cardiac cycle** refers to all cardiac events that occur from one heartbeat to the next. It is coordinated by electrical impulses which properly time **systole** (chamber contraction and emptying) and **diastole** (chamber relaxation and filling) of the myocardium.

Electrical activity begins at the **sinoatrial (SA) node** (considered the pacemaker of the heart and located in the right atrium) and spreads through the atrial walls; **depolarization** causes the myocardium to contract, **repolarization** causes the myocardium to relax. When depolarization impulses reach the **atrioventricular (AV) node**, located between the atria and the ventricles, the impulse is delayed slightly (shown by the PR segment on the EKG), allowing the atria to contract before the ventricles so that the ventricles can fill. The depolarization wave then spreads through **Purkinje fibers** located in the **septum** (the myocardial wall between the left and right sides of the heart) towards the **apex** or tip of the heart, where they spread upward along the outer walls of the ventricles, producing a smooth, upward rippling, milking-like contraction.

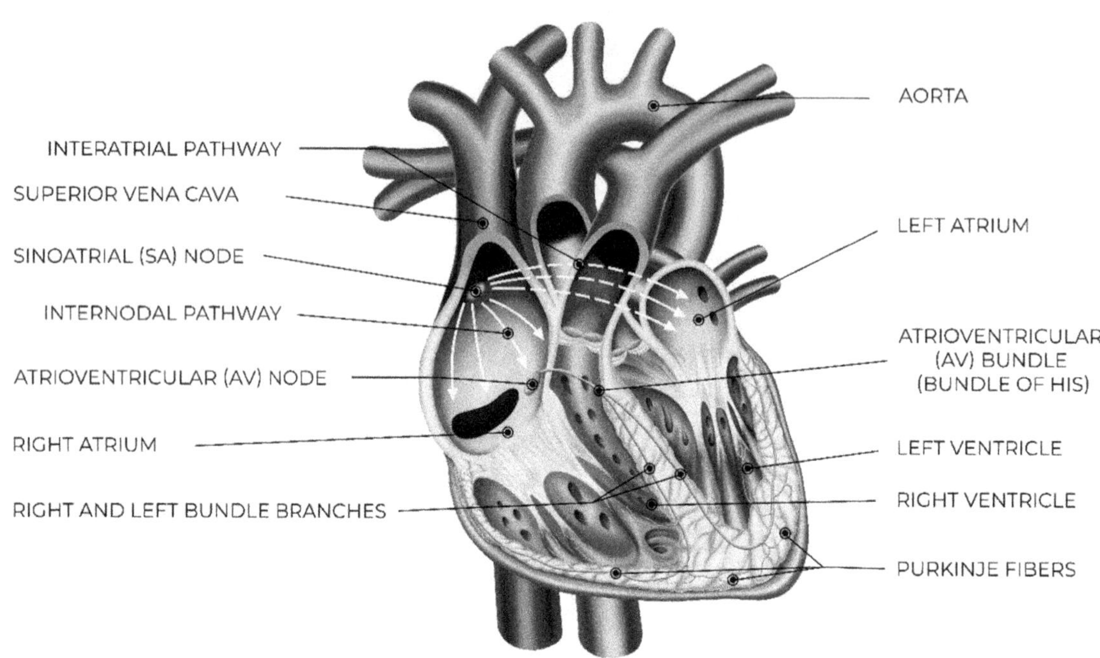

The Cardiac Cycle

Phase	Phase description	Heart sound	Ventricular S/D	EKG	Electrical activity
1	Atrial contraction	S4	Diastole (filling)	P Wave	Atrial depolarization (contraction)
				PR Interval	Partial atrial repolarization (relaxation), which is overshadowed by the QRS complex on EKG
2	Isovolumetric contraction (all valves passively closed)	S1 ("Lub" sound)	Systole (emptying)	QRS Complex	Ventricular depolarization (contraction)
3	Rapid ejection		Systole		
4	Reduced ejection		Systole	T Wave	Ventricular repolarization (relaxation)
5	Isovolumetric relaxation	S2 ("Dub" sound)	Diastole		
6	Rapid filling	S3	Diastole		
7	Reduced filling		Diastole		

Electrocardiography

The coordinated electrical system allows the heart to function properly so that blood can be pumped into the arteries for transport to the lungs for oxygenation (from the right side of the heart) or throughout the entire body for distribution (from the left side of the heart). Myocardial repolarization is similarly coordinated.

With a voltmeter, the **electrocardiograph (EKG or ECG)** gathers the electrical impulses through electrodes positioned on the outside of the chest. The signal is recorded or traced on a continuous roll of thermograph paper, which provides a permanent record of the electrocardiogram. The EKG is capable of measuring the amplitude or strength of electrical activity, and the duration or length of time associated with each electrical impulse. Normal heart contractions are recorded and viewed as normal rhythms on the EKG.

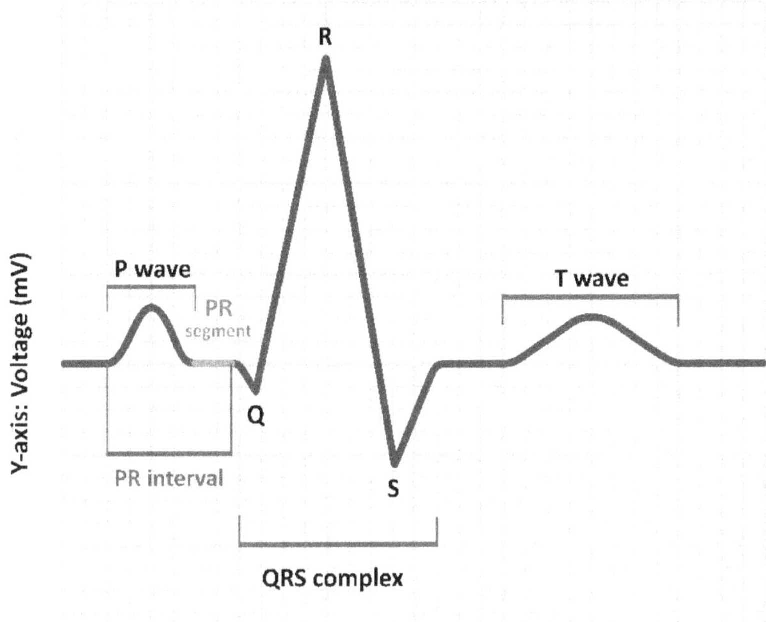

X-axis: Time (sec)

Obtaining an EKG

Electrical signals from the heart can be conveyed to the electrocardiograph in many ways, including: by wireless EKG devices positioned near the animal, by use of adhesive EKG pads, by rubber straps holding small metal plates to the skin, or by the subcutaneous placement of EKG wires. Each method has advantages and disadvantages. If pads are used, the pad is placed directly on the animal's bare skin. The animal's fur is clipped to allow complete contact. If alligator clips are used, they may be clipped directly to the animal's skin. However, this technique can be painful. Other techniques may provide the animal with a less traumatic experience. When necessary (particularly for long-term monitoring), EKG wires can be placed subcutaneously. The placement of surgical wire can be accomplished after cleaning the area. The wire is cleansed with alcohol. Then, a 20-gauge needle is used to introduce the wire under the skin. The ends of the wire are bent over, and adhesive tape is applied. This is done to prevent harm in long-haired animals. In addition, this method allows easy removal of the wire following the procedure.

During the EKG recording process the animal can be placed into a right lateral recumbent position. Some larger sized animals may remain in an upright position on their feet. Cats are normally more comfortable in a crouch position on the table. Regardless, the animal requires manual restraints.

When performing an EKG, the patient should be given a protective coverlet and cushion or mat to reduce the harmful effects associated with a steel table's ability to conduct electricity. The patient should be swabbed with alcohol, conducting gel, or paste. These substances increase signal conduction on the skin where contact is made. Some machines designed for taking human EKGs can be adapted for use with animals.

It is usually best to take a standard recording with the paper speed set at 25 mm/sec. Typically, 30 cm or 12 inches for each lead is recorded for an EKG that incorporates all the necessary information for proper evaluation. The paper speed is often set at 50 mm/sec for small dogs and cats. Various animals with faster or slower heart rates may require different paper speeds to provide adequate tracing differentiation and clarity. The EKG tracing should also incorporate pertinent patient identification and procedural information including: the date of the EKG, patient name and species, client name, and any other relevant information.

Pulse Oximetry Monitor

Pulse oximetry measures the percentage of hemoglobin in the blood that is oxygen saturated by passing light through the tissues using two wavelengths, red and infrared. Well-oxygenated hemoglobin will absorb more infrared light and allows more red light to pass through, whereas deoxygenated hemoglobin absorbs more red light, allowing more infrared light to pass through. The difference in this light absorption is calculated and gives a final percentage, which is the SpO_2.

The pulse oximetry probe must be placed on a hairless, unpigmented area where a pulse can be detected; common areas used include the ear, lip, tongue, prepuce, vulva, or in between the toes. The machine will either show a waveform that will represent pulse quality, or the machine will show just the pulse rate along with the SpO_2 reading. Normal SpO_2 values are 95–100% when the patient is getting 100% oxygen. Patients that are hypothermic or in shock will have a very low SpO_2 value due to vasoconstriction.

If the SpO_2 reading is low, there may be other factors affecting it, such as patient movement, skin pigment, or the tissue being too thin. It is best to evaluate the location and probe placement, as well as the patient's other vital signs, before determining if the low SpO_2 reading is legitimate.

Capnography

Capnography works by measuring the amount of carbon dioxide by the use of infrared waves in the breath at the end of expiration, also known as the **end-tidal CO_2**. Capnometry allows for the estimation of ventilation and how well the lungs are removing CO_2 from the body. A normal range is 35-45 mmHg. An elevated end-tidal CO_2 occurs with **hypoventilation**, whereas a lowered end-tidal CO_2 occurs with **hyperventilation**. The end-tidal CO_2 number gives information about cardiac output as well. If there is a decreased cardiac output to bring CO_2 to the lungs, then the amount exhaled will decrease. Capnography machines provide a waveform in which the height corresponds to the amount of carbon dioxide exhaled and the length of the waveform represents time. If the waveform is tall, that represents an increase in exhaled CO_2, and if the waveform is short, that indicates a fast respiratory rate.

Venipuncture

Venipuncture is an essential route of therapeutic administration and sample collection. Supplies that should be gathered when conducting a venipuncture include an appropriately sized, sterile syringe and hypodermic needle, cotton ball soaked in 70% isopropyl alcohol, and the appropriate phlebotomy tubes. Clippers may also be necessary if the animal's fur is thick.

Start by clipping the fur over the appropriate site, if necessary, and wipe with isopropyl alcohol on a cotton ball. The person restraining the animal should occlude the vein with their hand to improve its visibility. With the bevel of the needle facing up, the phlebotomist should insert the needle at a 25° angle and draw back on the syringe plunger, watching for a flash of blood. If the flash is present, the needle is correctly in the vein, at which point the person restraining the animal should stop occluding the vein. Draw back on the syringe plunger until the appropriate volume of blood is obtained and remove the needle from the vein. The person restraining the animal should be ready with a cotton ball to immediately apply pressure to the draw site until hemostasis occurs. The phlebotomist should immediately transfer the blood to the appropriate phlebotomy tube.

Phlebotomy Tubes

There are several different types of phlebotomy tubes used for blood samples in a veterinary clinic.

- The **purple-top tube** contains an anti-coagulant and is used for CBC (complete blood count), reticulocyte count, and hematocrit or PCV (packed cell volume). Purple-top tubes are not centrifuged.
- The **tiger top tube** has a red and grey top, contains a clot activator, and is used for chemistry panels, BUN, creatinine, and other serum sample tests.
- The **red-top tube** is used in immunology and can also be used for urine samples.
- The **blue-top tube** contains an anti-coagulant and is used to test for coagulation disorders.
- **Green-top tubes** contain heparin, an anti-coagulant, are PST (plasma separator tubes), and are used to collect plasma samples.
- **Grey-top tubes** are used to get accurate glucose measurements because they contain a glucose preservative which prevents glucose metabolism by red blood cells in vitro.

External Jugular Venipuncture

The left and right external jugular veins drain blood from the head and descend from the head superficial to much of the musculature on either side of the trachea and esophagus from the mandibular angle to the thoracic inlet. They are large and easily palpable.

For a canine blood draw, the person assisting should restrain a dog in a seated position, using one hand to elevate the head via the mandible gently out of the way, while the other restrains the animal's legs, if needed. Cats should be held in sternal recumbency; the restrainer should extend the forelimbs with one hand while elevating the cat's head gently back as the dog's would be. For venipuncture on a horse, the jugular vein is the preferred site; the animal should be properly restrained with a halter and a lead rope, at minimum. Bovine patients should be restrained in a headgate and squeeze chute for any type of blood draw, and the head may need to be haltered and tied off to the side to ensure proper and continuous access to the neck.

Cephalic Venipuncture

The cephalic vein drains the distal forelimb and runs dorsally over the forelimb. It is a common location for venipuncture on canine and feline patients. Dogs should be restrained in sternal recumbency, and the person restraining should occlude the cephalic vein on the opposite side of the animal from where they are situated by placing the thumb across the elbow joint and "rolling" the skin and underlying vein laterally, stabilizing and visually exposing the vein. The plunger should be drawn back slowly so as not to collapse the vein.

Medial Saphenous Venipuncture

The medial saphenous vein drains blood from the distal hindlimb and runs superficially on the medial side of the limb. Drawing blood from the medial saphenous vein is common in cats and should only be used when small amounts of blood are needed. The animal should be restrained in lateral recumbency, and the hand holding the hindlimbs should hold the top leg close to the animal's body while occluding the femoral vein. Firm pressure should be applied for longer than normal in order to prevent a hematoma.

Coccygeal Venipuncture

For small amounts of blood, coccygeal or "tail vein" venipuncture is helpful in cattle, especially when **preg-checking** them (blood testing to see if they are pregnant or **open** [not pregnant]). The cow should be restrained in a squeeze chute and headgate. Clean the underside of the tail and palpate the groove on the midline of the underside of the tail. 3-5 inches from the base of the tail, insert the needle perpendicularly into the groove. Apply pressure when the needle is removed.

Urine Collection Techniques

There are often unique requirements that should be followed in the collection of various kinds of urine samples. The urine is collected for inspection of solute concentration, physical properties, and chemical constituents. This unsterile urine sample should not be used for urine cultures.

In some situations, a specimen container should be opaque in order to protect the specimen from light. This keeps light from breaking down the components within the sample. Samples that should be protected from light include bilirubin and urobilinogen. Every container should be sterile to keep samples free from contaminants.

Tabletop samples (spontaneous micturition or voids on the examination table) are appropriate for use given the following conditions: a) the surface of the table is clean, and b) immediate testing of the sample is performed. However, tabletop samples do not meet the requirements for bacterial cultures, and usually a more specific urine collection technique is necessary.

Clean Catch

A **free-catch** or **voided sample** can be obtained by simply following the dog outside while the dog is on a leash. While the dog urinates, place a small, clean tray or container underneath midstream so the urine flows into the tray. This process is considered a **clean catch** if done properly because urine from the bladder is sterile; catching the urine midstream decreases the chances of bacteria being introduced to the sample, as the beginning and final release are not as free from contamination. In addition, the patient's vulva or prepuce (foreskin) should be sanitized beforehand. Clean catch samples cannot be used for bacterial culture.

Manual Expression

Urine can also be obtained through **manual expression**. This procedure involves the application of light pressure on the bladder, which is continued during the animal's mid-stream expulsion of urine. This procedure adheres to the criteria required for a clean catch specimen. The veterinarian should not attempt manual expression when it is suspected that the animal has some type of obstruction, as it could lead to bladder rupture. The veterinarian should not become impatient or apply too much pressure on the bladder.

The bladder can be found by palpating or applying a gentle pressure along the abdomen, beginning at the last rib. The examination should be carried out by moving from the front to the rear portion of the body in a caudal direction. Another technique used in locating the bladder consists of palpating along the upper portion of the rear legs. The movement starts at the back of the body and continues along toward the front lower portion of the body. Once located, pressure should be applied lightly over the bladder in a sustained or continuous manner to allow the urine to be expelled from the bladder. The expelled urine is collected in a sterile container.

Cystocentesis

Cystocentesis is a needle aspiration technique used to collect a sterile urine sample from a patient. This technique can be used on cats and dogs and is appropriate for the collection of a urine specimen for bacterial culture and sensitivity. The animal should be well-restrained or under sedation and placed in dorsal or lateral recumbency. To avoid harming the other abdominal organs, the animal should have a full bladder, and the process can be guided by palpation or ultrasound. Alcohol is wiped over the site where the needle is to be inserted.

One hand should prevent any shifting of the bladder, while the other inserts the sterile needle through the ventral abdominal wall in a caudodorsal direction toward the bladder. Once inserted, pull the plunger back slightly to see if urine is drawn into the syringe, and if not let go of the plunger and redirect the needle to try again using the ultrasound as a guide. Prevent any squeezing pressure from being applied to the bladder during this procedure so as to limit urine leakage into the peritoneal cavity. The needle and syringe should then be pulled out of the body as soon as the plunger is released.

Catheterization

The veterinarian may otherwise use **catheterization** to collect sterile urine from the urinary bladder. This is accomplished by using a rubber, plastic, or metal catheter (tube) to allow the passage of urine from the urinary bladder through the urethra with little risk of contamination. The animal's species and sex should guide the selection of the correct catheter type and size to be used in the procedure. Proper aseptic techniques should minimize the risk of infection in the animal and contamination of the sample taken. The veterinarian should also ensure that the animal does not experience any undue stress.

Catheterization is performed easily on male patients by a veterinary professional. To perform a catheterization, the dog will be placed in lateral recumbency while the restrainer extrudes the penis. Don gloves and clean the prepuce with a chlorhexidine solution, apply sterile lubricant to the end of the catheter, introduce the catheter into the lumen of the penis, and advance it until there is urine visible in the catheter. Connect a syringe (without a needle) to the other end of the catheter, and pull back on the plunger to draw urine into the syringe. Once the urine is collected, the catheter is pulled directly out of the penis.

Milk Samples for Bacterial Culture

The identification and treatment of mastitis is critical to an animal's good physical condition. **Mastitis** is inflammation of the animal's udder. This condition can have particularly detrimental effects upon a dairy herd. The dairy herd will have a sample of its milk taken for a culture. The samples are first tested for a simple positive or negative result, as this screening reduces the costs associated with more detailed laboratory testing. Any positive test result will indicate the need for further, more definitive testing. The samples should be collected from the animals before the milking process begins. However, samples may also be collected from an animal after milking has been completed, during the 6 or more hours that follow the prior milking episode.

In taking a sample, the udder should be thoroughly cleansed. Each teat should be wiped with alcohol beginning from the farthest point to the nearest in proximity. Then the teat should air dry. The initial milk stream must be thrown out. The midstream milk is collected and saved for the sample. The milk stream is aimed in a straight line towards the sample vial.

Fine Needle Aspiration

Collecting various blood and tissue cells for examination is often necessary. The veterinarian will use a **fine needle aspiration** to gather the cell samples from the skin, lymph nodes, and internal organs. The appropriate size includes a 22- to 25-gauge needle with a 3-12 mL syringe. Smaller gauge needles and smaller syringes should be employed with softer or more pliable tissues or cell accumulations. However, larger-bore syringes and larger gauge needles should be employed in gathering cells that are compact and solid when pressed. The veterinarian should release the suction pressure on the syringe before moving the syringe to another area. This allows multiple samples to be gathered from a wide variety of distances from the top to the bottom of a given mass or area of diagnostic concern. This also allows the veterinarian to take samples from different locations. The veterinarian will place the samples on a sterilized microscope slide. Next, the veterinarian will apply a staining solution. This will increase the ability of the veterinarian to carry out a thorough inspection of the cells.

Chapter Quiz

Ready to see how well you retained what you just read? Scan the QR code to go directly to the chapter quiz interface for this study guide. If you're using a computer, simply visit the online resources page at **mometrix.com/resources719/vtne** and click the Chapter Quizzes link.

Diagnostic Imaging

Transform passive reading into active learning! After immersing yourself in this chapter, put your comprehension to the test by taking a quiz. The insights you gained will stay with you longer this way. Scan the QR code to go directly to the chapter quiz interface for this study guide. If you're using a computer, simply visit the online resources page at **mometrix.com/resources719/vtne** and click the Chapter Quizzes link.

Producing Diagnostic Imagery

Diagnostic Imaging on a Patient

After collecting a patient history and presenting complaint as to why the patient is in the hospital, the veterinarian may need to take an inside look to gather more information on where the issue lies. For example, if the owner thinks that the pet has eaten an inanimate object and now will not eat or when the patient eats followed by vomiting, abdominal radiographs may be necessary to look for an obstruction. An ultrasound may be used as well to provide more detail of the organs. Another example is if the patient presents with limping, radiographs of the limb may be necessary to look for any fractures.

Safety Practices When Taking Radiographs

Radiographs should not be produced when a pregnant person is present in the room. When conducting radiological procedures, it is best to use nonmanual restraints on the patient, even if the state allows manual restraints, to avoid unnecessary x-ray exposure.

Persons in the room should wear the following: protective gloves, thyroid protectors, and aprons.

The x-ray machine itself should not be handled without protection. It is necessary to use a 2.5 mm aluminum filter to eradicate the lower-energy portion of the x-ray beam. The x-ray machine requires routine maintenance and calibration. It is important to keep body parts out of the path of the primary beam. This is necessary because of the primary beam's ability to transmit 25% of its radiation through a body shield. The technician should wear a dosimeter next to the outside collar of the apron. Ideally, diagnostic radiographs will be achieved with the fastest (i.e., lowest dosing) film-screen systems employed by the attending technician.

Personal Protective Equipment (PPE) Used for Taking Radiographs

Personal protective equipment (PPE) includes items that are worn to protect the person from health hazards. PPE used for personnel obtaining radiographs includes lead aprons, lead gloves, lead thyroid collars, and lead-rimmed glasses. Lead is an extremely dense material and serves as a barrier against scatter radiation. Lead aprons, gloves, and thyroid collars should be made of at least 0.25–0.5 mm of lead. Lead aprons should fit correctly, and there should be various sizes available. They need to have enough shielding from the neck to the middle of the thighs and wrap around the sides. Thyroid collars wrap around the neck, and lead gloves should be used during each exposure.

Dosimetry Badges

Dosimetry badges are worn to monitor the amount of exposure to scatter radiation for each individual. These badges have a radiation-sensitive film inside of a plastic holder with a clip to attach to the area on a person's body most at risk, such as the collar (thyroid). The badges are checked quarterly to evaluate each individual's radiation dose for that period of time, and the amount of exposure should not exceed 5 Roentgen equivalent man (rem) per year. A laboratory develops the film inside these badges and measures the level of radiation exposure. A control dosimetry badge is the same as a personnel dosimetry badge, but it is used to monitor the background radiation from shipment and storage at the location. The control dosimetry badge should be kept away from the radiology suite and is shipped back with the other personnel badges for dose readings. The control normally reads low, and that reading is subtracted from the other badges to obtain the occupational dose.

RADIATION DOSAGE AND HAZARDS

Radiation exposure standards are set to ensure patient and staff safety. The maximum radiation exposure allowed is defined in terms of dose rates and exposure time (dose = dose rate × exposure time). Thus, the maximum exposure time permitted is a function of the environmental and occupational dose rate. In clinical settings, the criteria are set according to guidelines issued by the **National Committee on Radiation Protection and Measurements** (the NCRP). These are derived from the recommendations produced by the **International Commission on Radiological Protection** (the ICRP).

The NCRP, and almost every province and state, has established radiological protection guidelines. These guidelines specify acceptable rates of exposure when, for example, one is holding an animal for an x-ray (some states, however, prohibit any type of manual animal restraint). To provide an extra measure of protection, staff will wear an individual dosimeter at the work site. It provides a cumulative record of radiation exposure over time and is evaluated by a federally approved laboratory on a routine basis.

CONTRAST RADIOGRAPHY

Contrast radiography allows hollow areas of the body (vessels, intestines, etc.) to be more meaningfully viewed. Two variations of the contrast medium include positive and negative contrasts.

Soluble contrast agents are found in products with iodine. These products are appropriate for the examination of the renal, articular, vascular, and gastrointestinal systems. It should be noted that some patients can exhibit toxic reactions to these agents, although these reactions rarely occur. Soluble iodinated contrast agents can be attributed to a hyperosmotic condition.

POSITIVE AND NEGATIVE CONTRAST AGENTS

Positive contrast agents, which are radiopaque, include barium and iodine. Radiopaque agents have the capacity to absorb x-rays more thoroughly than the absorption rate found in bones, causing the structure filled with the radiopaque agent to appear whiter on the film than any other structure in view. This allows for the identification of minor defects in the walls of an organ, and they will help identify a lesion or organ from the surrounding tissues.

Barium, an insoluble positive contrast agent, is typically employed when examining areas of the gastrointestinal tract.

Taking multiple radiographs throughout the day after administering positive contrast media will show how the organ in question is functioning; for example, if the barium is not passing through the intestines, there may be a foreign body present.

Negative contrast agents include air and carbon dioxide and are radiolucent; they will show up black in radiographs because they do not absorb x-rays.

POSITIONING FOR RADIOGRAPHIC VIEWS

COMMON RADIOGRAPHIC POSITIONING TECHNIQUES

To describe radiographic positioning, the terms used when the x-ray beam enters or exits the body or head are ventrodorsal or dorsoventral. To describe how the x-ray beam enters or exits a limb, the terms caudocranial or craniocaudal are used. A lateral (side) view is when the patient is placed with its side on the x-ray table and is defined as where the x-ray beam exits the body. For example, left lateral positioning is when the patient's left side is on the x-ray table. **Ventrodorsal views** are taken as the patient is on its back and are defined by where the beam enters through the ventral surface of the body and exits out of the dorsal surface. **Dorsoventral** is when the patient is sitting sternal and is defined as where the beam enters the body through the dorsal surface and exits through the ventral surface. **Craniocaudal** positioning is defined as where the beam enters the front side of the limb (cranial) and exits out of the back of the limb (caudal), whereas **caudocranial** is defined as where the beam enters the back side of the limb and exits out the front.

Thoracic Radiographic Views for the Small Animal

Dorsoventral (DV), ventrodorsal (VD), and lateral views are commonly taken for **thoracic radiographs**. If the animal is having trouble breathing, then a DV view may be taken instead of a VD, since VD has the animal placed on its back. To place the animal in right lateral recumbency, the animal will be laid on its right side with its front legs extended forward (cranially). The head should not be extended too much because this can create a false image of a narrow airway. Center the beam over the caudal dorsal aspect of the scapula, collimating the entire chest with the edge of the collimation being right in front of the scapula. To position for a VD view, the patient will lie on its back (dorsal) with the front legs extended and the head lying straight between the front legs. The other restrainer will hold the rear legs and extend them back so the patient is straight on its back. Collimate only to include the chest cavity, centering over the heart. Take both images upon inspiration. To perform DV positioning, the patient is sternal with the front legs extended out, and the head is straight between the front legs. Collimate over the area of the chest, centering over the heart, and take the image at inspiration.

Cervical Spine Radiographic Views for the Small Animal

When taking radiographs of the patient's spine, it is best to have the pet sedated because these images require specific positioning. Routine positions for **spinal radiographs** are lateral, including flexion and extension, and VD. For cervical lateral spine radiographs, place the patient on its side with the spine parallel to the table and the forelimbs will be pulled back toward the abdomen (caudally). An extension lateral view of the cervical spine is taken with the patient on its side, front legs pulled toward the abdomen and the head moved dorsally. The flexion lateral view of the cervical spine is taken with the patient on its side, with the front legs pulled caudally toward the abdomen and the head pulled toward the thorax. For a VD view of the cervical spine, the patient is on its back (dorsal) with the nose pointing up. The front legs are extended caudally and can be secured with a loop tie or tape. The base of the skull and the second vertebra of the thorax should be included in the VD view.

Pelvic Radiographic Views for the Small Animal

Common views requested for **pelvic radiographs** include extended-leg VD, lateral, and frog-leg VD. For lateral positioning of the pelvis, the patient will be lying on the side that is affected. The femur on the bottom will be pulled cranial with the stifle joint flexed, and the leg on top will be extended caudally. The beam should be centered on the greater trochanter, collimating for the pelvis. To position for the VD view of the pelvis, the patient needs to be in dorsal recumbency with the front legs extended with the head lying between. The other person restraining will extend the rear legs while rotating the stifles in so that the legs are straight and the sternum and spine are superimposed. Collimate for the crest of the ilium of the pelvis and down to the stifle joints. To position the patient for a VD frog-leg position, place the patient in the dorsal recumbent position, making sure that the sternum and spine are superimposed and the rear legs are left to fall into a normal flexed position with the femurs at a 45-degree angle to the spine. Collimate for the VD frog-leg position starting at the crest of the ilium of the pelvis, including the stifle joints, and centering on the greater trochanter.

Ultrasonography

Ultrasonography is noninvasive and records reflections of ultrasonic waves to allow internal organs to be seen in real time. A narrow beam with high-frequency ultrasound waves is directed into the area on the body that is of interest through the use of a probe and is transmitted through the tissues, or the waves may be reflected or absorbed. The waves that are reflected from the tissues come back to the probe and are called "echoes" that transfer to an image displayed on the monitor as a 2D image. Ultrasound waves do not pass through organs that contain air, such as the lungs, and they stop at bone, so bones are not seen in an ultrasound.

B-mode ultrasonography produces a 2D image and is used to diagnose pregnancy, examine the organs in the abdomen, and evaluate the function of the heart. **M-mode ultrasonography** produces a tracing of the structure in motion, and it is a good diagnostic tool to examine the chambers and valves of the heart, when combined with B-mode. The speed and direction of the blood flow in the vessels and heart can be viewed by Doppler ultrasound.

Basics of Sound Waves

A **wavelength** is defined as the span of distance that a wave travels in one repeating cycle. Wavelength is written in an abbreviated international symbolic or notation form as: λ (the lowercase Greek letter lambda). Audible sound has a longer wavelength than ultrasound.

A **transducer** is a device that converts one form of energy into another form. The defining features of the transducer may influence the wavelength.

The **frequency** is how many times the cycle occurred. Frequency is given the following symbol: (f). The wavelength will extend for a longer distance or increase as the frequency decreases. The frequency range for ultrasonic waves is 2-10 MHz. The frequency range for human auditory perception is approximately 0.02-20 kHz.

Sound velocity is defined as the speed at which a sound wave travels through a medium. The formula for velocity is given as the frequency multiplied by the wavelength.

Basic Ultrasound Concepts

Amplitude is the intensity or height of a wave. **Time period (T)** is the equivalent of one cycle of the wave.

Attenuation is the loss of vitality, amplitude, or power. With sound, this occurs when intensity is lost as an ultrasound beam passes through tissue. The loss can be attributed to the way the beam is absorbed into the tissue as it makes its way through. The absorption process creates heat and results in a loss of energy. Tissue that has sound refractory characteristics can scatter the sound in a multitude of directions.

Acoustic impedance is the capability of something to withstand or resist sound conduction. The density of tissue may be reflected in its degree of impedance. However, both air (not dense) and bone (very dense) will significantly obstruct the passage of sound. Thus, both bone and air have a high rate of acoustic impedance, despite their widely differing density. On the whole, however, tissues respond favorably to the passage of sound waves. Therefore, most bodily tissues have a low rate of acoustic impedance.

Sonographic Appearances

Echogenic tissues have the capacity to produce return echoes which are singled out by the transducer and displayed in a black and white image (with varying gray tones) that represents these tissues. Organs in proximity to each other will produce a larger echo reflection, indicating the gap between each organ.

Sonolucent (or **echolucent**) tissues do not reflect sound, and thus produce no echo.

Anechoic areas appear black as they do not give off echoes; chambers, spaces, and fluid-filled structures are anechoic and include vessels, cysts, and the urinary bladder.

Hyperechoic tissues are highly reflective of an ultrasound beam, thus producing a brighter or whiter appearance on the ultrasound image than the surrounding tissue. Examples of hyperechoic tissues include bone, tendons, and ligaments when perpendicular to the beam.

Hypoechoic structures create weaker echoes and therefore present as varying shades of grey. Examples include: muscle as compared to tendon fiber, soft atherosclerotic plaque, and some tumor tissue.

Isoechoic structures are more difficult to isolate because they produce echoes similar to the tissues around them, and they will appear to blend in on the monitor.

Spleen

The largest part of the **spleen** is hyperechoic. It has a standard granular profile. It is also surrounded by an illuminated capsule. The patient's spleen should be ultrasonographically imaged from the left side to minimize surrounding tissue interference. The spleen lies just below the skin and fascia, behind the stomach and under the diaphragm. Viewing the spleen from the trailing edge of the liver provides important imaging advantages. The liver's outer layer has a thick surface which presents an echogenic disparity that should be avoided.

Gallbladder and Kidneys

The **gallbladder** (or cholecyst) is located under the liver. The liver has a multitude of vessels and bile channels. Sonographic images of the gallbladder are displayed as anechoic, as it is largely fluid (bile) filled. Thus, it presents itself as an illuminated wall. Sludge or solid deposits can occasionally be found and visualized in the gallbladder. Animals that have not eaten before a sonogram often have large (i.e., dilated) gallbladder sonographic images.

The **kidney** will present as ovoid or egg-shaped. It will be enclosed by an illuminated capsule, as the cortex of the kidney is hyperechoic. The medulla of the kidney presents itself as anechoic. The pelvic fat will be displayed as an illuminated central zone. The sagittal view should be measured to determine the size.

Stomach, Bowel, Pancreas, and Adrenal Gland

The presence of gas or flatus in the abdomen and intestines presents a routine obstacle in ultrasonography. This is because air is hyperechoic and thus intestinal flatus limits the imaging of anything in the far field behind it. Even so, the intestinal walls on a sonographic image will look white or dark gray on the screen.

Depending upon its contents, the stomach may be hypoechoic. However, the rugal folds of the stomach are usually visible in the image created.

The **pancreas** is sandwiched between the spleen and the stomach. It is adjacent to the duodenum. The pancreas is a digestive and endocrine gland found in the body.

The **adrenal gland** appears as a standard (isoechoic) gray color. The adrenal gland is responsible for the secretion of hormones in the body. The adrenal gland itself is hypoechoic.

As reference points, the cranial pole of the kidney is situated toward the middle of the adrenal gland. The renal artery is next to the caudal pole found in the adrenal gland. The renal artery connects to the aorta.

Bladder, Prostate, and Uterus

A sonographic image of the **urinary bladder** is typically dark, as it is fluid filled and thus is relatively anechoic. However, the bladder walls present as hyperechoic, and it is not unusual to find debris in the bladder that aids in visualization.

In the male, the **prostate** can be ultrasonographically located by following the urethra to the pelvic inlet. The **urethra** is encircled by the prostate. The prostate is composed of 2 lobes and has an illuminated capsule in its ultrasonographic image.

In the female, the **uterus** is evident as the organ adjacent to an enlarged bladder. The wall of the uterus is hypoechoic.

The optimum time to discover an early uterine pregnancy in small animals is at about 30 days into gestation. In horses, the optimum early confirmation time is around 11-14 days into the gestation period. At these junctures, the sonographic equipment should be able to detect viable embryos in their gestational sacs.

However, it can often be hard to distinguish the exact number of fetuses inside the sac due to superimposition and the usual presence of gas in the intestines.

Heart

The heart is visualized using 2 types of sonographic imagery: M-mode or two-dimensional B-mode imaging. Sonograms of the heart require that 2 separate directional views be taken along both the long- and short-axis of the organ. The Doppler imaging technique can then be applied to determine the turbulence and velocity of red blood cells within the heart.

The walls and valves of the heart have a hyperechoic appearance.

Echocardiography

Echocardiography is a noninvasive ultrasound used to evaluate the heart's anatomy and function. A narrow sound beam is projected into the heart, and the echo pattern and strength are shown on the screen. The M-mode format provides the ability to evaluate fast-moving structures such as the heart's valves as well as the pattern of the heart chamber's wall movement due to its high resolution. M-mode is combined with B-mode to further evaluate the shape of the heart's chambers because it will help improve the beam's placement. Doppler echocardiography looks specifically at the heart's blood flow and will help to identify valve leaks or abnormal blood flow movement between the right and left sides of the heart. Doppler echocardiography can also detect any obstructions to blood flow to and from the heart.

Producing Echocardiograms

Most of the time, the patient does not need to be sedated to perform an **echocardiogram**. The patient will lie in lateral recumbency on a padded tray, and using the ultrasound transducer probe, the veterinarian will place it over the fourth and fifth ribs. There are specialized trays available to lay the patient in which allow the heart and lungs to be viewed from underneath the patient so there are fewer reflections from sound waves. The hair can be shaved if needed and must be wet to allow the transducer access to the skin. Ultrasound gel is placed on the transducer probe liberally and may be repeatedly applied throughout the analysis. The images show on the screen in real time, and the doctor can identify leaks in the valves of the heart as well as evaluate the movement of blood between the left and right sides of the heart. Echocardiography is commonly used to diagnose different forms of heart disease including valve abnormalities, dilated cardiomyopathy (dilation of the heart), and tumors in the heart.

Computed Tomography

Computed Tomography (CT) mainly examines the health of the central and peripheral nervous system, although it is also used for many other kinds of evaluations. A **CT scan** works as transmitted energy from x-rays is recorded by detectors on the opposite side of the patient producing a grayscale image. The brightness of a pixel in the image correlates to a tissue's ability to absorb the x-rays, helping to compare abnormal tissue to normal tissue. A CT scan only looks at one cross-sectional slice of the body at a time, and thinner slices produce better quality images. CT scans show the different levels in density of the tissues to produce a highly detailed image.

A CT scan requires the patient to be under general anesthesia; veterinary staff are separated by a large window where they can monitor the pet. The gantry table that the patient is lying on is slowly directed into the machine. The large x-ray tube that the patient is now in rotates 360° around the entire patient recording the x-rays from different angles. Every scan takes less than 30 seconds.

This imaging technique can detect numerous forms of disease in a variety of animals. However, it is very expensive.

Magnetic Resonance Imaging

Magnetic Resonance Imaging (MRI) uses a powerful magnet that surrounds the body of a patient lying on a table and produces cross-sectional images of anatomy. All soft tissues of the body can be viewed with MRI, but images of bone and air are difficult to produce.

MRI shares some similarities with computerized axial tomography. However, magnetic resonance imaging does not employ the use of ionizing radiation to create a likeness of the tissues. Enclosed coils in the device are able to transmit and receive magnetic field signals. Then the computer organizes those signals into high-contrast, detailed, cross-sectional images. All tissues have protons that have a charge and spin on their axis, naturally creating an electromagnetic field. During the MRI, the region of the body being imaged is inside of a large and powerful magnet that causes all of the protons to align with the magnetic field.

Magnetic resonance imaging provides an image resolution that has a better quality than other techniques used. Indeed, this device is sensitive enough to display detailed portions of an animal's anatomy and tissue makeup. Magnetic resonance imaging particularly lends itself to head and spine appraisals that require more intricate images to be produced.

Fluoroscopy

Fluoroscopy is an ongoing series of low-dose x-ray images that allow the viewing of internal organs in motion. The images produced are similar to that of an x-ray image, but because the images are continuously produced, it creates motion in real time similar to a movie. To perform a fluoroscopy, the patient is placed in a plastic box and a continuous x-ray beam is generated at the patient. The C-arm of the fluoroscopy machine has two sides with the patient in between, and the body of the machine along with the C-arm can move together if needed to be adjusted with the patient's height and position.

Swallow tests may be performed if a pet is having trouble swallowing food, an esophageal disorder is suspected, or they are having regurgitation issues. The patient is put into the plastic box, and a variety of different types and consistencies of food is prepared. The consistencies of the food should range from liquid to slightly formed, up to dry kibbles, and each type of food will have a contrast media added to it. As the continuous x-rays are produced, the veterinarian can easily watch the food travel through the esophagus and look for any abnormalities.

Nuclear Scintigraphy

In **nuclear scintigraphy imaging**, the patient can be given gamma emissions from radioactive material or radionuclides applied by a variety of methods. These methods include intravenous injections, transcolonic applications, or aerosol insufflation (i.e., blown into or onto the body). The radioactive material is picked up by sensors found in the gamma scintillation camera. The organ is then pictured on x-ray film, formatted in black and white shades of varying contrast.

Clinical nuclear scintigraphy is typically performed on the thyroid, bone, and liver. The results derived from this technique provide physiological, pharmacological, and kinetic data.

Nuclear scintigraphy is beneficial in many treatments provided to horses. However, the handler and persons coming into contact with horses having this procedure should use the recommended safety equipment to prevent undue exposure to the harmful effects of radioactive material. The animal will expel the radiopharmaceutical elements in its bodily waste. The contaminated urine and feces are normally expelled within 24-72 hours after the procedure was completed.

Equipment and Related Materials

X-Ray Machine

The x-ray machine must also include the following components: electrical circuits to control the x-ray tube, a control panel, and a tube stand. It has filters, collimators, and grids as part of its framework. The electrical circuits utilize high-voltage electricity to generate energy and speed. This speed allows the electrons to develop a high electromagnetic potential. The electrical circuits also supply a low-voltage electric current used for heating the cathode filament. A timer switch operates to measure exposure time in seconds. The rectification circuit is used to change the current supplied to the tube from alternating to direct current.

The control panel is utilized to manage and regulate the kilovoltage peak (kVp), milliampere (mA), milliampere-seconds (mAs), and/or seconds. This regulation is dependent upon the capacity of the x-ray machine. The kVp potential establishes the class of energy. The mA and involved time establish the intensity of the x-rays. The x-ray tube is set up on a foundation known as the tube stand.

X-Ray Tube

An **x-ray tube** consists of the following components: a cathode filament, an anode plate, a focusing cup, a target, a glass envelope (within which a vacuum is created), an aluminum filter, and a beryllium window. The x-ray tube generates the photons carrying the electromagnetic charge and directs them along a targeted pathway.

The entire x-ray device is encased within a tube-shaped Pyrex capsule that creates a vacuum. This is essential for x-ray generation. The x-rays are sent out through a small window fashioned from a thin section of glass which absorbs a small quantity of x-rays or electromagnetic radiation.

EM energy is measured as a kilovoltage peak or potential kVp, which dictates the penetration strength of the x-rays.

Cathode and Anode

The cathode filament is usually made from a coiled tungsten filament with a copper stem that releases electrons when heat is applied to its surface. The cathode filament is situated across from the focusing cup and the anode plate. The filament maintains a negative potential throughout the heating process. The electrons are drawn to the positively charged anode, which can be immobile or in rotation. Collision with the anode produces EM-charged photons; when EM-carrying photons crash into and pass through matter, the x-ray picture is created. Approximately 99% of the energy created is heat and 1% is x-rays (photons carrying EM energy).

X-Ray Film

Screens and Screen Speeds Used in X-Ray Film

The x-ray machine incorporates an **intensifying screen** made from a synthetic base covered in sheets of small **luminescent phosphor crystals** which function as a protective covering. Two intensifying screens are located on the interior fabric of the x-ray cassette. The film is packed in between these 2 screens. Visible light exposes the light-sensitive emulsion of the x-ray film when radiation connects with and illuminates the surface of the phosphor crystals, referred to as **indirect imaging**, and is responsible for more than 95% of the film's exposure to light.

Computerized x-ray machines rely on digital media, are much more versatile to use, and bypass the film development step altogether. Further, they have greater file-sharing and archival capacities. Thus, they are replacing the older film and intensifying screen-based processes. However, familiarity with traditional x-ray equipment remains important.

Screen Speeds and Exposure Time

Fair to good resolutions can be obtained with **medium-speed x-ray films**. These require relatively low exposure times. **Fast-speed films** allow a shorter exposure time and provide superior patient x-ray penetration. However, they trade speed for image quality. The poorer quality image is caused by the larger crystals and thicker layers applied in fast-speed screens. These blurred images show less detail than images taken with a medium or slow speed screen.

Film made with **silver halide crystals** or grains has a superior rate of sensitivity to the waves of light produced from the intensifying screens. This increased sensitivity allows a diagnostic radiograph to be created using a **shorter exposure time**. Greater resolution is obtained because of the finer image resolution grains on the film. This greater resolution is accomplished through longer exposure times. Shorter exposure times can only be achieved with larger grains on the films. X-rays performed on animals usually require only a medium-grain film. This medium-grain film is a concession made to obtain a reasonably good image resolution without an extended exposure time.

Non-Screen Film

Non-screen x-ray film does not utilize intensifying screens. It has improved sensitivity to direct ionizing radiation. However, the non-screen film will require a longer exposure time to work. Even so, it has the advantage of producing an image that has better detail-revealing resolution than that of an image gained via an intensifying screen. The film is packaged in a heavy envelope that does not allow light to pass through. This film is often used in dental offices, where the bulkiness of radiographic film coupled with an intensifying screen is prohibitive. The film speed is depicted by the label D or E. The faster non-screen film speed is the E label.

Manually Processing Film

Processing film involves the following steps: developing, rinsing (in a stop bath), fixing, washing, and drying. The chemicals must be diluted and mixed according to the manufacturer's directions. The chemical solutions are mixed at a temperature of 20 °C or 68 °F. The manufacturer lists detailed information about the time-temperature development of each chemical. The film should be shaken at regular intervals to prevent any air bubbles from forming while in the developing fluid. The oxidation of developing chemicals can be reduced by keeping lids securely fastened on the tanks. As the developer solution is used, the exposed silver halide crystals are changed to black metallic silver.

If the expected density or contrast does not appear, then the solution has weakened and should not be used. The fixer solution is used to remove unexposed, undeveloped silver halide from the image. It also hardens the film. It should be discarded if it takes longer than 2 or 3 minutes for this step to be completed. The process is finished when the image goes from a hazy, cloudy image to a clear image.

Appropriate Darkroom Conditions

Proper darkroom conditions must also be maintained in clean, well-ventilated, temperature-controlled facilities. The correct wattage should be used for a safelight. A filter for the safelight that matches the sensitivity of the film being developed should also be utilized. The light should be positioned at least 4 feet away from the workspace.

A **darkroom light switch** should have a delay to minimize any accidental light exposures. Wet and dark areas should be separated to prevent unintended exposures. The images should be processed by technicians wearing appropriate safety equipment. This includes proper gloves and protective eyewear. An eyewash bottle should be kept in the vicinity, in compliance with state, province, and/or federal regulations regarding timely treatment following an accident.

Light Leakage

Light leakage is defined as an event which leads to fogging of the images in the radiographs. A check for fogging can be accomplished by placing an open, unprocessed film cassette in the darkroom. Three quarters of the film should be covered with a lightweight paperboard for a period of 1 minute. The other portion of the cardboard should be covered for the second minute. The first section should be uncovered during this time. Continue in like manner, until the entire board has had 1 minute of covered exposure. This takes a total of 3 minutes. On the fourth minute, the film is left uncovered in its entirety so that the film can be totally exposed. After development, any darkened areas on the film will indicate conditions which permit film fogging to occur.

Factors That Influence Radiographic Density

Radiographic density relates to the degree of darkness present on the developed film's surface. This is directly correlated with the number of photons that have affected the film.

The density can vary according to the total number of x-rays that come into contact with the intensifying screen, a function of exposure time and temperature. The beam strength and exposure duration are measured in milliampere-seconds of x-rays that come into contact with the intensifying screen. The more x-rays that come into contact with the intensifying screen, the more densely activated (darkened) the film will be.

It can also be altered by the penetration strength of the x-rays, determined by the measurement of kVp (kilovoltage peak). The higher kVp settings produce higher energy x-rays, resulting in an improved film density.

Focusing filters and grids can make the beam weaker.

In addition, tissue density, patient coverings, and support pads can lessen the strength of the beam. Thicker or denser tissue causes a reduced film density (lighter film). In like manner, thinner tissue causes an increase in film density (darker film).

Automatic Film Processing

Mechanized film processors can be employed to provide automated film processing. The film is routed through the chemical solutions and out to a dryer on a roller assembly. The temperature ranges from 20-35 °C (77-96 °F). Mechanized film processing can take as little as 90 seconds or as long as 8 minutes. The procedures and chemicals are much like those used in the manual processing methods. However, these mechanical chemicals are mixed in a much more concentrated manner. The hardener is mixed directly into the developer solution. There is no rinsing step between the developing and fixing steps in this method. The mechanical process can only be accomplished by maintaining very clean equipment. The rollers, roller racks, and crossover rollers cannot be dirty. Chemicals should be replaced at recommended intervals to give optimum performance in the mechanized film development process.

Radiographic Image

X-rays are derived from the energy produced by electrons or negatively charged particles within an atom. This energy is converted to **electromagnetic radiation**. The radiation produces energy particles known as **photons**. Photons do not have any mass or electrical charge, but they can carry **electromagnetic (EM) energy**.

X-rays are forms of electromagnetic energy carried by photons with **high energy and a short wavelength**. Mineralized tissues of the body such as bones and teeth absorb the most x-rays, soft tissues like the spleen and kidneys absorb some x-rays, and air doesn't absorb any x-rays. The x-ray machine has a narrow beam of photons that aims at a specific area of the body with a cassette underneath that obtains the x-rays as they pass through to it. The areas that absorb the x-ray photons appear white, whereas areas that allow more photons to pass through will appear black. Areas that are fluid filled appear black or dark gray because those areas do not absorb many x-ray photons. For example, when taking a radiograph of a dog's front leg, the bones will appear white and the muscles and tendons will appear gray.

Radiographic Contrast and Subject Contrast

The degree of difference between the shades of black and white in a radiographic image is defined as the radiographic contrast. Radiographic contrast can be impacted by the following: kilovoltage, scatter radiation, processing features, and physical aspects, such as beam attenuation and fogging effects.

Kilovoltage peak or kVp has the strongest impact on radiographic contrast. The x-ray beam is polychromatic, with many wavelengths. Lower kVp ratings offer wider ranges of energy levels. Higher kVp ratings produce more consistent penetration and fewer disparities. Objects along the pathway of the beam scatter the effect. This creates a reduction in the film's contrast and is displayed by overcast shades of gray on the film.

Subject contrast distinguishes between the density and mass of two adjacent structures. A high subject contrast will produce a more prominent radiographic contrast. The thickness and density of the anatomic structures being imaged will also impact subject density. Higher tissue density is translated into higher subject density. Bones have high subject density, are more opaque to x-rays, and thus image as white or light gray on a radiographic image.

Radiation Safety

The practice owner is responsible for applying the appropriate radiological safety procedures in accordance with state or province requirements. These guidelines involve the use of **dosimeter devices**, efficient radiation detection devices, equipment registration, staff certification, and radiologically appropriate room design. The health department is normally responsible for regulating these devices and safeguards. Trained personnel are necessary to apply the appropriate radiation safety guidelines. Personnel must be able to use the devices correctly, according to instructions received.

Every cell in an organism can be affected by ionizing radiation, which is able to modify or disintegrate a molecule. This can dangerously interrupt the normal functioning of tissues but may not be immediately apparent. Intergenerational delays may occur when damage presents itself only in the genetic makeup of reproductive cells. Other alterations may not be readily apparent because of concurrent tissue restoration. Even so, somatic cell damage may take place throughout the body. The region of the cell most susceptible to the effects of ionizing radiation is the nucleus and those aspects central to cellular reproduction.

Proper Maintenance of Lead Aprons and Gloves

Lead aprons and gloves should be checked at least every 6 months to ensure there are no holes or tears. Lead gowns and gloves are inspected by using a fluoroscopy or radiographic machine set at 80 kVp and 5 milliampere-seconds (mAs) to check for any cracks, which would appear dense. If there are any signs of cracks or radiation leakage, the item must be replaced. There should be a rack, normally on the wall in the radiology suite, that the gowns and gloves can hang on so they do not get folded or stacked on top of one another. Hanging them will also keep them from accidentally getting punctured or cut by any sharp object. The gowns and gloves can be washed with mild detergent and warm water, but chemicals and machine washing are not recommended.

Ultrasound Transducers

The **transducer probe** is a handheld device that sends and receives sound waves by using the piezoelectric effect; this device will transform sound waves into electrical energy, from which an image can be obtained.

The transducer probe consists of many crystals that rapidly change shape when an electrical current is applied. The rapid shape changes produce sound waves that travel outward. There are a few different sizes and shapes of transducer probes, which will determine the viewing field. The transducer pulse control changes the frequency and length of the sound waves. The central processing center is the computer that performs the calculations and holds the electrical power for the transducer probes and the central station itself. The display screen will present the image received from the ultrasound data that the central processing unit has processed.

Types of Transducers

The sound waves produce echoes that can be received as they bounce back in return. The **pulsed-wave transducer** is a device that emits a short pulse of sound and works to send and receive these signals in a patterned sequence.

The **continuous-wave transducer** utilizes 2 transducers. The first transducer sends out a constant sound wave, while the second transducer continuously receives sound waves as they echo back.

The **linear array transducer** has a tiny row of crystals that operates in a regular rhythm and produces a composite image from many parallel lines. These lines form an image in a rectangular shape. Thus, the linear array transducer is often best applied to imaging a wide, near field such as transrectal and equine tendon examinations.

The **mechanical sector transducer** utilizes one or more crystals in its operations. The device will create an image that has the form of a pie wedge or circle segment. It is often a better choice when deep tissue penetration and a large, far-field view are needed.

The **phased array sector scanner** is a computerized device that guides ultrasound pulses from about 20 crystals through a particular area. Providing images of time-motion (TM) activity, the phased array sector scanner is best applied to echocardiography. However, this compact device can be an expensive purchase.

The **broad bandwidth transducer** utilizes a piezoelectric ceramic and epoxy material in the probe. It is a lightweight device with minimal acoustic impedance. Importantly, these transducers can operate on a variety of frequencies. These frequencies or short-duration pulses are available because of the transducer's ability to transmit over a wide range of bandwidths.

Transducer Crystals

Ultrasound devices function with **transducer crystals** to enhance the electrical energy conversion process. However, a transducer crystal cannot send and receive sound waves simultaneously. Thus, the transducer must perform these functions in an alternating pattern (unless a dual-crystal [continuous] wave transducer is used).

Natural crystals are often utilized as transducer crystals. These crystals include: quartz, tourmaline, and Rochelle salts. Some synthetic crystals are also utilized as transducer crystals. **Synthetic crystals** include the following: lead zirconate titanate, barium titanate, and lithium sulfate.

Sound vibrations are promoted via a piezoelectric effect. A dampener is applied to terminate the vibrations after they have been received. Then, new echoes received come into contact with the crystals and initiate the vibration again. These vibrating movements back and forth are subsequently transformed into electrical energy.

Doppler Imaging

Doppler imaging is beneficial in examining aspects of the body that remain in constant motion, such as the heart. This technique uses differences between sound wave frequencies received at a remote point as opposed to the frequency found at the sound's origin to analyze certain characteristics about motion. The difference is most pronounced when there is activity between the original sound and the receiver. Specifically, the sound wave frequency increases when the receiver moves towards the originating location of the sound, and it decreases when the receiver moves away. Thus, the frequency will increase or decrease in relation to any movement between the receiver and the originating source. The position-dependent wave amplitude changes between a stationary object and one in motion are referred to as a "Doppler shift."

Doppler imaging is beneficial in determining whether or not a lesion or a mass exists in a vessel. Doppler imaging can also help in locating portal systemic shunts and in assessing cardiac function and effectiveness in the body.

ULTRASONOGRAPHY RESOLUTION

A properly resolved image on an ultrasound is defined as 2 small objects in close proximity which can be individually recognized. The frequency of the transducer is critical to the resolution quality of the image. Resolution is increased when higher frequencies are applied. This is due to the shorter wavelength used to gain the image. Lateral resolution refers to the ability to properly resolve 2 objects that are both side-by-side and perpendicular to the beam. The beam functions to visually separate the 2 objects from each other. The degree of lateral resolution is also a function of the beam's width. Objects in parallel position to each other are best able to be identified when they are spaced farther apart than the diameter of the beam. Axial resolution is the ability to resolve 2 objects that are located one above another in the beam's pathway. In this situation, greater resolution and differentiation are obtained at lower frequencies.

SOUND BEAM ZONES

The size and design of the transducer control the ultrasound beam zones. The **near field** (also called the Fresnel zone) refers to the entire area of the ultrasound beam that precedes the focal point and is most proximal (nearest) the crystal. It is characterized by a narrowing, gradually converging beam shape. The shifting of the focal point closer to the image can produce a better resolution of the image. The transducer can be brought into focus by "shaping" (manipulating) the crystal. The focus can also be improved by adding a lens to the transducer. The section of the beam that gets broader and less intense as it moves away from the focal point is known as the far field (also called the Fraunhofer zone).

DISPLAY FORMATS USED FOR ULTRASOUND IMAGES

The different display formats for ultrasound images—amplitude mode, brightness mode, and motion mode—are essential to the ultrasound's ability to provide a useful image.

The **amplitude mode** (A-mode) provides the depth and dimensions of a target as a one-dimensional graph with a succession of rising points. Each rising point stands for a returning echo. Higher points on the graph indicate larger, more intense echoes.

The **brightness mode** (B-mode) produces a two-dimensional map of data represented by dots or small marks on a graph. The dots represent the returning echo. The deepness of the mirrored image is indicated by the location of the dot on the graph's baseline, used to reference the results found.

The **motion mode** (M-mode) is represented by a one-dimensional wave graph. Its vertical axis indicates the immediate position of the moving reflector. The horizontal axis represents the time. Objects in motion are represented by wavy lines on the graph. Stationary or immobile objects are represented by straight lines on the graph. The M-mode is best applied for cardiac examinations on a patient. The M-mode provides a beneficial evaluation of the condition of cardiac valves, walls, and chamber sizes.

PROPAGATION ARTIFACTS

Propagation artifacts: Reverberations, refraction, and mirror images. **Reverberations**, exhibited as linear echoes, are a result of sounds reflected between a strong reflector and the transducer in a continuous pattern. An example of a reverberation-prone surface is bone.

Refractions are a result of sound beams changing directions as they are bounced off one medium and strike another medium's surface. Refractions are to blame for the manifestation of organs in unusual positions. An example of this is when an image is duplicated and appears as if it exists on both sides of a reflecting axis. This phenomenon is often due to the close proximity of a strongly reflective organ to the reflector, such as the liver or the diaphragm.

Attenuation Artifacts

Attenuation artifact occurs when tissues in the near field reduce the intensity of the ultrasound beam, leaving tissues in the focal region and far field poorly imaged. Attenuation artifact may cause a lesion itself to be perceived as a hypoechoic mass or cyst.

Acoustic shadowing is found when an object reflects a sound wave in its entirety, producing an acoustic shadow of the actual structure. **Posterior shadowing** occurs when an object blocks sound waves from passing deeper into the tissue, which can be a result of calculi or gas in the intestines.

Objects located on the backside of organs filled with fluid may present with enhanced echoes, when compared to adjacent objects or tissues. This **acoustic enhancement** is a result of a fluid's anechoic nature, allowing sound waves to more readily pass through.

Maintaining and Caring for the Ultrasound Machine

The **transducer probes** must be wiped down and cleaned with a specific ultrasound cleaner to rid them of any excess ultrasound gel. All wires and connections must be inspected regularly, and any wires that are frayed or not working properly must be replaced. The central processing center must be regularly assessed to be sure that all buttons work correctly and that the image produced is of good quality. If the ultrasound machine contains a printer, it must be filled regularly with the correct paper to print the ultrasound images. The ultrasound machine itself must be stored in an area with low traffic that is dry so nothing leaks onto the machine. Some hospitals may even cover their machines to prevent dust and debris from accumulating.

Nuclear Scintigraphy

Nuclear scintigraphy is an imaging technique used to evaluate the kidneys, bones, the thyroid gland, and brain. It requires that **technetium** (a radionuclide or radioactive isotope) be infused intravenously. The animal will then be scanned to locate and track the radioactive isotope. The isotope appears as a radiographic "hot spot" approximately 2 hours after the injection has been given to the animal. The lower limbs of the animal should be scanned about 20 minutes after infusion of the isotope. The animal will be in a radioactive state for a period of 24-36 hours following the procedure. During this time the animal should be left alone except for feeding and watering. However, water should not be given to the animal whenever the pelvis is being examined, as the full bladder will obscure certain views of the pelvis. The veterinarian may administer a diuretic to reduce the size of the bladder.

Nuclear scintigraphy is an appropriate examination for tendon injuries, suspected suspensory injuries, and crippling injury or lameness. Of particular benefit is the ability to detect equine tibial stress fractures, condylar fractures, and pelvis, carpus, and hock injuries.

Chapter Quiz

Ready to see how well you retained what you just read? Scan the QR code to go directly to the chapter quiz interface for this study guide. If you're using a computer, simply visit the online resources page at **mometrix.com/resources719/vtne** and click the Chapter Quizzes link.

Anesthesia

Transform passive reading into active learning! After immersing yourself in this chapter, put your comprehension to the test by taking a quiz. The insights you gained will stay with you longer this way. Scan the QR code to go directly to the chapter quiz interface for this study guide. If you're using a computer, simply visit the online resources page at **mometrix.com/resources719/vtne** and click the Chapter Quizzes link.

Classifications of Anesthetic Drugs

Benzodiazepines

Benzodiazepines are controlled substances that can be used to treat epilepsy and anxiety, and they are used as muscle relaxants and anticonvulsants during anesthesia. Drugs containing benzodiazepines include the following: diazepam or Valium, zolazepam, midazolam or Versed, and lorazepam or Ativan. All of these variations of the drug may result in depression of the cardiovascular or respiratory systems. However, the remote risk has been determined to be acceptable for both geriatric and pediatric patients. Candidates found to derive the greatest benefits from the drug are elderly, depressed, and/or nervous patients. Benzodiazepines used in conjunction with ketamine may serve as an effective general anesthetic induction agent.

Diazepam is soluble when placed in oil. However, water does not dissolve diazepam. Diazepam may work faster when it is used in conjunction with other drugs. Opioids like butorphanol and oxymorphone easily mix with midazolam. Midazolam is a medication that is known to be water-soluble.

Phenothiazines

Phenothiazines act as sedatives and anti-emetics, and the most common are acepromazine and chlorpromazine. They are only approved for use in dogs, cats, and horses.

Acepromazine is contraindicated for any patient with a history of convulsions, epilepsy, or head injuries. Acepromazine is known to decrease the threshold level for seizure activity.

Phenothiazine-induced peripheral vasodilation in patients with symptoms of shock or hypothermia may cause hypotension (i.e., low blood pressure). Patients with depression or liver or kidney diseases should not be prescribed phenothiazines. These drugs should only be given to the very young or old if absolutely necessary, and with careful observation. A lower dose or alternate medications, such as benzodiazepines, may be given instead.

Unexpected antihistamine effects can occur when animals are not given a medication-specific allergy test beforehand. Some animals experience adverse effects from taking phenothiazines. These effects include abnormal heartbeat, an unexpected reaction of excitability replacing the desired effect of sedation, and personality changes. These side effects normally subside within 48 hours of taking the medication.

A_2-Agonists

Medications that are **α_2-agonists** (alpha-2 agonists) provide sedation, analgesia, muscle relaxation, and anxiolysis. Some α_2-agonists include xylazine, romifidine, detomidine, and medetomidine. Xylazine is also known as Rompun and AnaSed. Detomidine is also known as Dormosedan. Medetomidine is also known as Domitor.

Note that α_2-agonists are not to be used as preanesthetic medications. Instead, this medication is more suitable for general sedation purposes. The potential for side effects exceeds its benefits as a preanesthetic medication.

Aggressive animals destined to be euthanized can be given α_2-agonists to produce a sedative effect. This medication is also beneficial when given as an analgesic or pain reliever. However, the relief will only last for about 16-20 minutes. There is a 50% chance that dogs will become nauseated to the point of vomiting when given this drug. This chance increases to 90% when the medication is given to cats. There are 2 α_2-agonists employed for treatments in horses. These are xylazine and detomidine. Ruminants may be given a significantly lower dose of xylazine.

Phencyclidines

Phencyclidines are available under the following names: Ketamine or Ketaset, Ketalean, Vetalar, and tiletamine hydrochloride. Tiletamine hydrochloride is a combination of zolazepam and Telazol. Another name for phencyclidines is cycloheximide. Patients that need to remain immobile will benefit from the application of this drug in their treatment. This drug is a beneficial preanesthetic when applied to the mucous membranes in the mouth or oral cavity.

Cats are the only animals that can take phencyclidines as a solitary form of medication. Other animals should never have this medication in solitary form. Dogs do not respond well to phencyclidine as a preanesthetic medication. It is best to avoid its use in patients with a history of seizure activity, suspected brain herniation, or suspected perforation of the eye chamber. Visceral analgesia (pain relief for pain arising in the internal organs) is inadequate to justify its use. However, the response is much better when given for the purpose of peripheral analgesia. It should be noted that the animal's recovery period after being given this drug may be extensive and unpredictable.

Opioids

The following medications are opioids: morphine, oxymorphone or Numorphan, butorphanol or Torbugesic, Torbutrol, hydromorphone, meperidine or Demerol, Pethidine, and fentanyl. **Opioids** have the following effects on the body: analgesia, sedation, dysphoria, euphoria, and excitability. These effects are precipitated by the drug's interaction between one or more dedicated receptors in the brain and spinal cord in various reversible combinations.

Opioids can act as an agonist or antagonist against each dedicated receptor. Preanalgesia medication is given to the patient as an induction agent or for a more balanced anesthesia transition. It also aids in controlling pain after the surgery. The effects of this medication can be reversed by giving the patient a pure antagonist agent. Opioids are categorized as narcotics in Canada and as Schedule II drugs in the United States. Neither country allows the dispensing of these medications without a prescription from a licensed physician or veterinarian.

Two Classes of Opioids Used in Premedication Protocol

Opioids consist of two classes: **pure mu agonists** including morphine, hydromorphone, and fentanyl and **partial mu agonists** including buprenorphine. Because morphine and hydromorphone cause vomiting in most patients, they should not be used with patients who have obstructions of the esophagus or GI tract. They also should not be used in patients with eye issues because vomiting causes an increase in cranial pressure. Opioid agonists such as morphine are highly addictive with the potential for abuse and are classified as Schedule II drugs. Buprenorphine has a long duration of action and provides less analgesia than pure mu agonists, but it will provide less respiratory and cardiovascular depression. Butorphanol is an agonist-antagonist, meaning it is an antagonist at the mu receptor, preventing activation. Butorphanol is also an agonist at the kappa receptor meaning it activates these receptors. Therefore, because butorphanol is an agonist-antagonist, it partially reverses the effects of full agonists. Naloxone is used to reverse the effects of other opioids because it is an opioid antagonist.

Nonsteroidal Anti-Inflammatory Drugs

Nonsteroidal anti-inflammatory drugs are abbreviated as **NSAIDs**. These drugs include the following: aspirin, acetaminophen, carprofen, ketoprofen, and meloxicam. These drugs are not dangerous to use in combination with opioids. NSAIDs are appropriate for the treatment of musculoskeletal pain. They are frequently applied in the treatment of patients with arthritis and other joint diseases. However, long-term NSAID therapy should not be used by patients with chronic kidney problems. It is best to use meloxicam in long-term therapy for renal-compromised patients, as it has a lower risk for nephrotoxic results.

It is never appropriate to administer acetaminophen to a cat. Dogs should only be given acetaminophen on atypical occasions. Analgesics that are considered strong and safe can be given in direct postoperative orthopedic procedures. Pain medications are also particularly beneficial in the treatment of painful degloving injuries (where a large section of skin is severed from its underlying blood supply). Alternative medications include ketoprofen and carprofen.

Barbiturates

Barbiturates can be used for sedation, as anticonvulsants, and for general anesthesia. This drug can serve as an induction agent prior to endotracheal intubation. The drug may be given as an inhalant anesthetic for maintenance purposes. Barbiturates are considered sedative-hypnotic medications. This category of drugs can also be applied to depress respiration and the cardiovascular system in general. The effects of barbiturates are not reversible, and no other medication can fully counterbalance their effects. Barbiturates bind to proteins in the body. Thus, the rate and amount of absorption can change when the level of plasma protein is altered.

Phenobarbital and Pentobarbital

The most widespread use of **phenobarbital** in veterinary medicine is as a sedative for dogs, and it is also beneficial when used as an anticonvulsant. Varying the dosage may cause effects to last for shorter or longer periods of time, up to 24 hours. It can be administered intramuscularly with no negative effects upon tissue. The drug will reach its optimum effect about 5 minutes following the injection. Intravenous administration works more quickly, and the patient may respond after only 1 minute following administration. The patient should exhibit a strong response to the medication. Sheep take longer to recover from this medication than any other type of animal. The majority of animal species will respond quickly and have an easier recovery period when given this drug.

Pentobarbital has been replaced with ultra-short acting barbiturates. In the past, it was often employed for the purpose of anesthesia inductions. Pentobarbital may also be given with phenobarbital. While it is not an anticonvulsant, its sedative properties can reduce symptoms while waiting for the phenobarbital to take effect.

Neuroleptanalgesics

Neuroleptanalgesics are combinations of analgesics with a neuroleptic tranquilizer. Versions of this drug include oxymorphone and acepromazine. Neuroleptanalgesics are employed when it is necessary to produce a deep sedative effect. The dose can be reduced for less extensive procedures, resulting in shorter durations. These shorter time frames may include treatments involving the suturing of an injury or the removal of porcupine quills. Neuroleptanalgesics are beneficial in the treatment of patients with conditions resulting in cardiac distress or shock. Naloxone or nalbuphine are reversal agents for neuroleptanalgesics.

Some side effects include hyperactivity, auditory stimuli, defecation, vomiting, panting, and in some cases, bradycardia.

Propofol

Propofol is also known as Diprivan or Rapinovet. This drug is useful in veterinary medicine for the following purposes: sedation, anesthesia induction, and anesthesia maintenance. It is also effective as an anticonvulsant. Propofol usually results in an induction procedure that is relatively easy and stress free.

Propofol is a short-acting sedative that is rapidly dispersed throughout the body, including the brain. Although it is oil-soluble, the medication is not retained in the muscle or fat and is metabolized out of the body very quickly by the liver. Metabolic clearance of this drug is faster than required for barbiturates. This is also the preferred preanesthetic induction medication for the sight hound breeds (i.e., whippets, greyhounds,

Deerhounds, Irish Wolfhounds, Pharaoh Hounds, Afghan Hounds, Salukis, Borzois, Ibizan Hounds, Basenjis, Rhodesian Ridgebacks, and a select few others). It is also preferred for low body mass index patients. Further, it is useful as an injectable maintenance anesthesia due to its fast-acting properties. It should be noted that propofol may cause tachycardia, bradycardia, temporary arterial and venous dilation, and depressed cardiac contractility. Typically, however, this medication has no effect on the cardiovascular system.

Guaifenesin and Fentanyl

Guaifenesin is also known as glycerol guaiacolate. This drug is described as a decongestant and antitussive. Guaifenesin works on the central nervous system and skeletal muscles as a relaxant. It is most often used for treatment in large animals. This medication can serve well for anesthesia induction and recovery. The animal will experience only mild effects on the respiratory and cardiac systems. While the drug is able to cross the placental barrier, the fetus should not experience any harmful effects.

Fentanyl is most often used as an analgesic (pain reliever). Unconsciousness can result from the use of fentanyl. Mainly, this drug is employed in conjunction with a tranquilizer, sedative, or benzodiazepine. It is considered to be an injectable induction agent. This drug does not cause problems with apnea. While it can cause contractility or cardiac output changes, it is not contraindicated even for most high-risk patients. Fentanyl is usually classified as a neuroleptanalgesic.

Etomidate

Etomidate is also known by the name Amidate. This drug is used as an anesthesia induction agent. It is considered to be safe and fast acting. It is dispersed rapidly throughout the body and does not build up in any tissues or organs. An animal is administered the drug through a repeated bolus or continuous infusion. During this time the animal may suffer from vomiting, diarrhea, and excitement. This can be attributed to the drug, the induction process, and/or postanesthesia effects. The animal may show brief signs of apnea (a pause in breathing), and thus should be monitored carefully.

Etomidate is a medication that can cross the placental barrier. However, it is usually harmless due to the liver's ability to metabolize the drug quickly. Etomidate is able to mildly depress the respiratory system. It can also have a rare side effect that results in extreme muscle rigidity and seizures in horses and cattle.

An animal may experience a great deal of pain when given an IV injection of etomidate. Thus, some veterinarians also administer lidocaine for pain control. The injection can also result in phlebitis or inflammation of the veins. However, inflammation more often occurs in smaller-sized veins.

Inhalation Anesthesia vs. Injectable Anesthesia

Inhalation anesthesia has certain advantages over injectable medications. These advantages include the anesthetic depths achieved and the ease in regulation. The patient's recovery is also considered to be more rapid. Further, inhalation anesthesia provides a drug that is metabolized at a nominal rate. This is a result of the body's ability to easily expel the excess medication through the respiration process.

Inhalation anesthesia should be delivered in an initial dose that is considered a fully safe concentration, and then increased as needed. This will allow the induction of anesthesia without undue depression of the respiratory and cardiovascular systems. Inhalation anesthesia typically has both analgesic and muscle relaxant properties, and both will benefit the patient. Patient recovery is considered to be more rapid due to the capacity of these medications to be quickly eliminated from the body. Inhalation medications do not persist or accumulate within the body's tissues or systems.

General Considerations for Inhalation Anesthetic Medication

There are certain factors that should be recognized when using inhalation anesthetic medications. First, the lungs absorb inhalation anesthesia as either gases or vapors. The medication is rapidly carried from the alveoli to the brain and body. During initial dispersal, this medication remains in the same chemical form (it has not yet been changed by the liver or other metabolic events). The amount ultimately delivered to the patient can be impacted by variables such as vapor pressure, boiling point, and the anesthetic delivery system used. The medication has to be carried through the lungs subject to alveolar partial pressure, the inspired concentration, and the alveolar concentration. To be effective, the tissues must be able to readily absorb the medication. Delivery from the lungs to the brain is contingent upon the drug's solubility, the relative rate of blood flow in the arteries and tissues, the strength of the anesthetic, the tissue type, and the blood saturation of the tissues.

Minimal alveolar concentration (MAC) is the level of anesthetic vapor concentration in the lungs needed to prevent a motor response to surgical pain in 50% of all patients. The potency level rises as the MAC number is reduced.

ISOFLURANE

Isoflurane is known to induce only insignificant metabolic changes in the liver. Isoflurane is also considered to be a prudent treatment as related to the cardiovascular system. Indeed, this drug exhibits low arrhythmogenicity even while simultaneously enhancing cardiac productivity. Isoflurane is a medication that rapidly induces anesthesia, and with a shorter recovery period than many other medications. The dosage of this drug can also be adjusted easily, given the drug's low solubility characteristics. In fact, it offers a much quicker dosage adjustment and response time than that available through the drug halothane.

Even so, there are some problems associated with isoflurane. These issues pertain to respiratory depression, difficult recovery periods, and rising costs—as both halothane and isoflurane require an out-of-circle precision vaporizer to raise vapor pressures. Isoflurane produces blood pressures associated with normal rates when linked with vasodilation.

The minimal alveolar concentration (MAC) of isoflurane for canines is 1.2%. The MAC of isoflurane in cats is 1.6%.

HALOTHANE AND METHOXYFLURANE

Halothane has only modest respiratory depression effects, is not considered to be nephrotoxic, and can be mask induced. The minimal alveolar concentration (MAC) of halothane is 0.8%.

Some drawbacks of halothane anesthesia are found in the risk to the patient of cardiac arrhythmias, hypotension from cardiac depression, minimal analgesic or pain-relieving impact, and hepatotoxic effects. The patient should be given an out-of-circle precision vaporizer to maintain the required elevated vapor pressure. This practice provides the patient with the safest exposure to halothane.

Methoxyflurane has a lower solubility factor than halothane. This creates a faster rate of anesthesia induction and recovery level for the patient. The veterinarian can thus respond to adjustments needed in the concentration levels at a faster pace.

DESFLURANE

The MAC rating for desflurane is 7.2%. Desflurane promotes rapid anesthesia induction and recovery. This can be attributed to the drug's low solubility and consequent rapid dispersion. It does not display a tendency for either hepatotoxicity or nephrotoxicity.

Desflurane requires the use of a unique, electrically heated vaporizer in its administration. This type of vaporizer can be extremely costly to purchase. Further, desflurane has a pungent odor that can irritate the respiratory tract. Thus, patients tend to cough and hold their breath when being administered this drug. Some animal species will experience malignant hyperthermia from the use of this drug. Other patients may recover before treatment is finished. Patients that experience a premature recovery will need more sedation given immediately.

Sevoflurane

Sevoflurane is considered to have a very low solubility, and therefore provides speedy anesthesia induction and recovery periods. Further, it does not readily induce cardiac arrhythmias. The animal should also respond with a superior rate of muscle relaxation. The drug has an analgesic quality used to bring pain relief to the patient.

Sevoflurane is considered to be a particularly appropriate analgesic inhalant for the majority of avian or bird species. Sevoflurane is considered to be less overpowering than other inhalants. Thus, it leaves the patient with no symptoms resembling a hangover, as might otherwise be expected from the use of a psychoactive drug.

Sevoflurane and isoflurane both produce respiratory depression in the patient. Sevoflurane can also cross the placental barrier. This can result in concurrent fetal depression. Finally, this drug is typically more costly than either halothane or isoflurane.

Sevoflurane is MAC rated at 2.4%.

Nitrous Oxide

Nitrous oxide (chemical symbol: N_2O) is a very weak general anesthetic; however, it is very effective as a carrier gas for other more powerful anesthetics. Mixed in a 2:1 ratio with oxygen, it serves to increase the rate of inhalation induction in the patient. At the start of anesthesia induction, large quantities of nitrous oxide are distributed from the alveoli into the bloodstream. For some animals (depending upon the procedure), N_2O alone may provide sufficient anesthesia. Other animals may require further analgesics to be administered. Nitrous oxide has an immediate effect due to the body's inability to metabolize the medication (less than 0.004% of this gas is metabolized). The body's cardiovascular and respiratory systems suffer little effect from the application of this medication.

With a MAC rating over 100%, another medication must be used in conjunction with N_2O if general anesthesia is required. Further, the inspiration levels of O_2 drop to 33% when N_2O is administered. This drop in levels can endanger the patient. The patient may suffer from hypoxia if there is a history of respiratory problems. Further, N_2O is contraindicated in animals with gas-occupying conditions such as gastric dilation, intestinal obstruction, or pneumothorax.

Analgesics in Anesthesia

Analgesia will give the patient pain relief by inhibiting pain stimuli from connecting with the pain pathway so that the patient has no perception of the pain. Analgesia should begin prior to the surgical procedure as part of the premedication protocol. Every patient will have its own analgesic protocol after a full physical exam, blood work, and evaluation of medical history. Certain drugs may not be suitable for some patients. For example, Rimadyl (an NSAID) should not be given if the patient is taking prednisone because it is contraindicated. Alpha-2 agonists should not be used in patients with heart disease, and some drugs will need to be used in conjunction with other drugs to provide appropriate pain relief. A multimodal approach to analgesia is most effective, in which different classes of drugs are used or combined to block different areas of the pain pathway to provide adequate analgesia to the patient.

Pre-Medications and Postoperative Medications

The most common routes of administration for premedication drugs are IV, IM, and SQ. The first factor to consider when choosing a route of administration is which route the specific drug is labeled for because some drugs may not be given IV and others may not be given SQ or IM. For example, diazepam should only be given IV because of its solubility. Another factor to consider is the desired onset of action: the IV route is the fastest while the SQ route is the slowest. An antibiotic injection may be given perioperatively if needed, such as in an orthopedic surgery. You may be required to administer cefazolin, which is given IV slowly over the course of 10 minutes. An injection for pain is often required after any painful procedure. For example, carprofen (an

NSAID) is given SQ, and oral medications will be given by the owner at home starting the next day for continued pain relief.

Preanesthetic Medication

Preanesthetic medication lowers the stress level of an animal when it is given before a procedure because it supports a smooth induction and effective recovery period. The patient that receives a preanesthetic may have a reduced need for anesthesia induction and maintenance medications. It may also produce some intraoperative and postoperative analgesic effects. These medications have also been known to lower certain secretion levels and to reduce certain autonomic reflexes. This effect gives the handler a more manageable animal that is easier and safer to handle.

However, the application of preanesthetic medication can come with some drawbacks. Specifically, time and medication cost factors are involved. However, some of these costs can be counterbalanced through the reduced need for subsequent induction and maintenance agents.

Administering a Preanesthetic

Preanesthetic medication can remain effective for a period of up to 2 hours, and can be given to the patient by a variety of means. The most common administration is through an intramuscular (or IM) injection, and most preanesthetic medications will reach maximum effectiveness levels approximately 20 minutes after an intramuscular injection. An intravenous (or IV) injection works faster than other methods. However, an IV injection should be given with careful consideration, as administration via this route may induce certain temporary behavior and personality changes. Various side effects from preanesthetic drugs are associated with xylazine, acepromazine, opioids, and diazepam.

Anticholinergics in Anesthesia for Small Animals

Anticholinergics such as atropine or glycopyrrolate are used as part of the premedication protocol for small animals as a way to avoid the effects of the parasympathetic reflexes. These drugs block the vagal reflexes, preventing cardiac arrhythmias, drying out secretions, and reducing gastric reflux while under anesthesia. Dosing must be accurate because if given at a higher dose, these drugs can cause tachycardia, and low dosing can cause an AV block. They are contraindicated in patients that have a preexisting tachycardia, any cardiac disease, and patients that have GI stasis. Though generalizations cannot be made across all species, anticholinergics are at times recommended in pediatric patients (patients younger than 6 months of age) due to the fact that they rely on the heart rate to maintain CO, in any airway surgery because this can stimulate a vagal reflex, as well as patients who are brachycephalic breeds because they commonly have a high vagal tone. Anticholinergics can also be administered IV in emergency situations for a rapid onset of action.

Sedative and Tranquilizer Drugs Used in Premedication Protocol

Tranquilizers such as acepromazine or midazolam or **sedatives** such as medetomidine can also be added to the premedication protocol. Remember that tranquilizers and sedatives will sedate the patient, but sedatives provide analgesia as well. Acepromazine causes vasodilation leading to hypotension and decreases the patient's seizure threshold, but it is also an antiemetic and an antihistamine. Medetomidine is an α_2 agonist sedative and muscle relaxant that also provides analgesia and can be reversed with atipamezole (Antisedan). Medetomidine use will lower the amount of other anesthetic agents needed for the patient, such as inhalants and induction agents. Medetomidine is contraindicated for use in patients with cardiac or respiratory disorders because it has adverse effects on the cardiovascular system. Benzodiazepines such as midazolam are used for sedation and as anticonvulsants and anxiolytics. However, they do not provide analgesia, so they should be combined with a drug that does. Benzodiazepines are contraindicated in patients with kidney or liver disease because the drug is metabolized mainly through the liver and eliminated via the urine.

Pre-Procedural

ANESTHESIA PLAN

A veterinarian is responsible for supervising the veterinary technician. This includes overseeing the technician's collection of information regarding a patient's anesthesia risk factors. This information will be used to promote a comprehensive anesthesia plan. The **anesthesia plan** should be strictly adhered to during the performance of any procedure. Furthermore, it should be used to check the status of a patient's recovery following the administration of anesthesia. Medical record documentation should bear out adherence to the anesthesia plan. To this end, there should be an authentication process applied to all medical record entries.

The technician is responsible for consulting with and keeping the veterinarian informed of any irregularities or unexpected situations and occurrences.

MEDICAL HISTORY FOR DEVELOPING AN ANESTHETIC PLAN

A complete patient physical exam and medical history are necessary to be able to provide an appropriate anesthetic plan. Any chronic diseases that the patient may have, such as kidney or liver disease, must be noted because some anesthetic drugs are metabolized through the liver and excreted via the urine. These drugs should be avoided in this case. If the patient has a history of cardiovascular disease, certain premedications such as dexmedetomidine should not be used. Any medications that the patient is currently taking are necessary to know because some medications may not be taken together, such as steroids and NSAIDs. If the patient has a history of seizures, then certain anticonvulsant drugs may be added to the premedications.

ANESTHETIC PLAN FOR PEDIATRIC OR NEONATAL PATIENTS

Neonatal refers to patients younger than 4 months of age, and **pediatric** refers to those patients 6 months of age and younger. Pediatric and neonatal patients' cardiac output and blood pressure maintenance solely rely on the heart rate and stroke volume, so if the heart rate decreases (bradycardia), then the cardiac output decreases and so does blood pressure. Pediatric patients have a higher chance of hypoxia during apnea due to their reduced pulmonary reserve. Pediatric and neonatal patients have a more pliable rib cage and weak intercostal muscles; therefore, they use more energy and effort for breathing, which could lead to airway collapse and respiratory fatigue. Pediatric patients are prone to hypoglycemia because of their minimal glycogen stores, so their blood glucose should be monitored. They should fast only a few hours before an anesthetic procedure and be fed a couple of hours after recovery. Pediatric and neonatal patients are prone to hypothermia due to their immature thermoregulatory system, so monitoring temperature pre, peri, and post anesthesia is vital.

ANESTHETIC PLAN FOR GERIATRIC PATIENTS

A complete blood panel is recommended for geriatric patients to evaluate kidney and liver function, as well as a complete blood cell count and electrolyte panel. Lowered drug dosing will be used to lower cardiovascular effects and lower the amount of work on specific organs for elimination of these drugs. The geriatric patient should be placed on a warming device such as a heating pad with a blanket between the pad and the patient's body, an IV fluid warmer, and foot covers to prevent heat loss because these patients are more susceptible to hypothermia due to less body fat. Geriatric patients need to have their temperature monitored closely during the procedure as well as during recovery. Hypothermia leads to hypotension and arrhythmias, so the vital signs must be watched closely to protect the geriatric patient.

ANESTHETIC PLAN FOR BRACHYCEPHALIC PATIENTS

A complete physical exam must be done for brachycephalic patients (such as bulldogs, shih tzus, pugs, and boxers) prior to administration of pre-medications, including full panel blood work, auscultation of the heart and lungs, as well as an evaluation of the degree of upper airway obstruction. Any abnormal upper airway sounds or heart murmurs should be noted because this will affect the drugs used, as well as the monitoring of the patient. An SpO_2 reading should be taken in room air on the patient to get a baseline reading of the patient's normal reading because brachycephalic breeds normally have a lower SpO_2 reading (93–95%) than other breeds. Premedication should include an anticholinergic, which will prevent bradycardia and dry the patient's oral secretions, along with a sedative that provides analgesia and buprenorphine or morphine. The brachycephalic breed must be preoxygenated for 5 minutes prior to induction, and a laryngoscope must be used to intubate because it will be difficult to visualize the back of the throat. It is necessary to wait until these patients are alert and swallowing to extubate, and they must be closely monitored during recovery until they are standing and bright, alert, and responsive (**BAR**).

Preanesthetic Blood Work

Before a patient undergoes a surgical procedure, it is important to run preanesthetic blood work. Preanesthetic blood work may include a CBC, chemistry panel, and electrolytes. The major reasons these tests are important are that a **complete blood count (CBC)** can detect clotting disorders or an abnormally high WBC count indicating infection, which would put the patient at risk for an anesthetic procedure and surgery. Certain anesthetic agents will metabolize through the liver and be excreted via the urine, and a **chemistry panel** will indicate the kidney (blood urea nitrogen, creatinine, phosphorus) and liver (alanine transaminase, alkaline phosphatase, and bilirubin) function. If the chemistry panel shows an abnormal level of kidney and liver enzymes, this can mean that the patient could have a slower, abnormal recovery from anesthesia and the anesthetic plan may need to be altered. **Electrolyte** levels, including potassium, sodium, and chloride, may indicate signs of dehydration as well.

Fasting Before Anesthetic Procedures

The patient will need to be **fasted** (no food or water) commonly after 10 p.m. the night prior to the anesthetic event. The reason for fasting the patient is because most anesthetic drugs cause vomiting. While the patient is under general anesthesia, the larynx relaxes, which is the part of the body that prevents matter from going down into the trachea. If the patient were to vomit while anesthetized, the vomited material could risk going down into the trachea to the lungs (**aspiration**) rather than into the esophagus to the stomach. If the patient does aspirate, this can lead to pneumonia.

Overview of Anesthetic Procedures for Owners

When the patient arrives for an anesthetic procedure, the veterinary technician and the veterinarian will perform a full physical exam and evaluate the patient's medical history. Based on the patient's health status, species, and weight, a premedication protocol will be implemented. The patient will be premedicated prior to the surgery to sedate and provide analgesia preemptively. Once adequately sedated, the patient is induced with an IV agent to achieve general anesthesia. Once induced, the patient is intubated and maintained on a low level of anesthetic inhalant. From the moment of induction, the patient is continuously monitored by a licensed veterinary technician who will be adjusting the vaporizer and oxygen settings as needed and manually assessing vital signs including the heart rate, respiration rate, mucous membrane color, capillary refill time, pulse quality and strength, and temperature. Monitoring equipment will also be used, including blood pressure monitoring, EKG, capnography, and pulse oximetry. After the surgery is completed, the patient will be extubated once they show signs of waking up (swallowing). During the recovery phase, the veterinary technician will keep a close eye on the patient and continue to monitor vital signs until the patient is alert and standing.

Importance of an IV Catheter

An **IV catheter** provides direct access to the vein. It is important to place an IV catheter in every patient going under anesthesia as well as those hospitalized patients requiring intravenous medication or fluid administration. An emergency could happen at any time while the patient is under anesthesia, and emergency medications such as epinephrine or atropine may need to be administered intravenously. Placing an IV catheter prior to surgery is more efficient than having to place one during an emergency when circulatory collapse occurs most of the time, leading to low blood pressure and making it harder to place an IV catheter. An IV catheter is also useful when administering fluids to a patient under anesthesia to maintain blood pressure by allowing the movement of blood to the body's vital organs. While patients are hospitalized, it is ideal to have an IV catheter placed for fluid therapy and to ease administration of IV medications.

Placing an ET in a Patient

Endotracheal (ET) tubes are used when a patient is anesthetized to secure and protect the airway. The patient must be sternal with the head and neck extended in a straight line so the larynx is visible. The restrainer should hold the patient's head and place the thumb and forefinger behind the canines on the maxilla and pull the head up and out straight. The person who will be intubating will pull the tongue out of the mouth over the lower incisors and open the mouth wide. A laryngoscope should be used because it has a light to illuminate the area, as well as free up the epiglottis if it is hidden behind the soft palate. The ET is inserted into the trachea but not advanced past the thoracic inlet. Use a tie (either gauze string or an IV line) to tie around the ET and then behind the canines and tie behind the patient's ears or on top of their nose. To determine if the ET is placed correctly, watch for the reservoir bag to inflate and deflate with respirations, fog to appear in the ET from respirations, or confirm with capnography because the presence of CO_2 means that the ET is placed correctly.

Inflating an ET Cuff

In order to correctly inflate an ET cuff, you will need two people. The cuff is inflated with air from a syringe that attaches to the cuff. A 3 mL syringe should be used for cats, and a 10 mL syringe can be used for dogs with larger ET tubes. Once the patient is intubated, one person will close the pop-off valve and squeeze the reservoir bag up to 20 cmH_2O while the anesthetist listens closely to the patient's mouth for leaks. If a leak is heard while squeezing the reservoir bag, then a little more air may be needed to inflate the cuff. Open the pop-off valve when reinflating the cuff and after no leaks are heard. The person squeezing the reservoir bag should say "breathing" when they squeeze and "release" when the bag relaxes because a leak will only be detected on inspiration and the bag would empty when squeezed as the air goes past the tube into the oral cavity.

Anesthetic Ventilation

One form of mechanical ventilation is referred to as **intermittent positive pressure ventilation** or **IPPV**. It involves establishing a preset respiratory rate. Successful ventilation can help preserve normal acid-base levels by oxygenating the patient and reducing CO_2 retention. Assisted ventilation is usually necessary for overweight patients, patients in head-down recumbency, and patients with hypothermia or pulmonary disease. Ventilation is controlled in patients who receive neuromuscular blocking agents. In addition, patients with thoracic surgery, diaphragmatic hernia, gastric torsion, or hypoventilation should receive this same care. The veterinarian should note the respiratory rate, inspiration-to-expiration ratio, tidal volume, and inspiratory pressure. These outcomes should be reassessed continuously throughout the surgery. Ventilation is further checked by looking at the animal's chest motions from the breathing process.

A patient that demonstrates spontaneous breathing while receiving IPPV is being underventilated. Overventilation is not advisable, as it can cause the pulmonary alveoli to be harmed. A patient in an underventilated state will have a reduced cardiac output. Respiratory alkalosis can occur as a result of unwarranted levels of CO_2.

Reservoir or Rebreathing Bag

The **rebreathing bag** permits fresh and exhaled gas to accumulate and be available for the patient's next breath. It is important to have the correct-sized rebreathing bag for the patient because if the bag is too small the patient won't be able to make a full breath before using up the gas in the bag and deflating it first. If the rebreathing bag is too big for the patient, then the anesthetic system's volume increases, which prolongs the time to change the inspired anesthetic concentration. The rebreathing bag is also used to manually breathe for the patient that is not adequately breathing on its own under anesthesia or in emergency situations when the patient must be intubated and manually ventilated.

Calculating Reservoir Bag Size

To choose the correct size of reservoir bag, you take the patient's tidal volume and multiply that by six. The patient's tidal volume, which is the amount of inhaled and exhaled air with each breath, is normally around 20 mL/kg. For example, for a dog that weighs 10 kg: 10 kg $\times$ 25 mL/kg = 250 mL and 250 mL $\times$ 6 = 1,500 mL.

Then, to convert milliliters to liters, because rebreathing bags are weighed in liters: 1,500 mL ÷ 1,000 = 1.5 L. So, a 2-liter bag would be used for that patient as the rule of thumb is to round up to the nearest liter.

Preoxygenation

Preoxygenation can be done around 5 minutes prior to induction by delivering pure oxygen to the patient through a mask via the anesthetic machine. Preoxygenation aids in replacing nitrogen in the patient's lungs with oxygen, reducing the risk of possible hypoxemia that can result from induction agents. Hypoxemia is the insufficient oxygenation of arterial blood in the body resulting in poorly oxygenated vital organs, causing cyanosis in the patient. Brachycephalic breeds will benefit from being preoxygenated, especially given the fact that intubation may take longer to accomplish. Obese and pregnant patients will also require preoxygenation because they are at risk for oxygen desaturation.

Patients with **cardiac disease** should be preoxygenated and require IV fluid therapy. It should be given carefully to avoid fluid overload, which can cause congestive heart failure. Monitoring the patient's blood pressure, oxygenation, and lung sounds will need to be done to determine if fluid therapy should be stopped or slowed.

Anesthetic Process and Monitoring

Stages and Planes of Anesthesia

Stage I

The first stage of anesthesia is the voluntary excitement stage. The patient is conscious, has control of motor responses, and may display the fight-or-flight response.

Stage I of anesthesia encompasses initial anesthetic administration up to the point of the loss of consciousness. This is known as the stage of **induction**, early analgesia, and altered state of consciousness. The patient may experience the following: dulled sensations, pain loss, blood pressure elevation, vomiting, inspiratory struggling, and coughing. The patient's pupils will begin to dilate as Stage II approaches. The patient's breathing rate is usually high and irregular at this time.

Stage II

Stage two is labeled involuntary excitement, and it starts when the patient goes unconscious up until regular, steady breathing is established.

Stage II commences with the loss of consciousness. In Stage II, the patient may experience the following: excitement or delirious activity and vocalization, symptoms of involuntary struggling, and physiological agitation. During this time it is expected that the patient's eyes will remain closed and its jaw will be set. The patient's point reflexes may be amplified. The patient's pupils will be dilated and respond to light. Stage II does not last long.

Patients experiencing fairly uncomplicated inductions can move from stage I to stage III (the surgical stage) without incident.

Stage III

During **Stage III**, the surgical stage, the patient's pupils will constrict further and the patient will gradually lose the palpebral reflex. However, the patient's breathing will be full and regular. There are 4 planes associated with Stage III anesthesia:

- **Plane 1** is light anesthesia in which the patient is able to be intubated and short exams and surgical procedures can take place. The patient retains the palpebral reflex, swallowing reflex, and should be able to produce regular respirations with a respectable measure of chest activity.

- **Plane 2** is medium anesthesia in which most surgical procedures can take place. The patient will lose the palpebral reflex and will demonstrate a fixed pupil response. Respirations will continue to be regular and the chest and muscles in the diaphragm will continue to exhibit a good amount of movement.
- **Plane 3** is deep anesthesia and is not normally necessary for most surgical procedures. The patient's breathing becomes shallow due to a partial intercostal paralysis, limiting the patient's ability to breathe with its chest and abdominal muscles.
- **Plane 4** is an unstable and potentially life-threatening stage that should be avoided. This stage is formally reached when the patient ceases to breathe.

STAGE IV

Should the patient experience prolonged apnea, cardiac arrest, or brainstem or medullary paralysis, the "overdose" or fourth stage of the anesthesia will have been encountered. **Stage IV** of anesthesia is excessively deep, and if the patient gets to this stage, prompt remedial steps must immediately be taken because this can lead to cardiovascular and respiratory depression or death.

RESPONSE IF THE PATIENT WILL NOT REMAIN ANESTHETIZED

If a patient will not remain anesthetized, you must check their respirations. If they exhibit shallow respirations, this could lead to the patient being under a light stage of anesthesia possibly due to the gas anesthetic not entering the lungs. The patient may need to be given manual breaths with oxygen and gas anesthetic until adequate anesthetic depth is reached. The ET may be too short, or the cuff may not be properly inflated. Vaporizer settings and oxygen settings must be checked. If the gas anesthetic is too low, the patient could be too lightly under anesthesia and painful stimuli such as an incision could easily arouse the patient.

ADJUSTING THE VAPORIZER SETTING FOR THE ANESTHETIZED PATIENT

Directly after the patient is induced, the anesthetic vaporizer will be set at or higher than (~3%) for a few minutes to reach an adequate anesthetic plane. However, if certain drugs such as dexmedetomidine were given as a premedication, then the vaporizer setting may be lower (1.5%) right after induction because dexmedetomidine causes cardiovascular and respiratory depression. Every 5 minutes or more frequently, the vaporizer setting should be checked, along with the patient's vital signs, and adjusted accordingly. If the patient is under a light plane of anesthesia and is showing signs of an increased heart rate or is responding to the palpebral reflex, the vaporizer setting should be increased, and the patient should be reevaluated after a couple of minutes. If the patient appears to be too deep under anesthesia showing signs of a decreasing heart rate or lower respiratory rate, then the vaporizer setting should be turned down accordingly and the patient should be reevaluated continuously until the patient is at the appropriate depth.

REFLEXES USED TO DETERMINE ANESTHETIC DEPTH

There are **reflexes** that the technician can assess on the patient to determine anesthetic depth. A neurological reflex is an involuntary motor response to stimuli that should be instantaneous. They do not require consciousness, and delayed or absent reflexes indicate a disrupted **reflex arc**. Reflex arcs consist of the sensory receptor, afferent or sensory neuron, interneuron, efferent or motor neuron, and effector target. Reflexes used to determine anesthetic depth include: palpebral and corneal reflexes, pupillary light reflex (PLR), and the pedal reflex.

A muscle relaxant-assisted surgery will mask some of the usual signs used to monitor depth of anesthesia. In this case, regularly checking the depth of anesthesia takes on additional importance.

PALPEBRAL REFLEX

The **palpebral reflex** is tested by lightly touching the medial or lateral canthus of the eye to stimulate blinking. If the patient still displays the palpebral reflex, the patient may be too lightly sedated for certain procedures. The patient's medial palpebral reflex will fade away after the lateral reflex becomes more intense. In stage III, plane 2 of anesthesia, the medication causes the patient's reflex to grow slower and weaker. The only acceptable reflex is found in that of a mild medial palpebral reflex that can be viewed after an analgesic has been given to the patient. This reflex is also present when an injectable anesthesia is used as a solitary medication. It may also be present when methoxyflurane is used.

Corneal Reflex and Eye Movement

The **corneal reflex** can be tested by gently tapping the lateral aspect of the cornea to induce eyelid closure if the reflex is still intact. If reflex closure of the eye does not occur with this stimulation, then the patient is moving into a deep plane 2 state and may be over-anesthetized. This reflex is more difficult to determine if the eyeball is significantly rotated downward, as occurs with dogs and cats.

Minimize use of this reflex test to avoid injury to the cornea. Other monitoring devices should be more frequently relied on.

Patients that are in stage III, plane 2 of anesthesia will not exhibit eyeball movement, and the pupils will begin to dilate and the eye will rotate to a ventral medial (central) position. In dogs and cats, the eyeball rotates down when under halothane, isoflurane, barbiturate, and propofol anesthesia and does not revert to a central position until deeper in plane 3. Patients that exhibit any eye movement or blinking are not sedated heavily enough for surgery to commence.

Pupil Size and Pupillary Light Reflex

During stage I, the patient's pupils should be a normal size. During stage II, they may be dilated, but they should return to normal in stage III, plane 1. Surgical anesthesia (plane 2) patients will have slightly dilated pupils. Pupils that are more than slightly dilated are a cause for concern and may indicate excessively deep anesthesia.

When a patient has a normal **pupillary light reflex (PLR)**, both pupils will constrict when bright light is shone on one eye. Under light and medium (non-surgical) anesthesia, the PLR will be intact. The pupillary light reflex is delayed under surgical anesthesia (stage III, plane 2).

Pedal Reflex

Another way to evaluate the depth of anesthesia is to check for the **pedal reflex**. This requires the technician to firmly squeeze or modestly pinch the patient's skin—specifically, between the toes in dogs and cats, squeezing together the claws in cattle and swine, or applying firm pressure on the pastern of a horse. This action stimulates the animal's pedal reflex. The usual reaction is for the animal to pull the leg away. However, if properly anesthetized, the anesthetic plane greatly reduces the animal's response and reaction time. Patients considered to be within a surgical plane will not be able to respond to the stimulus at all.

Jaw Tone

Jaw tone is resistance given when opening the patient's mouth, and presence of jaw tone means that the patient is too lightly anesthetized to intubate. The test is conducted by grasping the lower jaw of the animal and attempting to open the animal's mouth gently and widely, up to 3 times. This test is given to the animal prior to endotracheal intubation. The animal will usually resist the mouth-opening efforts. This response diminishes when the animal reaches a light surgical plane. However, there are occasions when the addition of a strong analgesic or methoxyflurane can produce some signs of response. This does not indicate that a suitable plane of anesthesia has not been reached.

Pharyngeal and Laryngeal Reflexes

The pharyngeal reflex enables swallowing, and the laryngeal reflex enables coughing and closing of the larynx. The **laryngeal reflex** causes the epiglottis and vocal cords to close when the larynx is touched, such as by an endotracheal tube. If an animal is not sufficiently anesthetized, the laryngeal reflex can make intubation difficult. The **pharyngeal reflex** is an animal's normal response to food or liquid in the pharynx, triggering swallowing. It is lost under surgical anesthesia, but it returns when the animal is waking up, signaling the time to remove the endotracheal tube.

Fluid Therapy During Anesthesia

The decision to have a patient receive **fluid therapy** during anesthesia depends on the patient's age, physical condition, as well as the length and type of anesthetic procedure. Fluid therapy during an anesthetic procedure makes up for the ongoing fluid loss as well as provides cardiac support and allows the body to maintain fluid volume for longer procedures. While the patient is under anesthesia, the anesthetic gases and premedications can lower blood pressure, whereas IV fluid therapy will offset this decrease. Low blood pressure can result in kidney damage, so IV fluids are critical in keeping blood pressure up so the vital organs are properly oxygenated. IV fluids also help to protect the kidneys and hydrate the patient because fasting for surgical procedures can lead to dehydration as well as blood loss from certain procedures. Sometimes the patient's body temperature will decrease while under anesthesia, and administering warm IV fluids can keep the patient at an ideal body temperature. IV fluids also aid in the excretion of anesthetic from the kidneys and liver, which leads to a smooth recovery.

Replacement Fluids for Stable Anesthetic Cases

The sedated and stable patient can be given IV fluid replacement crystalloids like Normosol R or Plasmalyte 148. Maintenance crystalloids include Normosol M or Plasmalyte 56. Replacement crystalloids are comparable to plasma because they have high sodium and chloride levels with a reduced potassium concentration. These medications can be administered 5-10 mL/kg/hr for dogs and 1-5 mL/kg/hr for cats. Longer applications will require that the first hour be run at no more than 10 mL/kg/hr, with additional hours reduced to 5 mL/kg/hr.

Monitoring Anesthetized Patients

Once the patient is induced, the technician should hook up the patient to the anesthetic machine with the gas and oxygen flow and check the patient's heart rate and respiratory rate, adjusting the vaporizer setting as needed. The monitoring equipment used will include blood pressure, EKG, capnography, and pulse oximetry. Every 5 minutes while the patient is under anesthesia, the technician should manually check the patient's heart rate, respiratory rate, pulse strength and quality, mucous membrane color, capillary refill time, temperature, and lung sounds. The oxygen and vaporizer settings should also be checked every 5 minutes and adjusted according to the patient's depth and status. If there is a decrease in the patient's temperature, steps should be taken to stabilize it.

The patient's EKG reading should be monitored for abnormalities. If the patient is experiencing a sinus arrhythmia under anesthesia, the EKG monitor may not be able to catch every beat, so taking a heart rate using a stethoscope is important. The respiratory rate given on the monitor may pick up inaccurate movements, so manually measuring the patient's respiratory rate is important, as is listening to lung sounds with a stethoscope to make sure that they are clear.

Body Temperature

When the patient's metabolism slows down while under anesthesia, the demand for anesthesia sufficient to maintain the surgical plane lessens as well. This is also true when the body temperature is reduced, so body temperature should be carefully watched when a patient is under anesthesia to prevent complications. The patient may require additional body temperature support starting with induction and during the recovery period as well.

Using large amounts of scrubbing solutions or using alcohol for EKG lead contact can cool a patient, so limiting scrub solutions and using gel instead of alcohol for EKG lead contact will help keep the patient's body temperature from decreasing. The patient should be placed on top of a towel, warming blanket, or a forced-air warming device such as a Bair Hugger, and should not be placed directly onto the cold surgery table. If the patient is undergoing a dental procedure, their face must be kept as dry as possible by placing towels under the neck and switching out damp towels often because this can quickly lower their body temperature.

Anesthetic-Induced Hypothermia

Hypothermia is a drop in body temperature below the normal range. Hypothermia affects several different areas of the body, including the cardiovascular, respiratory, and metabolic systems, as well as decreasing immune function, which in turn increases the risk of infection. While under anesthesia, if the patient becomes hypothermic, their metabolic rate decreases, causing slower drug metabolism and elimination, leading to longer recovery times. When the body temperature gets as low as 95 °F, vasodilation occurs and leads to hypotension (low blood pressure); at temperatures any lower than this, the body can't regulate its own body temperature. When a patient is hypothermic, the blood thickness and PCV increase, which increases the work for the myocardium.

	Ranges (°F) for Adult Cats and Dogs
Normal	100-102.5
Mild hypothermia	98-99.9
Moderate hypothermia	96-98
Severe hypothermia	92-96
Critical hypothermia	Less than 92

Heart Rate and Respiratory Rate

Heart rate should be carefully monitored during general anesthetic procedures using a stethoscope to obtain an accurate assessment of rate and heart sounds. Mechanical monitoring equipment with a digital readout can also be employed. Dogs under anesthesia should have a heart rate ranging from 70-140 beats per minute. Cats under anesthesia should have a heart rate ranging from 100-140 beats per minute. The animal's heart rate may slow down when the anesthetic plane deepens in the patient. Bradycardia can be caused by a number of drugs, hypotension, end-stage hypoxia, and vagal nerve stimulation. In such situations the heart may still maintain a constant rate even when the patient falls into a dangerously deep state of anesthesia.

The pulse rate can be monitored by digital palpation along its artery. Pulse deficits and diversions between the actual heartbeat and a palpable pulse response must be recorded on the patient's chart. Arterial palpation and electrocardiograms should be used together to monitor the patient for arrhythmias.

Normal respiratory rate for an anesthetized patient is 8–12 breaths per minute.

Blood Pressure

Normal blood pressure ranges vary by species. In most cases, the animal will be in deeper anesthetic planes when exhibiting a drop in blood pressure. Blood pressure can rise with hypercapnia (high levels of blood carbon dioxide, usually due to hypoventilation). However, blood pressure may sometimes be reduced with hypercapnia. Thus, the animal's rate and depth of ventilation must be carefully monitored.

Species	Systolic	Diastolic	MAP
Dogs	90–140 mmHg	50–80 mmHg	60–100 mmHg
Cats	80–140 mmHg	55–75 mmHg	60–100 mmHg

Mucous Membrane Color

Check the patient's **mucous membranes** easily by lifting the lip and looking at the gums. The mucous membrane color represents the blood flow to the tissues. Unpigmented areas of mucous membrane are seen as pink when in a normal state; the discoloration of these tissues can be attributed to pathophysiology. If the patient's mucous membranes appear pale, this could mean that the patient is anemic, and it represents poor perfusion. Mucous membranes that appear blue or purple may indicate a decreased amount of oxygen in the tissues (cyanosis); this is a medical emergency. If mucous membranes are yellow, this commonly indicates a liver problem. The bile is not being excreted by the liver but is instead accumulating in the tissues, giving them a yellow color. A brilliant pink coloration can be attributed to the condition known as hypoventilation and high CO_2 levels within the body caused by incomplete respiration and/or CO_2 retention.

Capillary Refill Time

The **capillary refill time (CRT)** is calculated as the amount of time it takes for blood flow to come back to an area after digital compression has been applied to an unpigmented mucous membrane (gingival tissue is a common site). A normal CRT is <2 seconds, and if the CRT is more than 2 seconds, the patient could be experiencing hypotension, vasodilation, or hypothermia. During general anesthesia, the CRT levels also require observation. In addition, the patient's blood pressure should be monitored concurrently. Blood pressure and CRT levels are both indicative of the quality of peripheral perfusion arising from cardiac output. CRT indices are expected to become more protracted as the anesthetic plane deepens and if hypovolemia (loss of blood volume) ensues in the patient.

Troubleshooting Problems with Anesthetized Patients

Perioperative Sinus Bradycardia

Heart abnormalities, hypothyroidism, or hyperkalemia can cause **sinus bradycardia**, measured as a heart rate less than 60 bpm in large dogs, 80 bpm in medium to small dogs, and 100 bpm in cats. Common causes of sinus bradycardia are a result of low body temperature and the patient being too deep under anesthesia, which is why diligent vital sign monitoring is important. A patient with sinus bradycardia can exhibit hypotension and poor tissue perfusion. Sinus bradycardia should be treated with atropine or glycopyrrolate; otherwise, it will result in a longer recovery time due to decreased drug metabolism through the kidneys.

Perioperative Sinus Tachycardia

Sinus tachycardia is defined as an abnormally high heart rate of more than 180 bpm in cats and more than 150–190 bpm in dogs, depending on the animal's size. Elevated heart rate can cause hypotension. If the heart cannot compensate for the decreased stroke volume caused by sinus tachycardia, then the oxygen perfusion increases. Certain drugs, such as anticholinergics, can cause sinus tachycardia, as well as the patient becoming stimulated during a surgical procedure due to inadequate anesthetic depth. Constant monitoring of the patient's anesthetic depth is vital, and the vaporizer setting may need to be adjusted accordingly if the patient is not under a correct anesthetic depth. Adequate pain control will need to be administered as well to prevent the patient from having an increased heart rate in response to a painful stimulus.

Ventricular Premature Complexes (VPC)

Ventricular premature complexes (VPCs) happen before the heart has time to fill, making it harder for the heart to pump blood effectively. During ventricular tachycardia, less blood is pumped to the body as a result of ventricular tachycardia because of the VPCs making it harder to pump effectively; therefore, the heart can stop if the abnormal beat happens at the wrong time. VPCs can be treated with a lidocaine bolus when the VPCs cause hypotension or when many occur at once.

Dyspnea and Cyanosis

Dyspnea is labored breathing or shortness of breath, and **cyanosis** is the discoloration of skin or mucous membranes due to inadequate tissue oxygenation (the patient's tissues will appear bluish-purple or grey). Common causes of respiratory distress while under anesthesia could be an empty oxygen tank, the oxygen flowmeter may be turned all the way down, or it could be a damaged circuit. An airway obstruction or respiratory disease such as pulmonary edema may be a cause as well. The anesthetic depth must be evaluated as well. If the patient is inhaling an excessive amount of gas anesthetic, they may be too deep. If respiratory distress is noticed, the first step is to deliver 100% oxygen to the patient and turn the vaporizer off. Ventilate with oxygen until the patient has a normal mucous membrane color (pink/moist) and the SpO_2 reading is within normal limits (>95%). Always alert the attending veterinarian in this emergency situation.

Perioperative Hypotension

If the MAP under anesthesia is less than 60 mmHg, this can lead to delayed recovery from anesthesia, decreased metabolism of drugs via the kidneys, renal failure, and CNS abnormalities. Severe untreated hypotension can lead to cardiac and respiratory arrest. The first step is identifying the cause of hypotension in the anesthetized patient. Many anesthetic drugs affect blood pressure, so if the patient is otherwise healthy with normal vital signs other than BP, then anesthetic drugs are the likely cause. If the drug has a reversal agent, then it should be administered, or the anesthetic depth should be lowered. IV fluids are to be administered at no more than 10 mL/kg/hr for the anesthetized patient in order to compensate for vasodilation and replace the patient's ongoing losses. If hypovolemia is the cause, then a bolus of IV fluids should be administered, and the patient's BP should be reevaluated. If the patient is experiencing blood loss, this should be replaced at 3 mL crystalloid fluids to 1 mL of blood loss, whereas hetastarch may be required for extreme blood loss.

Cardiac Arrest on a Patient Under Anesthesia

If the patient under anesthesia has no heart rate and is not breathing, the first thing to do is turn off the vaporizer and alert the veterinarian. Signs that could indicate oncoming cardiac arrest include low blood pressure and weak or irregular pulse, cyanosis, and a trend in a decreasing respiratory rate that is noticed during 5-minute-interval monitoring. **Cardiac arrest** is when there is no pulse or heartbeat, apnea, and a loss of certain reflexes such as the palpebral reflex. The patient's eyes will appear fixed and wide open with dilated pupils that are unresponsive to light. In order to respond quickly to this emergency, it is critical that the person monitoring take manual heart rates and respiratory rates and check the mucous membrane color and capillary refill time, as well as feel pulses for the duration of anesthesia to notice trends such as a slow decrease in respirations. Monitoring equipment is helpful, but can be unreliable; for example, an EKG will appear normal even if the heart is not contracting.

Interpretation of Blood Gases

The veterinary technician should always monitor a patient's pH and blood gas levels while the animal is under anesthesia. Lower rates of pH are indicative of metabolic or respiratory acidosis; higher rates are indicative of metabolic or respiratory alkalosis.

The **$PaCO_2$**, or partial pressure of carbon dioxide in the alveoli, can also be used to determine the patient's respiratory condition. The **adjusted base excess (ABE)** levels can be used to determine the patient's metabolic condition. The patient's pH can be indicative of the direction in which the changes are taking place. The metabolic state is determined by the ABE levels, despite the presence of irregular levels of CO_2. This can be attributed to the changes in $PaCO_2$ that are assessed along with the ABE level. Normal levels of CO_2 suggest that the metabolic state can be determined through analysis of the HCO_3^-. Normal blood gas values:

	Dogs	Cats
pH	7.36 to 7.42	7.24 to 7.44
PaO_2 (mmHg)	95.3 to 108.9	87.9 to 117.9
$PaCO_2$ (mmHg)	34.1 to 39.5	26.6 to 40.6
HCO_3^- (mmol/L)	19.8 to 23	14.5 to 20.5
ABE (mmol/L)	-3.4 to -0.2	-11.4 to -1.4

Acidosis

Metabolic acidosis can be caused by a low adjusted base excess (ABE), low HCO_3^- as confirmed by blood gas analysis, lactic acid gain, renal failure, diarrhea, and losing and not reabsorbing HCO_3^- rich body secretions. Higher levels of H^+ can be detected when HCO_3^- is lost. Metabolic acidosis can be detected when HCO_3^- is less than 20.

Respiratory acidosis is a result of hypoventilation, where CO_2 excretion is lower than the CO_2 produced, leading to elevated blood levels of CO_2. Conditions that contribute to hypoventilation include: a state of deep anesthesia, pulmonary disease, or respiratory obstruction.

Hyperventilation or an IV alkalinizing solution can correct acute, anesthesia-induced acidosis. Sodium bicarbonate can be administered to patients to restore more acute imbalances.

However, this can be a deadly approach for patients with metabolic acidosis secondary to dehydration. The blood gas results should be noted and interpreted according to the factors associated with both the primary and secondary disorders.

ALKALOSIS

Respiratory alkalosis is a result of a patient's excreting more CO_2 than is produced, which may occur as a result of mechanical respiratory hyperventilation. It can also be caused by spontaneous hyperventilation in patients suffering from extreme pain or some other source of overstimulation.

The patient suffering from respiratory alkalosis may exhibit tachycardia and other electrocardiographic anomalies. The kidneys may be able to counteract the effects, if given enough time. Further, a mechanically ventilated patient can be given a lower minute volume of ventilation to reduce the effects of respiratory alkalosis.

POST-ANESTHETIC RECOVERY

The patient should receive continued ventilatory support for a few minutes after the inhalant anesthetic is turned off. This additional ventilatory support will be essential to the patient's speedy recovery as it assists in ridding the body of residual inhalant anesthetic.

Patients must be monitored closely during the recovery phase of the anesthetic procedure. Once the patient has swallowed twice, the ET can be removed (**extubation**) while the patient is in sternal recumbency (in case of vomiting). The patient's vital signs must be monitored during the recovery phase including the heart rate, respiratory rate, mucous membrane color, and capillary refill time. The patient's temperature should be monitored every 15 minutes until it is within normal range. To promote circulation during the recovery phase, the patient may be walked around or moved around to provide stimulation. If the patient becomes hypothermic (lower than a 98-degree body temperature) during recovery, place a heating pad covered with a towel under the patient and place towels on top of the patient. Also make sure a reversal agent was given if needed. Check the patient's temperature frequently and remove heat sources as necessary to prevent the patient from becoming hyperthermic.

Maintaining, Cleaning, and Preparing Equipment

PARTS OF AN ANESTHESIA MACHINE

An anesthesia machine is fashioned from the following: medical gas cylinders, a regulator, flowmeter, vaporizer, inhalation or exhalation flutter valves, check valves, y-connector, a rebreathing bag or reservoir bag, carbon dioxide absorber, soda lime canister, exhaust valve, manometer, oxygen flush valve, scavenger system, and a negative pressure relief valve.

The **gas cylinders** hold compressed gas which is subjected to extreme pressures. Full containers of oxygen are pressurized at around 2,000-2,200 psi (pounds per square inch). Full containers of nitrous oxide are pressurized from 750-770 psi. A **regulator** can reduce the pressure of the gas exiting to around 50 psi. The **flowmeter** sets the gas delivery at a certain rate. The flowmeter can further reduce the pressure to approximately 15 psi. Animal size is a crucial variable that must be accounted for in the gas flow rate. Thus, minimum gas volume requirements are around 60 mL/kg of patient weight. The liquid anesthetic is changed to a vapor with the **vaporizer**. It regulates the quantity of anesthesia combined with the carrier gas.

PRECISION AND SIMPLE VAPORIZERS

A **precision vaporizer** incorporates an anesthetic vapor concentration that is regulated independently, and based on the time, temperature, and fresh gas flow rate. An anesthetist can compensate for the temperature and flow rate manually. This can be accomplished with a vaporizer. The percentage of the anesthetic is fixed according to dials, charts, and/or mathematical calculations. It is impossible for the patient to physically extract gases out of a precision vaporizer. This is due to the internal resistance inherent in the device. The problem is alleviated with an out-of-circle position. The complexity of this device requires particular skill when it is being serviced.

Simple or **non-precision vaporizers** are not appropriate for the administration of a specific, continuous percentage of anesthesia. This is because non-precision vaporizers are unable to accommodate the following variables: changes in temperature, fresh gas flow rates, ventilation changes, liquid and wick surfaces, and the volume of liquid anesthetic. Thus, these vaporizers do not lend themselves to an accurate calculation and consistent maintenance of the percentage of anesthetic given to the patient. Even so, the low internal resistance allows an in-the-circle application, and this application can include an out-of-circle operation. The nonlinear concentrations given make it hard to regulate the anesthesia depth. However, this simple device does not require as much maintenance as the precision vaporizer requires.

Rebreathing Circuits

Rebreathing circuits are recommended for patients weighing more than 10 pounds. They operate by circulating a combination of expired and fresh gases and work to push the expired gas through the soda lime canister, which absorbs the carbon dioxide. It is then rebreathed by the patient. The amount of CO_2 in the inhaled gas is regulated by the flow rate of the fresh air and the presence or absence of a CO_2 absorber. A rebreathing system requires the patient to open the one-way valves, which provide slight resistance, so the patient must work to overcome that.

The fresh gas flow rate should not exceed the metabolic oxygen expenditure of the patient. This rate is typically 5-10 mL/kg/minute with a closed rebreathing system. The pop-off valve can be in the closed position during operation of the system.

If the CO_2 absorber is not working effectively, then the patient can be exposed to unhealthy levels of CO_2. It is important to consistently monitor the operation to keep the O_2 flow at the desired metabolic levels. This monitoring will prevent undue pressure from developing in the rebreathing system's operation.

Circle System

The **circle system** is a rebreathing system that utilizes a check valve to ensure and control the unidirectional flow of gas. The circle system's **inspiration and expiration tubes** are linked to the endotracheal tube with a **y-connector**. The **reservoir bag** achieves an improved form of breathing with its gas reservoir. The circle system's **carbon dioxide absorber** removes the carbon dioxide from the expired gas. The tanks must be replaced every 6-8 hours when in use.

The **exhaust valve** is utilized in extracting the exhaust gas from the machine into the scavenger system. The **manometer** can detect the amount of pressure of gas in the lungs and airway of the patient. It measures the pressure using the following increments: millimeters of mercury (mmHg) or centimeters of water (cmH_2O). The system can be cleansed with pure oxygen by releasing the **oxygen flush valve**. The waste gas is accumulated and directed out of the building. A second alternative allows the waste anesthesia to be extracted by a charcoal or soda lime **canister** in the **scavenger system**. The **negative relief valve** is described as a safety valve that releases to allow room air in when a negative pressure is formed.

Universal F-Circuit System

Another rebreathing system is the modified circle system that contains a **universal F-circuit** with the inspiration hose on the inside of the expiration hose. This system requires the following: a CO_2 absorber, rebreathing bag, unidirectional valves, pop-off valve, and a scavenger. The expired gases heat the inward-bound fresh gases. The universal F-circuit is lightweight and less cumbersome than the circle system version. It also incorporates safety measures through an end-of-the-inspiration hose and end-of-the-expiration hose pull-away connection. This juncture disconnects when the circuit is stretched. The empty space of this system is fashioned like the one found in the circle system. However, the empty space does increase when the hoses stretch.

Nonrebreathing Circuits

In a **nonrebreathing circuit**, the oxygen flows through the flow meter and into the vaporizer, and then the gases leaving the vaporizer flow through the hose straight to the patient. Exhaled gases in a nonrebreathing circuit pass through another hose and flow to the reservoir bag but not a CO_2 absorber, and then this gas is released into the scavenger system. Because the gas flows in and out in the nonrebreathing circuit, there is no resistance for the patient to overcome. A higher fresh gas flow is required with the nonrebreathing circuit because the fresh gas has to push the expired gas away from the patient so that it is not rebreathed.

The Bain System

The **Bain system** is also known as the Bain coaxial anesthesia circuit. It holds a tube inside another tube. The interior tube allows fresh gas to flow in, and the exterior tube conducts exhaled gases away. The Bain system does not incorporate a CO_2 absorber and is a non-rebreathing system. The following is drawn from the interior tube during the patient's inspiration or inhalation process: fresh gases, either 100% fresh gas or a mixture of fresh and expired gases. A **nonrebreathing system** utilizes the fresh gas flow rate of 200-300 mL/kg/minute in the mechanism. A **partial breathing** system can utilize a flow rate of 130-200 mL/kg/minute in the system. The Bain system is compact and light. It has a minimum amount of empty space, which promotes effortless breathing. This is an ideal system for a patient that is under 7 kg or 15 lb. The Bain system is also ideal for treatments that are applied to the head or where there is a need for a great deal of physical manipulation of the patient during a procedure.

Maintenance of an Anesthesia Machine

The oxygen tanks should be turned off when not in use. This reduces any additional pressure on the oxygen tank regulator. Removable parts of the anesthesia machine can be cleaned with a gentle soapy solution. Any parts that have come into contact with the patient should be cleaned and sanitized. Removable parts should be placed in a tub of cold disinfectant solution to soak. Following the soak, the parts should be thoroughly rinsed and left to air dry. Cleaning should be performed following each anesthesia induction. Vaporizers should be turned off when not in use. In addition, these appliances should be emptied to prevent any undue buildup of preservatives or residue. A good rule is to check the color of the barium hydroxide or soda lime granules. A color change is a good indication that it is time to change the solution. If the substance becomes rigid or brittle, then it should be replaced. It is important to note that rubber does require replacing, as it wears out with use.

Maintenance of Soda Lime

Soda lime is a mixture of calcium hydroxide and potassium hydroxide. Soda lime is an important part of the anesthetic machine because it absorbs carbon dioxide (CO_2). Soda lime contains ethyl violet, which turns purple when the granules have reached their limit on absorbing CO_2. You must change the soda lime granules after every 8–12 hours of use. If 8–12 hours of use is not reached in approximately a week, the soda lime should be replaced because moisture is required for the chemical reaction to occur, so it could be drying out if it is not used. If the soda lime is exhausted and has reached its capacity to absorb CO_2, gases recirculate to the patient, which can lead to hypercapnia, and the patient will require more gas anesthetic and oxygen to stay in the right plane of anesthesia. This can lead to hypotension, poor organ perfusion, renal failure, and even death. To replace the soda lime, unscrew the soda lime canister from the anesthetic machine, dump out all of the used granules, fill the canister with new granules, and attach it snugly to the anesthetic machine.

Maintenance of Scavenging Systems

Scavenging systems collect, remove, and dispose of up to 90% of waste anesthetic gases away from the building and staff members. Three passive scavenging systems include the floor drop, absorption via charcoal, or a scavenge hose directed out of a window. Passive scavenge systems work on the oxygen flow creating positive pressure during exhalation. Active scavenging systems have a central vacuum using negative pressure that connects to an interface near or on the anesthetic machine.

There should be regular inspection and maintenance of the scavenge system. Active systems should be regularly checked for leaks and should be repaired when needed. An activated charcoal canister, such as an Fair canister, must be replaced after 12 hours of use or once it reaches 50 grams of use, whichever comes first. The F-air canister should be weighed on a gram scale after each use and discarded after it reaches 50 grams.

Finding a Leak in the Anesthetic Machine

Certain areas of the anesthetic machine must be checked to see where the leak may be coming from. If the pressure check shows a large leak (500 mL/min), then a few areas must be checked including the pop-off valve, rebreathing bag, soda lime canister, and the breathing circuit. The rebreathing bag should be inspected for holes, as should the breathing tube. The soda lime canister should be removed, and the anesthetic machine should be checked for loose granules that may be preventing the canister from making a proper seal. Thoroughly clean the area of granules and soda lime dust, replace the canister, and pressure check the machine again. A soap solution can be sprayed around common areas on the machine that may leak, and bubbles will rise during the pressure test to show where the leak is coming from.

Performing a Leak Test

Prior to each anesthetic procedure, the veterinary technician must perform a **leak test** on the anesthetic machine. First, close the pop-off valve along with the end of the breathing tube with your thumb so it is sealed. Push the O_2 flush valve to fill up the reservoir bag. Hold the pressure at around 20 centimeters H_2O on the pressure gauge for up to 45 seconds, and if the pressure holds and the reservoir bag stays full, then there are no leaks. If the reservoir bag slowly deflates and the gauge shows a decrease in pressure, then there is a leak that may be coming from the reservoir bag or the rebreathing tube. If neither of these is causing the leak, then take a spray bottle with soapy water or glass cleaner in it, close the pop-off valve, hold off the end of the rebreathing tube, and flush the O_2 to fill the reservoir bag. Spray certain areas of the machine such as the neck of the bag, areas where hoses connect to the machine, and areas where the soda lime connects to the machine. Squeeze the reservoir bag, look for bubbles to form on the machine, and listen for leaks.

Equipment Troubleshooting

Some problems associated with anesthetic delivery can be traced to mechanical dysfunction. The problem can be as simple as a disconnected endotracheal tube, rebreathing bag, or breathing hose. The problem may also be found in leaking or blocked equipment. These issues can contribute to the poor oxygenation of a patient.

Sometimes such a problem will lead directly to medication overdosing or under-dosing. For example, anesthesia under-administration may be traced to an empty vaporizer. A broken or ineffective setting on a vaporizer can also cause this problem. In addition, sometimes the problem is found in hoses that are not securely fastened, poorly connecting the patient to the device.

Too much carbon dioxide can be the result of an exhausted CO_2 absorbent or a stuck unidirectional valve. Sometimes, the mixture of anesthesia administered to a patient may be in a hypoxic form. This happens when the nitrous oxide levels are too high when matched with the O_2 flow. The higher settings on the vaporizer can result in a patient that has been over-anesthetized. The patient may then suffer from acute hypercapnia or hypoxia. Consequently, all mechanical equipment must be examined prior to use, and maintained regularly.

Chapter Quiz

Ready to see how well you retained what you just read? Scan the QR code to go directly to the chapter quiz interface for this study guide. If you're using a computer, simply visit the online resources page at **mometrix.com/resources719/vtne** and click the Chapter Quizzes link.

Emergency Medicine and Critical Care

Transform passive reading into active learning! After immersing yourself in this chapter, put your comprehension to the test by taking a quiz. The insights you gained will stay with you longer this way. Scan the QR code to go directly to the chapter quiz interface for this study guide. If you're using a computer, simply visit the online resources page at **mometrix.com/resources719/vtne** and click the Chapter Quizzes link.

Triage

Medical Trauma

Trauma that commonly causes bleeding in the abdomen, fractures, and ruptured organs is categorized as **blunt trauma**. **Penetrating trauma** is specific to the path of the object that penetrated the body such as bite wounds. A patient presenting with any form of trauma should be thoroughly examined for any obvious fractures or hemorrhaging. The veterinarian will listen to the patient's heart for any abnormalities, as well as the lungs to make sure that they sound clear. During the overall exam, the patient should be supported in case of spinal injury or a fractured extremity. The veterinarian will palpate the abdomen to feel for any free fluid or see if the patient is in pain in that area. Close monitoring of the patient is essential because an underlying injury may be present even if the patient is seemingly normal. The hospital should have a triaging scale created for trauma cases. There should also be categories set for triaging trauma cases, such as cardiac or skeletal.

Trauma Triage

Triage is the assignment of the degree of urgency to a presenting illness or injury to determine the order in which it should be treated. The first person to communicate information to the client would be the person who answers the phone when they call. If unsure of the severity of the call, the veterinarian must be notified so they can take the call. Once the patient arrives, they must be assessed quickly by the front-desk staff. To quickly but efficiently assess the patient, check the eyes for dullness or a sunken appearance, check the ears for any blue or pale color, and check for respirations to see if the patient is having difficulty breathing. Also check to make sure the patient is alert and responds to you. If the patient exhibits these signs, they must be triaged as STAT or urgent and brought to the veterinarian immediately.

Triage Scale

First-priority cases need to be treated immediately upon arrival and include patients who are having difficulty breathing; have excessive bleeding; are in shock; have allergic reactions; have ingested any form of poison; have abdominal distention; or have been hit by a car.

Second-priority cases involve patients who are currently stable but need to be monitored closely because their status could change quickly, including patients with excessive vomiting and diarrhea, seizing patients, and a possible urethral obstruction.

Third-priority cases are nonurgent, completely stable patients that can be treated in a few hours such as patients with a fever, ear hematoma, or small wound.

Mentation

The veterinary technician will review the patient's medical history and current status, along with any medications being administered, and nutrition. After reviewing the patient's history, the technician can perform the physical examination. A TPR and the patient's mentation should be noted, along with the patient's hydration status. The patient's **mentation** status will be noted as **bright**, **alert**, and **responsive** (BAR), quiet, alert, and responsive (QAR), dull, or depressed. The veterinary technician should evaluate the patient for any signs of pain. Signs of pain include a fast heart rate, vocalizing, abdominal pain upon palpation, hunched posture, trembling, and depression. The technician will also note how much the patient is eating and drinking or will be administering food via a feeding tube and recording the time and amount. The technician will also note and evaluate any urine and bowel movement output as well. The technician must make sure that the patient is provided comfort with blankets and make sure that they are clean and dry at all times. If the patient is a cat, make sure that the litter box is being cleaned.

Evaluate the Patient's Behavioral Status in Critical Status

When a client brings their pet in for an emergency or critical event, probing questions should be asked about the **patient's behavior**. Asking questions such as if the owner has noticed any sudden behavior changes recently and what the behaviors are can aid in diagnosing the issue. Certain sudden behavior changes, such as hiding, aggression, and anxiety, can indicate pain. If the owner acknowledges that their pet has acted aggressively lately, further questions should be asked such as the following. When does the pet show aggression? Does the pet show aggression if you touch a certain area of its body, indicating it is in pain? If the patient is being hospitalized, their behavior must be monitored throughout their stay along with vital signs. Watching for trends in behavior while in the hospital can prove whether supportive care and medications are helping if the animal seems more relaxed and is resting. If the patient is restless and panting, this could also be due to stress, so ongoing behavior evaluation is vital to have a baseline of how the patient has acted since they presented to the hospital.

Triaging a Patient That Has Been Hit by a Car

If an owner calls and says their pet has been hit by a car, the triage begins with the receptionist who should tell the owner to bring the pet in right away and alert the veterinarian. If an owner walks in with their pet without calling, this is a level 1 on a scale of 1–5, with 1 being the most urgent. The veterinary technician will need to immediately bring the pet to the treatment area and obtain a TPR. If the patient has no heart rate, CPR will begin, but if the patient is breathing and alert, then further assessment can begin. The veterinarian may have the technician place an IV catheter and administer IV fluids along with taking radiographs of the dog's chest and abdomen to check for internal bleeding.

Common Eye Injuries in Dogs

Proptosis is when the eye bulges due to an eye injury that disconnects the eyeball from the orbit, and the eyelid spasms, keeping the eye from going back into the socket. Foreign objects can become lodged in the patient's eye causing irritation, swelling, and tearing. Foreign objects may be dislodged by flushing the eye with saline and obtaining the object with forceps. **Glaucoma** is an increased pressure in the eye, which results in fluid buildup in the eye, bulging, and pain if the pressure gets too high. Lowering the pressure in the eye is the first thing to address when dealing with glaucoma, which can be done with medication or surgery. **Corneal ulcers** are caused by scratches or other injuries to the eye. Corneal ulcers can cause the eye to bulge if the cornea becomes weak, and surgery may be required. Triaging an eye injury will be done by initial assessment; if it is a case of proptosis, this will need to be addressed immediately, whereas a patient that presents with a possible eye infection or dry eye will be less urgent. Any suspected eye injuries should be seen the same day the owner calls.

Ethylene Glycol Toxicity

Ethylene glycol toxicity is caused by the ingestion of ethylene glycol, which is lethal in small doses and is the main component of antifreeze (95%). Ethylene glycol tastes sweet, and in most instances, patients willingly ingest it off of a garage floor or driveway. In smaller doses and at lower concentrations, ethylene glycol can be found in motor oils, brake fluid, paints, and printer cartridges. The minimum lethal dose of undiluted ethylene glycol in cats is 1.4 mL/kg and 4.4 mL/kg in dogs. Ethylene glycol is absorbed through the GI tract, and within a few hours the concentration of ethylene glycol is at its highest in the blood. Metabolic acidosis and renal tubular epithelial damage result from the toxic metabolites of ethylene glycol. Ethylene glycol produces glycolaldehyde from the enzyme alcohol dehydrogenase, which is metabolized to glycolic acid. Glycolic acid is metabolized to oxalic acid, which forms calcium oxalate crystals when bound to calcium. The buildup of these crystals causes acute kidney failure.

Clinical Signs of Ethylene Glycol Toxicity

The first noticeable clinical signs of ethylene glycol toxicity are that the patient appears intoxicated as well as having vomiting, polyuria, polydipsia, a low body temperature, and seizures. Neurological signs normally appear within the first half hour post-ingestion. These symptoms may improve after 24 hours, but then the patient may become very dehydrated and could develop an increased heart rate and respiratory rate. Two to three days after a dog ingests ethylene glycol, acute renal failure develops (24 hours in cats) and the patient may have virtually no urine output. They also will appear lethargic, anorexic, may have seizures, and possibly die. Patients that ingest ethylene glycol must be treated within a few hours of ingestion for the best possible outcome.

Treating Ethylene Glycol Toxicity in Dogs and Cats

To treat a patient with ethylene glycol toxicity, absorption must be decreased. This must be done in addition to preventing the toxin from further metabolizing, attempting to remove the already metabolized toxin, and correcting metabolic acidosis resulting from metabolized ethylene glycol. Inducing vomiting will prevent ethylene glycol from being absorbed, but it must be done within 2 hours of ingestion to be effective. IV fluid therapy will help hydrate the patient and increase urine output while aiding in the excretion of metabolized ethylene glycol. The compound 4-methylpyrazole is used to inactivate alcohol dehydrogenase, which will prevent the metabolism of ethylene glycol. Metabolic acidosis that results from the metabolism of ethylene glycol can be corrected with sodium bicarbonate.

Chocolate Toxicity in Dogs

Theobromine is the toxic chemical found in all chocolate, but the darker the chocolate, the more theobromine is found, which dogs are unable to metabolize. Baking chocolate and dark chocolate can contain up to 130–450 mg of theobromine per ounce, whereas milk chocolate only contains up to 58 mg per ounce. Agitation, hyperactivity, diarrhea, and vomiting can be seen at concentrations as low as 20 mg/kg of theobromine. At 40 mg/kg, a racing heart rate, high blood pressure, and arrhythmias can be seen, and at a concentration of greater than 60 mg/kg, neurological signs are seen, including seizures. Fatalities are rare but can occur at concentrations of around 200 mg/kg. Early treatment for chocolate toxicity is vital and can be achieved by administering medications such as Apomorphine to induce vomiting and giving activated charcoal orally to block the theobromine from being absorbed from the body, along with IV fluids to help with the removal of theobromine from the body.

Emergency Nursing Procedures

Types of Circulatory Shock

Circulatory shock is the result of a decrease in adequate circulating volume in the body. In order for the body to have effective circulating volume, it must have normal blood pressure and blood volume. Circulatory shock is put into three categories: hypovolemic, cardiogenic, and distributive shock. **Hypovolemic shock** occurs when blood volume is low due to a traumatic injury, resulting in excessive blood loss. **Cardiogenic shock** happens when circulating blood volume drops even though there is normal blood volume. Cardiogenic shock happens when the stroke volume decreases and is seen in patients with heart failure. **Distributive shock** is a result of an issue with peripheral blood vessels causing blood to flow away from central circulation, normally due to serious infection of the body. A fast heart rate, pale MM, low blood pressure, and weak pulse are all signs of shock that can progress to a drop in oxygen delivery to the tissues that can lead to organ failure and death.

Control Acute Blood Loss

Preventing shock with severe internal or external hemorrhage requires adequate hemoglobin, oxygen, and substrate levels, as well as a functional heart, sufficient blood volume, and patency and tone of vessels.

When controlling external hemorrhage, apply pressure to the site of bleeding and clamp injured arteries, if needed. Oozing wounds may require a compression bandage, and aggressive bleeding may require a tourniquet or pneumatic cuff temporarily (for less than 10 minutes).

Intra-abdominal and intrathoracic bleeding may be detected with sonography to identify free fluid in those regions. Internal bleeding may worsen with restoration of blood pressure and circulation. Intra-abdominal bleeding can be controlled with packing, while preventing further contamination. While ruptured organs or neoplasia will likely need to be removed, anesthesia time should be minimal. Intrathoracic bleeding can be managed with thoracocentesis to evaluate volume of lost blood; exploratory surgery may be required.

Types of IV Catheters

Butterfly catheters have wings on the end with the needle in between so you can hold the wings during placement, and there is a line of tubing with an adaptor end to connect a syringe. Butterfly catheters are not for long-term use, but they are more commonly used to obtain blood samples or administer IV medications in cats and small dogs, ideally using the medial saphenous vein. Over-the-needle catheters are over the needle when placed, and then the needle is pulled out while the catheter is pushed into the vein. **Over-the-needle catheters** can be placed in any accessible vein, but they are normally placed in the cephalic vein and are used to administer IV fluids and medications and to administer emergency medications. Over-the-needle catheters can be placed and kept patent for up to 72 hours. **Through-the-needle catheters** are longer catheters used for critically ill patients requiring long-term venous access, and they must be placed using sterile technique in the jugular or lateral saphenous vein.

Catheter Use for Critically Ill Patients

The catheter type and vein to use for placement will depend on what the patient is presenting with. If the patient will be hospitalized for the next couple of days, then an over-the-needle catheter can be used because it can be maintained for up to 72 hours. If a critically ill patient requires central venous access for parenteral nutritional supplementation, numerous blood draws, and long-term medication administration, then a through-the-needle catheter must be placed. When trying to determine which vein to use for catheter placement, you should consider if there is any injury to the limb and avoid using that limb. **Intraosseous catheterization** (meaning directly into the marrow of the bone) is used in critical situations especially in neonates with limited IV access due to vascular collapse. Intraosseous catheterization can be used to administer fluids as well as emergency medications when a vein is not accessible in critically ill patients.

Blood Transfusions and Administration

Blood transfusions can be given to treat anemia, coagulopathies, and acute blood loss. Packed RBCs, fresh frozen plasma, whole blood, frozen plasma, and synthetic blood substitutes are **blood products** that are available for use. Blood products are administered intravenously through an IV catheter. Blood products should be administered through an IV set designed solely for blood transfusions because they have fibers that remove blood clots and debris. A blood transfusion should be complete in less than 4 hours at up to 4 mL/kg/hr, and plasma transfusions can be given at up to 6 mL/kg/hr. Bolus amounts may be given if the patient is having severe hemorrhaging, which could result in death. If the patient reacts to the transfusion, they will have vomiting, diarrhea, and respiratory distress. The patient's vital signs need to be carefully monitored throughout the entire process.

Requirements for Dogs and Cats to be Blood Donors

In order to be able to be a blood donor, the dog must be at least 1 year old but not more than 8 years old and weigh at least 55 pounds, allowing for around 450 mL of blood to be drawn without causing harm. If the donor is a cat, then it also must be at least 1 year of age and younger than 8 years of age, weighing at least 10 pounds, allowing for at least 60 mL of blood to be drawn without causing harm. The PCV of the donor must be checked prior to blood donation to make sure it is within the normal range, which is between 37% and 55% in dogs and 30% and 45% in cats. The donor should have up-to-date vaccines and should not be ill. Cats should be tested for FIV/FeLV to be sure that they are negative, and only indoor cats should be considered to be donors. Dogs and cats can donate blood every 5 weeks if they meet the requirements. Routine blood work, fecal checks, and heartworm tests should be done for regular donors.

Collecting Blood from a Donor

The procedure for preparing a blood donor begins with a sedative. The patient is placed in lateral recumbency with its neck stretched out to allow easy access to the jugular vein. The jugular vein is ideal for withdrawing the blood from the patient. The cephalic vein is also concurrently used to give the animal needed replacement fluids. Both the cephalic vein and the jugular vein are in need of preparation before commencing the blood withdrawal. The preparation includes clipping the hair in the area of venipuncture. A catheter is a thin tube that is used to inject fluid into the cephalic vein. The blood is drawn out of the jugular vein by means of a 16-gauge needle. The blood is collected in a bag that holds an anticoagulant.

Additional Procedures Used in Collecting Blood from a Donor

A **scale** is applied to gain an exact measurement of the blood collected. This exact measurement is used to ensure that the collection bag is not filled too much or too little. A full collection of blood is measured at 450 mL (for dogs) and 60 mL (for cats). There is a risk to the animal of developing a **hematoma** (a clotted mass of blood) at the jugular venipuncture site, which can be diminished by placing a firm, but gentle force directly on the jugular vein for 2 minutes following the closing stages of blood withdrawal. In addition, it is advisable to only take a maximum of 10-20 mL/kg at an interval of at least 3 weeks. The veterinarian should make every effort to replace the blood extracted with fluids given at rates measuring 3x the volume of blood lost. The replacement fluids should be administered to the patient via a catheter through the cephalic vein in the region of the patient's head.

Feline Blood Collection

The first step in preparing the cat is to clip the hair away from the jugular and the cephalic vein regions. The next step involves providing an aseptic cleansing to the regions involved. The animal should next be given a sedative. The cat is then placed in lateral or sternal recumbency. A 19-gauge butterfly needle is inserted into the jugular vein. To diminish the movement associated with the needle in the jugular vein, the staff should utilize a 60 mL syringe with 8.5 mL of anticoagulant joined with a flexible phlebotomy tube to the butterfly needle. In addition, the staff should maintain a focus on the animal's vital signs, including its pulse, respiration, and blood pressure throughout the procedure. Partway through, the cat should be given replacement fluids. The blood and anticoagulant should be mixed often. The withdrawal should be finalized at the time that the 60 mL syringe is measured in its fullness. This is followed by the removal of the butterfly needle. Then, the staff places pressure on the jugular vein to prevent a hematoma or blood clot from developing. The replacement fluid is completed at 180 mL, or 3 times the amount of blood extracted.

Nutritional Support

Nutritional support is a vital part of managing a critically ill patient, and patients without it can have an impaired immune system, making them more prone to infection. A lack of nutritional support can also lead to dehydration, muscle weakness, fatigue, organ failure, and death. With appropriate nutritional support in the hospital, wound healing will be enhanced, organ function will be maintained, and body mass will be sustained for critically ill patients. The enteral route (feeding tubes) for nutritional support is the method of choice if the patient will not tolerate syringe feeding or eating on its own. The type of food will be chosen based on the patient's degree of malnutrition and the calorie and protein requirements.

Four Types of Feeding Tubes

A **flexible PVC catheter** is normally used as an orogastric feeding tube and is placed through the mouth, down the esophagus, and into the stomach. **Orogastric feeding tubes** are good for short-term use, but they hold a risk of the patient biting the tube as well as possibly causing gastric reflux. **Nasogastric tubes** are passed to the stomach through the patient's nostril, and a nasoesophageal tube is put through the nostril and passed just to the thoracic esophagus. Nasogastric and nasoesophageal feeding tubes run the risk of the patient developing irritation and swelling of the nose (rhinitis) and nosebleed (epistaxis). An **esophagostomy tube** is placed while the patient is under anesthesia, and while the patient is on its right side, a surgical incision is made on the left side of the neck and the tube (red rubber or silicone) is pulled into the esophagus, then into the mouth and turned around to be placed directly down to the distal esophagus and sutured in place on the neck.

NASOGASTRIC INTUBATION

A **nasogastric intubation** is the process of inserting a tube through the external nares, the nasal cavity, the pharynx, and the esophagus and into the stomach region to supply hydration, liquid nutrition, medications, or contrast medium to the animal. A nasogastric tube can be left in place over a long period of time, whereas an orogastric tube cannot. Animals that are anorexic may require lengthy nasogastric feedings if they are extremely thin or unhealthy. This may be particularly effective for an anxious animal that is a poor candidate for forced feedings.

Nasogastric intubation should only be performed on alert patients. Sedation is usually not necessary.

PROCEDURE FOR A NASOGASTRIC INTUBATION

The tube is measured first. The tube's length is estimated by measuring from the nares to a point between the ninth and thirteenth ribs. A topical anesthetic and lubricant are applied to one nostril. More anesthetic drops are applied in the same nostril after 2-3 minutes. The animal's head is then held in one hand. The other hand should be used to introduce the tube into the anesthetized nostril. The animal must be checked to find out if the tube is properly positioned (stomach versus lungs). This is accomplished by inserting 1 mL of sterile saline into the tube. The animal will cough if the insertion is incorrect. Optionally, gentle suction may be applied until frank stomach contents are aspirated and visualized. Prompt extubation and reinsertion of the tube is necessary if pulmonary intubation has occurred.

The tube requires a cap to prevent aspiration of air into the stomach. Recheck the location of the tube and aspirate it before each feeding. A finger can be placed over the top of the tube when the tube must be extracted. This keeps any seepage from occurring in the pharynx or throat while the tube is being withdrawn.

EQUIPMENT NEEDED

The equipment needed for nasogastric intubation includes a nasogastric feeding tube, a topical ophthalmic anesthetic, lubricating jelly, a syringe, sterile saline solution, injection cap, and any medications or substances needing to be introduced into the patient's stomach. The tube that is employed in the procedure can be of various sizes and materials. For instance, an infant feeding tube can be made from either red rubber or polyurethane. However, the critical elements of this tube are its small diameter and its composition from a flexible material that is soft. Animals that are under 5 kg or 12 pounds require a size 5 F feeding tube. Animals that range in size from 5-12 kg or 12-33 pounds require a size 8 F feeding tube. The insertion of the nasogastric intubation also requires a topical ophthalmic anesthetic (to reduce nasal insertion discomfort), lubricating jelly, a syringe containing sterile saline (1 mL), an injection cap, and any medication or liquid to be introduced into the animal's stomach. In some cases, the need for the tube to remain in place for an extended time necessitates that securing dressings be used.

OROGASTRIC INTUBATION

Orogastric intubation is employed to purge stomach contents with gastric lavage; to dispense food or nutrients to orphaned neonates, usually less than one month of age; and to distribute medications or radiographic contrast agents, such as barium, into the abdominal and gastrointestinal regions.

A variety of supplies are needed, including: an appropriately sized stomach tube, speculum, adhesive tape, a permanent marker, sterile saline in a syringe, and a lubricant. Smaller animals such as puppies and kittens will require a 12 F to 18 F infant feeding tube. Larger dogs, ranging over 10 kg or 22 lb, will require an 18 F foal stomach tube.

Usually, an orogastric intubation does not require sedation. However, in some cases a light tranquilizer can be employed. The animal can remain standing or be positioned in sternal recumbency. The tube should be measured against the length of the animal (typically from the mouth to the ninth intercostal space), giving an approximate length needed to gain access into the stomach, and marked with a permanent marker. The oral tip of the tube (i.e., that which will remain immediately outside the mouth) should be designated with tape. Then, the speculum should be introduced into the animal's mouth.

Performing an Orogastric Intubation

The animal's jaws should be held tightly shut against the speculum by the staff member assigned to the job of restraining the animal. The lubricated tube should be inserted into the mouth opening through the speculum and down to the pre-marked location on the tube. Proper placement should be verified before any fluids or other materials are inserted (typically by withdrawing stomach contents using gentle suction, or by putting 1 mL of sterile water into the tube to cause coughing if pulmonary intubation has occurred). If the tube is found to be located in the trachea, then the tube must be promptly taken out to avoid respiratory compromise and introducing fluids into the lungs. The procedure will have to be repeated until the location is verified as accurate. Once an accurate location has been reached, then necessary fluids and substances can be inserted into the tube. This is followed by a flush with water, using approximately 6 mL. The tube should not produce any seepage. If this occurs, the seepage can be stopped by placing a thumb over the tube. If this still does not work, then it should be kinked or bent over to stop backflow.

Performing CPR on Dogs

To perform CPR, the animal is laid in lateral recumbency and 100–120 chest compressions are given per minute for all sizes and species. The person performs chest compressions by placing the hands flat with the palm of one on top of the other, locking elbows, and pushing in a downward motion onto the compression point. Compressions must be forceful enough to compress the chest 1/3–1/2 of its normal width. For deep-chested dogs, compressions will be given over the widest part of the chest, and for narrow-chested dogs, compressions are given over the heart. The patient will be ventilated (if intubated) at 10 breaths per minute. If the patient is not intubated, a veterinary team member must put their mouth around the patient's snout, holding their mouth closed, and give 2 breaths per 30 compressions. To maintain the strength of compressions, it is recommended to switch people giving compressions every 2 minutes. Also, vasopressors should be administered every 5 minutes during CPR.

Function of the Respiratory System

The **respiratory system** starts with oxygen entering the body through the nose or mouth and into the trachea. The oxygen travels down the trachea, which divides into two bronchi and into the lungs. Once it enters the lungs, it ends up in the alveoli where gas exchange occurs, which provides the tissues of the body with oxygen taken in with inspiration, and removes carbon dioxide with expiration. The oxygen taken in at inspiration that enters the alveoli will attach to the hemoglobin in the body's RBCs and then is carried to the tissues. The oxygen molecules detach from the hemoglobin to enter the tissues to provide them with energy. Carbon dioxide is then sent back to the alveoli where it leaves the body via exhalation.

Laryngeal Paralysis

A patient presenting with **laryngeal paralysis** may exhibit stridor on inspiration, noisy respirations, exercise and heat intolerance, dyspnea, and cyanosis. Patients with severe laryngeal paralysis will be hyperthermic and experience coughing, vomiting, and anxiety. Certain activities may cause these symptoms to become worse, such as going on a walk in hotter temperatures. Laryngeal paralysis happens when stimulation of the laryngeal muscles is disrupted, causing the arytenoid cartilage and vocal folds to open at inspiration and close at expiration.

Oxygen Supplementation Techniques

Any patient experiencing hypoxemia will need oxygen supplementation, and there are a few ways to do it. The blow-by oxygen supplementation method is done by holding oxygen up to the patient's nose either by a breathing tube hooked to the oxygen tank or one with a mask attached. The **blow-by technique** will deliver oxygen concentrations of around 35% if given at 5 L/min. An oxygen cage will be able to deliver greater than 50% oxygen concentrations to patients, and the oxygen concentration in the cage can be regulated as well as the temperature and humidity inside the cage. **Intranasal oxygen catheters** can be placed inside the patient's nostril for oxygen delivery. **Transtracheal catheters** can be placed by passing a catheter into the trachea to deliver oxygen, and this method can deliver the highest oxygen concentration to the patient.

Urethral Obstruction in a Cat

Male cats can develop **stones** and/or debris in their urine that can obstruct their urethra, which is the pathway from the bladder to the penis, preventing urine from leaving the body. This is an extremely painful condition and is considered a medical emergency that must be treated as soon as possible because it can lead to complete blockage, causing damaged kidneys and even death in a matter of days. Signs and symptoms to look for include frequently going to the litter box to urinate with only tiny amounts of urine produced (or none at all), vocalizing in pain while using the litter box, decreased appetite, and licking at his hind end. These are signs that an owner may report when calling to request an exam. Occasionally the owner may think the cat is constipated and trying to have a bowel movement when in actuality the cat is straining to urinate and should be seen immediately to be checked for a **urethral obstruction**.

Splinting a Fractured Limb

To apply a splint to a fractured limb, stirrups, which are strips of nonporous white tape, are placed on the dorsal and palmar sides of the foot and then stuck together off of the paw onto a tongue depressor so the ends of the tape don't stick to each other while the leg is wrapped. Cast padding is applied over the fracture to stabilize the leg. A second layer of synthetic cast padding is then applied around the leg with extra padding over areas that can develop pressure sores from the splint such as the proximal and distal ends of the injured limb. On top of the padding, a type of elastic or roll gauze is placed to create a smooth surface to place the splint on. The stirrups are then removed from the tongue depressor and folded back so that the sticky side secures the cast. This prevents the bandage from slipping down the leg. The splint is then secured to the limb with a layer of roll gauze followed by a layer of vet wrap.

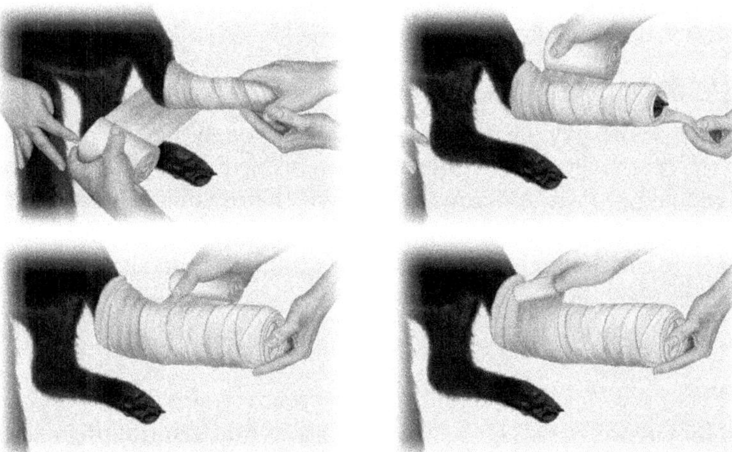

TREATING A DOG WITH HEATSTROKE

If a patient presents with **heatstroke**, the first thing to accomplish is cooling the patient down by use of cool water or towels applied to the patient's body and alcohol on the patient's feet. Cold water and ice are NOT recommended because they can cause vasoconstriction, moving the blood flow toward the body's main organs rather than to the body surface to help cool it down. If the patient is cooled too quickly, the body will not be able to regulate its own temperature due to heatstroke, so it is recommended to cool down to about 102.5 °F over the course of an hour. Cooling methods must be stopped after the patient's body temperature reaches around 102.5 °F to prevent them from shivering because that will increase their muscle activity and can raise their body temperature again. Oxygen supplementation must be administered to the patient via a mask to improve tissue perfusion, and room-temperature IV crystalloid fluids will be administered to help fight dehydration.

Chapter Quiz

Ready to see how well you retained what you just read? Scan the QR code to go directly to the chapter quiz interface for this study guide. If you're using a computer, simply visit the online resources page at **mometrix.com/resources719/vtne** and click the Chapter Quizzes link.

Pain Management/Analgesia

Transform passive reading into active learning! After immersing yourself in this chapter, put your comprehension to the test by taking a quiz. The insights you gained will stay with you longer this way. Scan the QR code to go directly to the chapter quiz interface for this study guide. If you're using a computer, simply visit the online resources page at **mometrix.com/resources719/vtne** and click the Chapter Quizzes link.

Assessing Pain

In order to effectively evaluate a patient's level of pain, you must first be familiar with the patient's normal demeanor and activity level. Questions to ask the owner include: How active is your pet on a normal day? How has their activity level changed recently?

When the pet comes into the hospital, they may hide in the corner and not move because they are scared, not necessarily because they are in pain. Monitor the animal passively without interacting with them by observing their movements, checking whether they are eating or drinking, and noting whether they seem to become more relaxed. Interactive evaluation involves manipulating joints that may be causing pain to elicit a response to pain or palpating different parts of the body suspected to be causing pain for the patient. An ongoing evaluation of pain should include documenting any changes in the patient's pain level or any medications administered and how they helped alleviate the pain.

Nociception

The four components of pain transmission include transduction, transmission, perception, and modulation. Nociceptors, found throughout the body, change the chemical, thermal, or mechanical energy, referred to as a stimulus, into electrical impulses at the site of pain during **transduction**. That electrical impulse travels through a three-neuron chain through the **transmission process**. During transmission, the first-order neurons travel to the dorsal horn of the spinal cord, second-order neurons send pain signals to the brain from the spinal cord, and third-order neurons take the pain signals to the cerebral cortex. Finally, the internal analgesic systems inhibit the dorsal horn cells in the spine from processing the pain with natural analgesics in the **modulation phase**.

Excitatory neurotransmitters will continue to send the signal to the brain, and **inhibitory neurotransmitters** will inhibit the signal from traveling any further.

Perception of pain includes noticing the pain, expecting it, and anticipating it.

Catecholamines

Once the patient experiences a painful stimulus, the body releases **catecholamines**. The release of catecholamines will cause high blood pressure, increased heart rate, and it may even lead to left ventricular dysfunction, ischemia, and infarction. The patient can become insulin resistant and hyperglycemic due to the release of cortisol and glucagon resulting from the pain response. If the patient is experiencing abdominal pain, they may have difficulty resting and getting comfortable or they may experience ileus. Patients that experience neck pain may be hypersensitive to slight movements and will exhibit signs of stress and irritability as well as difficulty getting comfortable. Patients that are experiencing chest pain may have difficulty breathing. All forms of pain will cause stress, and therefore immune suppression.

Pain Classifications

The four most common types of pain are acute, chronic, cancer, and neuropathic pain. **Acute pain** is the body's sudden response to a harmful stimulus or injury to the tissues, such as a burn or wound that causes pain described as throbbing, aching, or burning. **Chronic pain** lingers longer than the usual healing time and is a result of a disease such as osteoarthritis, which will need to be managed for the duration of a patient's life. Pain associated with cancer results from the actual tumor or from the cancer if it has metastasized, and it also encompasses painful effects from chemotherapy and radiation. Damage to the CNS causes **neuropathic pain**, which can be hard to detect in animal patients.

Assessing Acute Pain

Acute pain refers to the sudden onset of pain resulting from surgery, sudden trauma, or a medical issue; it ranges from mild to severe and can last up to a few days but can be managed with analgesic drugs if the pain is assessed regularly. Each patient should have the same pain assessment protocol in place whether they are a hospitalized patient or have just had surgery. The first step would be to visually assess the animal, particularly its posture. If the patient appears hunched over or standing rather than lying down and relaxed, this is an indication of pain that should be addressed right away. Visual assessment should be followed by physical examination, specifically palpation of the area suspected to be painful, such as a wound or surgical incision, to observe the patient's response. If the patient tries to bite, move away, whine, or flinch, this is an indication of pain that would need to be addressed.

Assessing Chronic Pain

The owner is normally the first to recognize if their pet is having chronic pain issues because they will notice certain behavior changes, such as insomnia, restlessness, or excessive panting. Even if the patient is not presenting with a specific problem, it is important that the veterinary staff asks questions relating to possible behavior issues that could indicate chronic pain. If the pet is becoming aggressive, hiding, or acting lethargic, these can be signs of chronic pain. Also, if the pet is moving around slower than normal, having trouble going up or down the stairs, or even having trouble jumping up and down, these would be possible signs of osteoarthritis. Asking the client probing questions is the key to catching pain issues early so that a therapy plan can be started to help the pet live a long and healthy life with well-managed pain control.

Neuropathic Pain

Neuropathic pain stems from an injury to the central nervous system. Intervertebral disc disease (IVDD) is common in dogs and affects the spinal cord, and depending on which part of the spinal cord is affected, different areas of the patient's body will experience pain. A tumor in the spinal cord or limb amputation may also cause neuropathic pain, and patients may experience phantom pain. When one of these possible causes damages the body tissues and nerves, it creates chronic pain that has heightened sensitivity and pain perception with any contact with the affected area.

Treating Pain

Preemptive Analgesia for Surgery

Blocking the pain pathway prior to a painful stimulus during surgery is considered **preemptive analgesia**. Blocking the pain pathway decreases postoperative pain for the patient. Preemptive analgesia will decrease the amount of induction agent and maintenance drugs needed, which lowers the cardiopulmonary effects of general anesthesia on the patient. Using analgesic drugs from more than one analgesic class is a multimodal approach that will increase the success of treating pain because the pain impulse can be blocked at several areas in the pain pathway, reaching a synergistic effect in which the drugs will interact and work together for the end result of preventing pain.

The Wind-Up Phenomenon

The **wind-up phenomenon** occurs if pain is not adequately treated. The prolonged stimulation of nociceptors causes the CNS to adversely adapt to repetitive pain impulses, causing the nervous system to change the way it is processing the pain. **Hyperalgesia** results, meaning that there is less stimulation needed to initiate a pain response. Wind-up is also a result of nerve fibers that would normally carry nonpainful information that are now recruited to the pain transmission process, resulting in harmless information being interpreted as pain, and this is called **allodynia**. The presence of hyperalgesia and allodynia together is known as **wind-up pain**.

Assessing the Response to Pain Treatment

There must be a protocol in place that is used on every patient to assess pain based on the normal behaviors of animals compared to how they behave if they are in pain and to what severity. Once the patient arrives at the hospital, there should be an assessment of pain if the patient is presenting with acute trauma or a medical issue. After administering pain control medication, for the duration of the hospital stay, the patient's pain can continue to be assessed compared to the initial exam as to whether it is getting worse, improving, or remaining the same. If the patient appears to still be in pain after pain control medication has been administered, then a different medication may be used or an extra dose may be given. Pain assessment following acute pain, such as from surgery, should be done every half hour, and then after 8 hours the patient can be assessed every hour depending on the type of surgical procedure.

NSAID Use

NSAIDs are effective at treating the patient's long-term pain by decreasing inflammation and stiffness. Common prescription brands of NSAIDs include Rimadyl, Previcox, and Metacam. While taking long-term NSAIDs, the patient should have annual blood work done to evaluate kidney and liver enzymes because NSAIDs can have a negative effect on these organs. NSAIDs are very effective pain management medications that work to alleviate inflammation and pain so the patient will be more active, allowing for muscle strength to build up so the patient can have more sturdy control over its joints. NSAIDs are much more effective when given daily, so they get ahead of the pain rather than being given only when the pet shows signs of pain.

Hydrotherapy

Hydrotherapy strengthens the patient's muscles and allows for joints that are normally painful to move freely. Hydrotherapy stimulates the cardiovascular system as well. While the patient is walking or swimming in water, they feel weightless. This workout is painless because there are no hard surfaces to step on and there is a reduced effect of gravity. Goals of hydrotherapy, whether it be in underwater treadmills or pools, are to increase the patient's range of motion, improve the strength of the muscles, stimulate circulation of the lymph system, and work out the cardiovascular system. Patients suffering from osteoarthritis benefit greatly from hydrotherapy, as well as patients with hip dysplasia, torn cruciate ligaments, and other musculoskeletal injuries.

Prescription Medications

Opioids work on the CNS to relieve pain and are mainly prescribed for acute pain management. Local anesthetics such as lidocaine are used to numb the area for certain surgical procedures such as debriding and suturing a small wound. Glucosamine and chondroitin supplements can help to rebuild cartilage in the joints. Glucosamine hydrochloride is a part of the cartilage and will stimulate the growth of cells within the cartilage. Chondroitin sulfate is a molecule that works by stopping the enzymes attempting to destroy the cartilage.

Epidural Single-Injection Technique for Administering Analgesia

An **epidural single injection** should be performed once the patient has been induced and is in sternal positioning. The **epidural space**, where the spinal needle is placed, is between the spinal processes of L7 and S1 (the lumbosacral space), and it must be surgically shaved and scrubbed using sterile gloves. The needle with the stylet pierces the skin to almost 1 inch deep, and then the stylet is removed. The hub of the needle is filled with sterile saline, and the needle is advanced until a "pop" is felt as it passes through the ligament; saline is drawn through the needle as it enters the epidural space. If blood enters the hub of the needle, the needle should be removed, and the procedure attempted again. If the needle is passed into the subarachnoid space, then cerebrospinal fluid will flow into the needle and the epidural will need to be redone. The agent to be administered is given slowly, and once it is given, the spinal needle can be slowly pulled out and removed. Morphine is a common analgesic administered via the epidural technique, and it has a slightly slower onset of action (up to 1 hour), so it is best given directly after induction.

Chapter Quiz

Ready to see how well you retained what you just read? Scan the QR code to go directly to the chapter quiz interface for this study guide. If you're using a computer, simply visit the online resources page at **mometrix.com/resources719/vtne** and click the Chapter Quizzes link.

Communication and Veterinary Professional Support Services

Client Education

Booster Vaccines

Young puppies and kittens are at risk for acquiring infectious diseases because of their immature immune systems. Antibodies from the mother's milk provide protection but do not last long, and there can be gaps in protection because the antibodies in the milk decrease before the pet's immune system matures. The first vaccine given is to jump-start the puppy or kitten's immune system against the virus or bacteria, and then **booster vaccines** are needed to further stimulate their immune system to produce antibodies to protect the animal. Vaccines for puppies and kittens are given 3–4 weeks apart, starting at 8 weeks, with the final booster given at around 4 months of age. The rabies vaccine will be given after 12 weeks of age and is given as a booster in one year. An incomplete or missed vaccine in a puppy or kitten series leads to incomplete protection and leaves the pet vulnerable to infection.

It is important to educate owners when an administered vaccine requires a booster so that they don't miss follow-ups and have a partially immunized pet.

Animal Nutrition

Discussing pet nutrition with owners is an important part of preventing disease and obesity in animals. Food brands, portion frequency and size, and specialty feed varieties should be discussed with owners, emphasizing the importance of not overfeeding pets and choosing a reputable food brand. Food portion and type should reflect an animal's species, age, activity level, and sometimes even breed, as large and small dogs can have varying nutritional needs. The animal clinic may have brands they recommend.

Owners should also be taught how to switch animals between types of food. They should start adding in small amounts of the new food, cutting back an equal amount of the old food, and gradually adding more and more of the new food each day so that the mixture changes slowly enough for the digestive system to acclimate.

Canine Socialization

Dogs build relationships with people as a result of handling in the early stages of life, socialization, genetics, as well as learning. In the first 3 weeks of a puppy's life, maternal care and handling are crucial. Attentive maternal care leads to a dog that can better handle stress as well as a more mature nervous system, so puppies that are bottle fed may have a harder time socializing. The transition period is when interactions with litter mates are crucial to social skills. Puppies do not make social attachments as easily after the **socialization phase**; therefore, it is crucial for puppies to have adequate socialization during the first 4–12 weeks, or it can lead to an increased response to stimuli through fear and aggression, as well as an inability to communicate. When an owner comes in with a new puppy for an exam, it is important for the veterinary technician to discuss how to introduce the puppy to other dogs, children, and other adults. Telling the owners to handle the puppy constantly and to play with its paws, ears, and mouth is crucial because this will get the puppy used to being handled and not to be fearful.

Dosage Measurement

When instructing the owner of an animal on measuring dosage, be sure to stress the need for accurate measurement tools. Measurements in teaspoons and tablespoons are not accurate, especially when using common kitchen silverware. A household teaspoon can range from 2–7 mL, resulting in **overdosing** or **underdosing**. A syringe or measured dropper is commonly used to measure and administer liquid medication to a patient. Common quantities are converted such as 1 tsp = 5 mL and 1 T = 15 mL, 1 liter converts to 1,000 mL, 1 fl oz = 30 mL, and 1 gal = 3,785 mL. Solid measurements are often used in veterinary medicine. For example, the veterinarian may need the technician to convert an animal's weight in pounds to kilograms to calculate a dosage. Conversions of solids include 1,000 g = 1 kg, 1 kg = 2.2 pounds, 1 lb = 16 oz, 1,000 mg = 1 g, and 1,000 μg = 1 mg.

Diabetic Pets

Insulin must be kept in the refrigerator. Prior to administering insulin, the pet must eat because if they receive an insulin dose without eating, this can lead to hypoglycemia. The veterinary technician must educate the client on what signs to watch for that can indicate hypoglycemia, such as shaking, seizures, weakness, and lethargy. If any of these signs occur, the owner should always have some light corn syrup available and can give a little amount by mouth as long as the pet can swallow. The veterinary technician needs to make sure that the owner knows to always double-check the amount of insulin they drew up and the syringe type before administering. Human insulins are made in different concentrations than veterinary insulins; therefore, they each require their own dosing syringes. Veterinary insulin (Vetsulin for dogs) is made at 40 units per mL and requires U-40 syringes, whereas human insulin (Humulin N) is made in 100 units of insulin per mL and requires U-100 syringes.

Demonstrating How to Administer Insulin

To demonstrate to the owner how to administer insulin at home, use an insulin syringe and sterile saline instead of insulin for the demonstration. Demonstrate with the sterile saline vial how to roll the vial between the palms of your hands to mix (instead of shaking). Show the owner on the insulin syringe how the units are marked and how many units their pet is going to be receiving. Draw up sterile saline to the amount they are directed to give, and have the owner watch you draw it up. Also, show the owner how to hold the patient and to lift up on the skin behind the neck to form a tent. Insert the needle into the subcutaneous (SQ) tissue up to the hub and push the plunger of the syringe to inject the saline. Pull the needle straight out and place it in a sharps container that the owner should have as well. Let the owner practice with saline with you until they are comfortable.

Home Dental Care

Home dental care can be managed by conscientious animal owners. Instruction regarding the importance of managing plaque and tartar buildup can support and encourage proper home dental care. The caregiver should be instructed on how to brush the animal's teeth using a finger brush or pet-friendly toothbrush and toothpaste (avoid human toothpaste). Owners should check the mouth before brushing. This oral examination may detect painful or problematic areas in the mouth. The caregiver should not brush the teeth if problems are detected to prevent further trauma from occurring to diseased areas, and brushing should not be done along teething gums as this can be painful on the animal. Veterinary products can be applied in daily tooth brushing and home care applications can include antibacterial or fluoride products. Daily cleaning that emphasizes the crown of the teeth can help prevent problems from developing.

Food and Food Additives

Hard food should be given to the animal to reduce the soft food debris that can adhere itself to the teeth. Food additives work by preventing further plaque buildup on the teeth, and they can be administered by sprinkling the correct amount per body weight of the pet onto their food once daily. Water additives work by reducing the bacterial count in the pet's mouth, administered by adding the correct amount of additive per body weight of the pet to their water daily. There are a variety of dental chews and specialized dental diets that are designed to scrape plaque off of the teeth as the pet chews. Product decisions should be made based on advice from the Veterinary Oral Health Council.

Chew Toys

Chew toys help maintain a healthy mouth with clean teeth as they reduce buildup on teeth and periodontal ligaments. Dense rubber toys or rawhide strips remove plaque and calculus from the teeth, and rawhide absorbs the animal's saliva during the chewing process. Consequently, the strip becomes soft and removes further debris from among the teeth's crevices. The dog can safely swallow the rawhide pieces, though they should be closely observed to prevent choking.

Dogs should not be given chew toys or chew bones that are harder or more resilient than the dog's teeth, as these could cause undue trauma or fractures. The dog should not be given any dried hooves or nylon chew bones. These types of products have been associated with injuries involving slab fractures in the animal. Nylon rope toys can also cause injury to gingival tissue. Tennis balls can lead to the exposure of dental pulp.

Assessing Feline Pain Level

Educate clients on the fact that feline patients hide pain well and that they must be able to notice the signs and symptoms of pain. The owner should be looking for subtle signs that are outside of the cat's normal behavior and daily habits. If the cat is normally very active, playful, and interactive, then a sign that something is wrong would be if the cat was sleeping more, hiding, or uninterested in toys. Inappropriate urination or bowel movements outside of the box could be a sign of pain once a UTI is ruled out. Aggression can also be a sign that the cat is in pain as well as fast/shallow breathing patterns and an increased heart rate. Physical characteristics of the cat's facial appearance such as dilated pupils, squinting eyes, and ears down or back could indicate pain as well. Educate the client that all of these signs could be pain from a variety of reasons or another serious medical issue and that the cat should be evaluated by the veterinarian. If the cat is currently being given long-term medications such as NSAIDs for chronic pain, then the owner will want to be aware of any changes in the pet's pain level to see if medication adjustments are necessary.

Managing Osteoarthritis Pain in Dogs

Nonsteroidal anti-inflammatory medications (NSAIDs) are often prescribed to a patient with osteoarthritis, and they work by blocking the inflammatory process, which in turn blocks the pain. An opioid such as tramadol may be given to the patient as well for added pain relief or if the patient cannot take NSAIDs due to kidney or liver issues. Maintaining a healthy weight, limiting exercise, and providing cushion and support in the sleeping area are crucial for managing osteoarthritis pain. Weight management is important because any extra weight puts more pressure on the bones and joints, causing further deterioration of the cartilage. Patients with osteoarthritis pain will need to move around and get exercise but cannot overdo it because this can add strain to their joints. Exercises should include short leash walks and physical therapy such as a water treadmill to improve the patient's range of motion, proprioception, and to build muscle mass.

Alternative Therapies

Alternative treatment options such as cold laser therapy, acupuncture, and shockwave therapy are available to use along with other forms of treatment for the management of osteoarthritis pain. Cold therapy lasers work by sending red laser and infrared laser light wavelengths to promote cell metabolism and enhance the health of the cells through increased circulation. Acupuncture is a form of therapy that stimulates areas of the body to release certain neurotransmitters, including beta endorphins and serotonin, by inserting tiny needles into areas composed of free nerve endings, blood, and lymphatic vessels. If certain points are stimulated at the same time, this creates pain relief and promotes healing. Shockwave therapy uses sound waves to work on specific areas in the body and to trigger the repair mechanisms of the body to reduce inflammation, promote the healing and overall health of bones, and to develop new blood vessels.

Communication

Professional Communication

Overcoming communication failures is paramount to maintaining good working relationships within the veterinary team as well as with clients. Whether it is in a mentor-mentee relationship or as equal colleagues, the same communication skills are effective. When communicating, it can be helpful to keep in mind the nine Cs of effective communication:

- **Clarity**: Say what you mean.
- **Conciseness**: Avoid overspeaking or using more words than are necessary.
- **Credibility**: Have a factual message that can be supported by research.
- **Creativity**: Use creative methods to create a lasting impression.
- **Correctness**: Use the proper pronunciation and grammar.
- **Coherence**: Have a logical and relevant flow.
- **Completeness**: Be sure to finalize your thought to provide full communication.
- **Courtesy**: Kindness and politeness should be present in words and in body language.
- **Concreteness**: Use specific words to convey the intended meaning.

Finally, feedback should be provided in a constructive manner. New veterinary technicians are building their experiences and should not be discouraged. Positive reinforcement is a more effective method for obtaining a desired behavior than is any form of punishment.

Addressing Inappropriate Behavior from a Client

Clients may exhibit a variety of inappropriate behaviors from complaining about finances to questioning medical decisions. A variety of de-escalation techniques exist at the veterinary technician's disposal. It may be advisable to have another staff member present in the room to act as a witness for discussions with an upset client.

- **Active listening**: Active listening is a method of communication in which the listener demonstrates their participation in the conversation using nonverbal cues and by naming the feelings that they understand the client is explaining and the reason for those feelings. This makes the client feel heard.
- **Preemptive strike**: The veterinary technician may recognize that a situation is at risk for being emotionally charged and mitigate the damage by early recognition and intervention. For example, if the patient is being rechecked for an ongoing issue, making an empathetic statement acknowledging the client's frustration may prevent an angry outburst.
- **Venting**: Clients may have frustrations and need to blow off steam. It may be beneficial to let them express their feelings uninterrupted before offering a solution. However, if the client is becoming increasingly agitated, a change in approach is needed.
- **Apologizing**: Offering a sincere apology can defuse a situation. When apologizing on behalf of the practice, keep the apology short and to the point. One can avoid admitting culpability but still express concern for the client's feelings.
- **Explanation of action**: Clients may perceive an offense that was unintended by the veterinary technician, such as a delay in receiving results. Often, explaining to clients that there was a plan in place for the veterinarian to consult with a specialist will appease them and let them know that they were not forgotten.
- **Offering choices/Providing alternatives**: Putting the situation in the hands of the owner will allow him or her to choose the most desirable option and feel like a more active part of the solution. For example, if a client is upset about a prolonged wait, the choice could be given of continuing to wait or to reschedule.
- **Refocusing**: If the client begins a tangential rant, gently redirect them back to the primary issue at hand and the plan for its resolution.

- **Setting limits**: If the client continues to escalate, set a limit by starting with an if-then statement and then offering a choice. For example, if a client is yelling and swearing, the veterinary technician might say, "If you don't stop swearing, then I am going to have to end this conversation. It's your decision if you want to continue." The technician should be familiar with the organization's policies regarding ending conversations and which conversations are appropriate to end. Most practices will not permit their staff to participate in inappropriate behavior.
- **Involving a supervisor**: In the event that the situation is unable to be deescalated, the veterinary technician should know which supervisor to refer the client to. This may be the veterinarian, practice manager, owner, or a member of the human resources department. It is important to know this information before a situation arises.

Regardless of the outcome of the situation, documentation is essential. Documentation should be included in the record by all involved parties, including those who may have witnessed an event.

VETERINARY TECHNICIAN CODE OF ETHICS

The veterinary technician code of ethics states that veterinary technicians should provide excellent care to animals with compassion and competence. Veterinary technicians should commit to lifelong learning through continuing education and educate the public about disease control and zoonotic diseases, as well as assisting with the control of such diseases. Technicians will keep client information confidential unless this information should be disclosed as required by law. Veterinary technicians should act responsibly and uphold the laws and regulations that apply to their position. Veterinary technicians are held accountable for their actions and must protect the public and the profession against other individuals within the profession who lack competence and ethics.

Collecting Patient Information

HISTORY AND PHYSICAL EXAMINATION

SIGNALMENT

The patient's **signalment** includes their age, breed, sex, and reproductive status (if the patient is intact, spayed, or neutered). Age is an important factor for determining which vaccines an animal is due for and it may help indicate the cause of the presenting problem. The breed is an important factor because certain breeds may be predisposed to certain diseases. For example, boxers can be genetically predisposed to cardiomyopathy, so annual EKG monitoring may be necessary. The sex of the patient is important, as is whether the patient is neutered or spayed. If a female is not spayed, then watching for signs of pyometra and mammary cancer is crucial.

PATIENT HISTORY

A thorough patient history is important and can provide insight into current and potential medical problems. An animal clinic should have standard forms for obtaining a patient history, and the history should include:

- How long the owner has had the pet
- Where the owner got the pet
- The pet's living and playing environment (indoor, outdoor, woods, water)
- The pet's normal daily routine
- If the pet has travelled or been boarded recently
- Type and quantity of food the pet eats, including vitamins, supplements, people food, and table scraps
- The pet's normal behavior

Past Medical History

After discussing the pet's general history, move on to the pet's past medical history, including:

- Vaccination history
- Active parasite prevention routine/protocol (fleas, ticks, heartworms)
- Known allergies
- Reproductive history, including whether the animal is spayed or neutered, whether it has ever had a heat cycle, and whether it has had any litters
- Past surgeries
- History of recurring medical problems
- Presence of chronic illness
- Current medications, dosage, and frequency, including topical preparations and medicated products used

History of Present Illness

If an animal presents with an emergency, obtain the history of present illness (HPI) first. Information to gather about the history of present illness includes:

- Owner's detailed description of the chief complaint (CC), assisted by questions from the technician, including appetite and energy level
- How long the problem has been occurring
- How each problem has changed or progressed over time
- Systems review
- Presence of vomiting, diarrhea, polyuria, polydipsia, and recent, noticeable weight loss or gain

Euthanasia

Euthanasia

Euthanasia is when death is medically induced. A drug is administered intravenously to cause loss of consciousness immediately followed by cardiac and respiratory arrest resulting in loss of brain function and death. The drug used for euthanasia is pentobarbital, which is a barbiturate and has a depressive effect on the CNS. Pentobarbital is actually a seizure medication, but when given in large doses, it leads to complete loss of heart and brain function in less than 2 minutes. When a pet is brought into the hospital for euthanasia, an IV catheter is placed and the animal is sedated first. After the patient is fully sedated, the euthanasia solution is administered via the catheter at the appropriate dose for the patient's weight and the patient is checked for a heartbeat. Once no heartbeat is detected, the animal is pronounced deceased.

Role of the Veterinary Technician

When an owner comes in with their pet to be euthanized, the hospital staff must have a protocol in place to ensure that the process goes smoothly. Once the owner arrives with their pet, it is best to get them into a room quickly so they do not have to sit in the waiting area very long. The veterinary technician or receptionist will have the owner sign a euthanasia consent form documenting that they provide consent to "put their pet to sleep." The veterinary technician will explain the process: an IV catheter will be placed, and a sedative will be administered first so that their pet is under no stress. The patient is commonly taken into the treatment area for the IV catheter to be placed and the sedative to be given. The veterinary technician will make sure that there is a soft blanket in the room for the patient to lie on and plenty of tissues for the owners. The veterinary technician usually is the shoulder to cry on and can give support to the owner, which may mean giving them a call a few days later to see how they are doing or creating a clay pawprint for them.

Proper Handling of the Deceased Patient Post-Euthanasia

Normally, there are two options for pet owners for cremation services. They can choose from general cremation or private cremation. **Private cremation** means that their pet is cremated alone, and they will receive the ashes back in an urn of their choice. With **general cremation**, the owner does not get the remains back because the pet will be cremated along with other pets that are to be generally cremated. Cremation services are normally performed by an outside service. The body of the deceased pet is kept in a freezer in the hospital until the cremation service picks up the body. The body is placed into a bag, and the bag is labeled with the patient's name, client's name, and the hospital name. The proper form filled out with the patient's name, breed, weight, and color will be needed for identification purposes as well.

VTNE Practice Test #1

Want to take this practice test in an online interactive format?
Check out the online resources page, which includes interactive practice questions and much more: **mometrix.com/resources719/vtne**

1. When an emergency situation arises, it is important to determine the degree of urgency to properly prioritize the most critical patients. This process includes providing an initial assessment of the patient with a primary survey and a brief medical history, which is called:

a. Triage
b. Stabilization
c. Staging
d. Resuscitation

2. A 10-year-old male neutered Shih Tzu has been repeatedly administered prednisone for chronic otitis. The owners now report that he is polyuric/polydipsic and polyphagic and has a pot-bellied appearance. Which of the following conditions is likely causing these signs?

a. Iatrogenic hyperadrenocorticism
b. Iatrogenic hypoadrenocorticism
c. Cushing's disease
d. Addison's disease

3. Aerosolization of intraoral bacteria during dental prophylaxis poses a significant risk to those within what distance of the dental scaler?

a. 12 feet
b. 10 feet
c. 8 feet
d. 6 feet

4. A 3-year-old thoroughbred filly has undergone colic surgery within the past 24 hours. What is an important part of your follow-up physical exam that should be monitored to identify laminitis?

a. Distal digital pulses
b. Fecal output
c. Packed cell volume
d. Gastric reflux

5. You have assisted in the resection of a large, vascular mammary mass. During postsurgery recovery, you notice that the patient's mucous membranes appear pale. The veterinarian asks you to run a packed cell volume value. The result is 20%. What does this value indicate?

a. The total cells within the blood sample
b. The percentage of white blood cells within the sample
c. The percentage of red blood cells within the sample
d. The total protein within the sample

6. Which of the following would NOT be an example of parenteral drug administration?

a. Intramuscular (IM)
b. Subcutaneous (SC)
c. Per os (PO)
d. Intravenous (IV)

7. Animals poisoned with ethylene glycol (antifreeze) often have large numbers of these crystals in the urine:

a. Struvite
b. Ammonium biurate
c. Cystine
d. Calcium oxalate

8. An 8-year-old intact male Labrador retriever presents after having multiple seizures for greater than 5 minutes over the past 2 hours. The owners administered midazolam intranasally, which was ineffective. Which of the following medications should be added if this patient has been diagnosed in stage 3 status epilepticus?

a. Ketamine
b. Dexdomitor
c. Propofol
d. Isoflurane

9. A newborn calf is suspected to have failure of passive transfer (FPT). What is an inexpensive, cow-side test that would support this diagnosis?

a. Total protein
b. Glucose
c. Temperature
d. Packed cell volume

10. Which of the following indicates atrial depolarization?

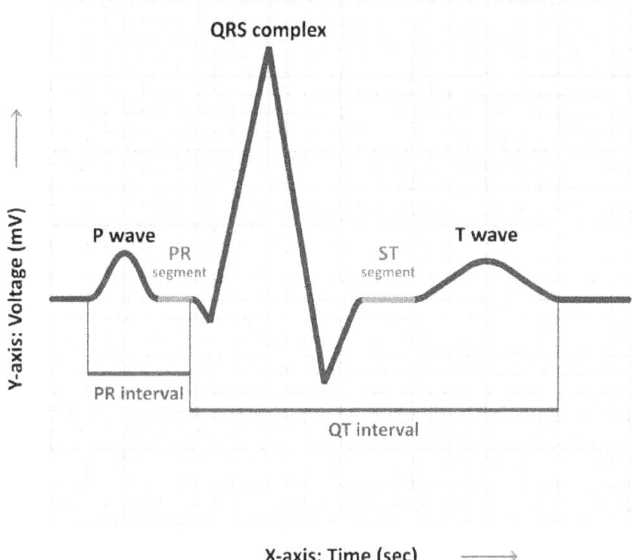

a. P wave
b. PR interval
c. T wave
d. QRS complex

11. Which type of substance requires a Drug Enforcement Administration license for purchase and diligent logs kept daily in addition to the prescription directions typically noted in the medical record?

a. Antibiotics
b. Anticonvulsants
c. Opioids
d. Anticonvulsants and opioids

12. Ruminants are typically castrated within the first few weeks of life. Which life-threatening infection that ruminants are specifically predisposed to is most commonly seen related to this procedure?

a. Tetanus
b. Botulism
c. Rabies
d. Listeria

13. You are preparing a 12-year-old neutered male Shih Tzu for an enucleation. After clipping the surgical area, which type of scrub would be most appropriate for cleaning the area?

a. Alcohol
b. Chlorhexidine gluconate
c. Povidone iodine
d. Peroxide

14. Urinary reagent strips are used to identify the presence of blood in a sample. Which of the following will NOT cause a positive result on the test pad?

a. Myoglobin
b. Hemoglobin
c. Erythrocytes
d. Leukocytes

15. What is the name of the anatomical structure that holds the tooth to the alveolar bone and appears as a radiolucent line between the two structures radiographically?

a. Apex
b. Periodontal ligament
c. Crown
d. Cementoenamel junction

16. Organophosphate compounds are commonly used in agriculture for pest management. Organophosphate toxicity results in stimulation of the muscarinic receptors of the parasympathetic nervous system. Which of the following is a characteristic sign of organophosphate toxicity?

a. Decreased tear production
b. Miosis
c. Tachycardia
d. Decreased saliva production

17. Where would one find guidelines to handle an isoflurane spill?

a. OSHA
b. EPA
c. SDS
d. FDA

18. You are assisting in an animal shelter that has noted a high number of upper respiratory infections in the cats and kittens. It is determined to be feline herpesvirus complex. What is the most important factor in mitigating such an outbreak?

a. Stress reduction
b. Vaccination
c. Antibiotic
d. Lysine supplementation

19. You are tasked with determining which instruments should be included in a surgery pack to be used for feline ovariohysterectomies. The veterinarian will not have a sterile assistant for these procedures. Which needle driver would be the most appropriate to include?

a. Olsen-Hegar
b. Mayo-Hegar
c. Allis
d. Mosquito

20. Orthogonal refers to what when taking radiographs?

a. Oblique view of a limb
b. An image with a focus on the bones
c. Two views at right angles to each other
d. A view of the limb of interest and the contralateral limb for comparison

21. You are monitoring an anesthetized patient, and the capnograph tracing resembles a shark fin with the expired CO_2 increasing during a single expiration. What severe situation does this indicate?

a. An obstruction of the endotracheal tube
b. Leaking around the endotracheal tube cuff
c. A leak within the system
d. A blocked valve within the circuit

22. A 9-year-old neutered male beagle presents with concerns for "slowing down." The veterinarian scores him as a 7/9 on the Purina Body Condition Tool. She also notes thickening of both stifles with a decreased range of motion and muscle wasting of the quadriceps. In addition to anti-inflammatory medication, what is a critical part of reducing arthritis pain in this patient?

a. Weight loss
b. Nutraceutical joint supplements
c. Grain-free diet
d. Cage rest

23. Cross-training is

a. Continuing education through in-house training, online training, and outside seminars
b. Training provided by a superior who is not a technician
c. Learning tasks that are the responsibility of other staff members
d. Training with another species

24. You are assisting the veterinarian with an exploratory laparotomy in a 3-year-old recently fresh dairy cow for suspicion of a displaced abomasum. When the procedure is performed standing, where should you secure the cow's tail to prevent contamination?

a. To the gate
b. To the post
c. To her leg
d. To the ground

25. At which stage of the respiratory cycle should thoracic radiographs be taken?

a. Peak inspiration
b. Peak expiration
c. Early inspiration
d. Early expiration

26. Which of the following client behaviors is NOT consistent with an animal hoarder?

a. Reluctance to identify the number of pets in the home
b. Client presenting a large number of pets in inconsistent patterns
c. Client having five pets that are consistently seen
d. Client attempting to get medication refills without bringing pets in

27. Which of the following is an acceptable abbreviation meaning three times a day with regard to medication administration?

a. SID
b. TID
c. BID
d. QID

28. Poultry and swine producers are often required to medicate large populations. Which of the following is a common route to administer medications in these two species to reduce labor needs and assure herd-wide compliance?

a. Medications are dissolved into the drinking water.
b. Oral tablets are given individually.
c. Topical application is performed.
d. Individual injections are given.

29. You are recovering an 8-year-old spayed female domestic shorthair cat from a prolonged dental procedure. The patient is experiencing a delayed recovery. What is your immediate concern as a cause for the delayed recovery?

a. Deep anesthesia
b. Anemia
c. Pain
d. Hypothermia

30. You are giving postsurgery discharge instructions to the owner of Bella, a 6-month-old Labrador, who was admitted for an ovariohysterectomy. During the patient's discharge, the owner is insistent that Bella will not need an Elizabethan collar (E-collar). What is the most compelling reason for the use of an E-collar?

a. To prevent overactivity
b. To prevent postoperative hemorrhage
c. To prevent postoperative infection
d. To prevent wound dehiscence and subsequent evisceration

31. You are assisting with nasogastric intubation of a 12-hour-old female horse. Which of the following should NOT be used to confirm proper placement of the tube before administering water?

a. Confirming negative pressure through aspiration of the tube
b. Auscultation of the abdomen while an assistant blows/pumps air through the tube
c. Visualization of the end of the tube passing through the esophagus externally
d. Aspirating air back through the tube

32. The process of using multiple analgesics from different classes is referred to as what type of pain management?

a. Matching analgesia
b. Multimodal analgesia
c. Preemptive analgesia
d. Local analgesia

33. You are assisting with tuberculosis testing of a herd of dairy cattle. The farm is equipped with headlocks as a restraint system. What vein would be the most convenient for sample collection?

a. Jugular
b. Ventral coccygeal
c. Subcutaneous abdominal
d. Auricular

34. A 3-month-old thoroughbred foal presents as dyspneic and cyanotic with severely enlarged submandibular lymph nodes, fever, and nasal discharge. What emergency procedure should be performed to restore airflow?

a. Endotracheal intubation
b. Nasal canula with oxygen
c. Thoracocentesis
d. Tracheostomy tube placement

35. Chloramphenicol is an antibiotic that is known to cause aplastic anemia in humans via bone marrow suppression. For which category of animal is the use of this drug prohibited in the United States?

a. Horses
b. Cats
c. Dogs
d. Cows

36. The condition in which CO_2 production is greater than CO_2 excretion resulting in a lowered blood pH is called what?

a. Metabolic acidosis
b. Metabolic alkalosis
c. Respiratory acidosis
d. Respiratory alkalosis

37. If a certain drug has a half-life of 2 hours, what percentage of the drug will be left in circulation after 4 hours?

a. 95%
b. 75%
c. 50%
d. 25%

38. A technician is about to administer an intramuscular injection of antibiotic to a box turtle suffering from an aural abscess. Where should the technician administer this injection?

a. Front leg
b. Back leg
c. Base of the tail
d. Neck

39. You are assisting with a dystocia in a dairy cow. The veterinarian determines that the calf is unable to be delivered vaginally and that a Cesarean section is the safest approach for the calf and the cow. What anatomical area should you clip in preparation for a standing procedure?

a. Ventral midline
b. Left paralumbar fossa area
c. Right paralumbar fossa area
d. Left paramedian abdomen

40. Which of the following is NOT an appropriate reason for compounding a medication?

a. The available concentration of the commercial product is not appropriate for the patient.
b. An alternative route of administration is needed.
c. A Food and Drug Administration (FDA)-approved product does not exist to treat the specific ailment.
d. The FDA-approved product is more expensive than a compounded alternative.

41. A 3-year-old thoroughbred stallion presents for a laceration repair on his distal forelimb. The owner voices a concern for development of proud flesh. What is proud flesh?

a. Infection of the tissues
b. Dehiscence of the laceration repair
c. Exuberant granulation tissue
d. Excessive scar tissue

42. A 1-year-old spayed female Himalayan presents for evaluation after his owner was diagnosed with ringworm. The cat does not have signs of alopecia. Which of the following diagnostic procedures would be advised?

a. Wood's lamp evaluation
b. Skin scrape and microscopic examination
c. Dermatophyte test medium (DTM) fungal culture
d. Hair pluck with microscopic evaluation

43. Which of the following imaging modalities will result in increased levels of radioactivity of an animal?

a. Magnetic resonance imaging (MRI)
b. Computed tomography (CT)
c. Positron emission tomography (PET) scan
d. Ultrasound

44. Which of the following drugs has historically been used to provide local anesthesia but has also been found to have significant systemic analgesia when used intravenously?

a. Acepromazine
b. Lidocaine
c. Ketamine
d. Buprenorphine

45. Which of the following would be a contraindication to obtain a urine sample via cystocentesis?

a. Suspected bladder neoplasia
b. Obese patient
c. Suspected renal disease
d. Suspected uroliths

46. A 5-year-old intact female golden retriever presents with a suborbital swelling below her right eye. The owner mentions that she has a habit of retrieving rocks in addition to tennis balls, sticks, and Frisbees. Fracture of what tooth is most commonly associated with an abscess in this location?

a. Upper right canine
b. Upper right first premolar
c. Upper right carnassial
d. Upper right first molar

47. An 8-year-old Shih Tzu presents with severe pyoderma, and the veterinarian prescribes a medicated bath with chlorhexidine-based shampoo. What is the ideal time frame to let the shampoo make contact with the patient?

a. 40–50 minutes
b. 30–40 minutes
c. 20–30 minutes
d. 10–20 minutes

48. Which of the following medications may lower the seizure threshold?

a. Acepromazine
b. Hydromorphone
c. Diazepam
d. Propofol

49. What is the most common dental issue for lagomorphs, such as rabbits?

a. Dental caries
b. Crown fractures
c. Tooth overgrowth
d. Retained deciduous teeth

50. Equine and bovine species have teeth that continue to grow throughout their lifetime. What is the term used to refer to this type of tooth?

a. Permanent
b. Deciduous
c. Hypsodont
d. Diphyodont

51. What is the preferred technique for performing a fecal flotation?

a. Gross examination
b. Centrifugation using Sheather's sugar solution
c. Direct smear
d. Flotation with sodium nitrate solution

52. Which of the following viruses causes neurologic signs and is almost 100% fatal if contracted by either humans or animals?

a. Distemper
b. Rabies
c. West Nile
d. Eastern equine encephalitis

53. When performing a dental cleaning, what is the step that will smooth microcracks and ensure complete removal of plaque?

a. Ultrasonic scaling
b. Polishing
c. Hand scaling
d. Gingival probing

54. Identify the pictured tissue forceps:

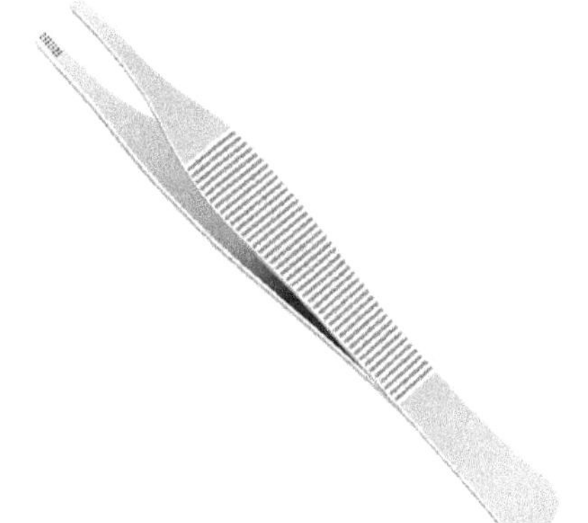

a. Rat-tooth thumb forceps
b. Olsen-Hegar needle driver
c. Kelly hemostatic forceps
d. Adson-Brown thumb forceps

55. A 2-year-old neutered male standard poodle presents for sudden collapse. In addition to hemoconcentration, hyperkalemia, and hypochloridemia, he is hypoglycemic. The veterinarian diagnoses an acute Addisonian crisis. What is the preferred resuscitative IV fluid choice?

a. Lactated Ringer's solution
b. Normal saline
c. Hypertonic saline
d. Normosol-R

56. A call comes into the facility about an 8-month-old Jack Russell terrier that ingested rat poison approximately 20 minutes prior. The owners are instructed to come in immediately with the animal and bring what important information?

a. Insurance information
b. Vaccine records
c. The packaging for the poison
d. Medical history

57. A 5-year-old spayed female Great Dane was diagnosed 3 days previously with infectious bronchitis, and a course of doxycycline at 10 mg/kg was prescribed. Today, she presents as tachypneic with labored respiratory effort. Thoracic auscultation reveals harsh lung sounds in the right lung field. What should your immediate concern be?

a. Hypoxia secondary to parenchymal disease
b. Sepsis secondary to pneumonia
c. Pyothorax secondary to pneumonia
d. Heart failure secondary to endocarditis

58. You are assisting a surgeon performing a gastrotomy on a 6-month-old female kitten who has ingested a small rubber ball. Based on the risk of contamination, how would you classify this procedure?

a. Clean
b. Clean-contaminated
c. Contaminated
d. Dirty

59. Which of the following restraint objects should never be used to restrain a fractious cat?

a. Rabies pole
b. Cat muzzle
c. Towel wrap
d. E-collar

60. Which of the following induction agents is known to produce apnea and potentially respiratory arrest when administered rapidly?

a. Ketamine
b. Tiletamine and diltiazem (Telazol)
c. Propofol
d. Dexdomitor

61. Which of the following is not required attire for all staff when in the surgery suite?

a. Gloves
b. Hair cover
c. Mask
d. Shoe covers

62. A 55 lb female dog is to receive 2 mg/kg of carprofen every 12 hours. How many milligrams of carprofen will the dog have received after 24 hours?

a. 100 mg
b. 75 mg
c. 50 mg
d. 25 mg

63. Which of the following cell types routinely appears artificially decreased on an automated count?

a. Neutrophils
b. Platelets
c. Monocytes
d. Red blood cells

64. You are attempting a nail trim on an extremely aggressive German shepherd. The owner has brought it in wearing a basket muzzle. Which type of restraint would provide the safest scenario to continue this task?

a. Standing restraint
b. Lateral restraint
c. Sternal restraint
d. Minimal restraint

65. A 7-year-old neutered male Dachshund presents with a history of being attacked by a larger dog. He is found to have puncture wounds along his dorsum, and the veterinarian decides to allow them to heal on their own. This is an example of what type of healing?

a. First intention
b. Second intention
c. Third intention
d. Debridement

66. Basic cardiopulmonary resuscitation (CPR) includes which of the following interventions?

a. Defibrillation
b. Electrocardiographic evaluation
c. Administration of emergency drugs
d. Chest compressions

67. A 6-year-old male neutered Chihuahua presents for dental prophylaxis. During the procedure, several teeth are noted to have significant gingival recession and tooth mobility. Extraction is required. Which of the following would be the most appropriate radiographs to take?

a. No radiographs are necessary if there is visible dental disease.
b. Pre-extraction radiographs for teeth with gross pathology.
c. Postextraction radiographs only to identify incomplete extraction.
d. Pre-extraction radiographs of the entire oral cavity followed by postextraction radiographs of the extracted teeth.

68. You are assisting with a dental prophylaxis, and the veterinarian asks you to make a note regarding the pathology noted on the upper left permanent canine tooth. Using the Triadan system, what number would you assign this tooth?

a. 104
b. 204
c. 304
d. 404

69. An increase in heart rate that is accompanied with normal P-QRS-T complexes on electrocardiogram (ECG), and occurs as a result of increased activity of the sinoatrial (SA) node is termed:

a. Ventricular tachycardia
b. Atrial fibrillation
c. Sinus tachycardia
d. Atrial tachycardia

70. A 2-year-old intact male pit bull presents as a suspected hit by car. He displays tachycardia and hypotension. The veterinarian requests that an IV catheter be placed in preparation for a fluid bolus as well as a complete blood count and serum chemistry. Which vein would be preferred for the blood draw?

a. Cephalic
b. Lateral saphenous
c. Jugular
d. Medial saphenous

71. You are assisting with a blood draw on a 14-year-old spayed Pomeranian with a history of polyuria/polydipsia. You obtain a small amount of blood using a 25-gauge needle. The resulting sample is described as 3+ hemolysis. Which of following chemistry values will be affected by this degree of hemolysis?

a. Glucose
b. Creatinine
c. Potassium
d. Albumin

72. When recovering an animal from anesthesia, the return of what reflex would indicate it is appropriate to extubate the patient?

a. Palpebral
b. Pain withdrawal
c. Respiration
d. Swallow

73. A 5-year-old intact male feline presents as an emergency situation. The patient is awake but recumbent. He does not respond to noise or light, but he does respond to the initial needlestick when blood is taken for the minimum database. How would you classify his mentation?

a. Alert
b. Stuporous
c. Comatose
d. Delirious

74. Which of the following is an example of an absorbable suture material?

a. Nylon (Dermalon)
b. Polyglactin 910 (Vicryl)
c. Polyester (Ethibond)
d. Silk

75. A 3-year-old black Lab presents for sudden collapse after chasing a tennis ball for an extended period of time on a hot summer day. Its temperature reads 105 °F. What action should be taken immediately?

a. Blood should be drawn for a minimum database.
b. The animal should be completely submerged in cold water.
c. An IV catheter should be placed for fluid administration.
d. Oral fluids should be offered.

76. A 17-year-old spayed female domestic shorthair has been diagnosed with hyperthyroidism. The owner is unable to regulate the disease with oral medication and reports that the patient will not eat the prescription diet. What nuclear medicine procedure may be recommended for this patient?

a. Nuclear scintigraphy
b. Iodine-131 treatment
c. 18F-FDG scan
d. Fluoroscopy

77. Furosemide is often administered to patients to promote fluid loss. Which electrolyte should be monitored with chronic furosemide use?

a. Potassium
b. Sodium
c. Calcium
d. Magnesium

78. Which of the following bandage layers provides padding and absorbs exudate?

a. Primary
b. Secondary
c. Tertiary
d. Fortified layer

79. A 4-year-old intact terrier mix weighing approximately 45 lb presents for porcupine quill extraction. There are approximately 10 quills visible on his lips and nose, and about 5 can be seen intraorally when he opens his mouth to pant. What would you choose for a short-acting sedation protocol for this patient?

a. Tiletamine and diltiazem IM
b. Dexmedetomidine and butorphanol IV
c. Acepromazine and hydromorphone SC
d. Propofol IV

80. You are tasked with wrapping surgery packs for sterilization. What is the minimum amount of sterilization indicators that should be used and in what location?

a. One: the indicator strip should be located inside the innermost pack wrap.
b. One: the indicator tape should be located on the outside of the pack.
c. Two: the indicator strip should be located between the folds of a drape and indicator tape on the outer pack wrap.
d. Two: the indicator strip should be located on top of the instruments and indicator tape on the outer pack wrap.

81. Which of the following leukocytes is the most abundant in the blood of cattle?

a. Monocytes
b. Neutrophils
c. Erythrocytes
d. Lymphocytes

82. Which small mammal has a high risk of dystocia if bred after 6 months of age?

a. Chinchilla
b. Rabbit
c. Guinea pig
d. Ferret

83. A 10-year-old intact female collie has been diagnosed with mammary masses that are rapidly growing, red in appearance, and painful when palpated. The veterinarian would like radiographs to perform a "mets" check before moving forward with surgical resection. What is the most likely area to experience metastasis of neoplastic cells?

a. Lungs
b. Liver
c. Spleen
d. Skin

84. Which type of monitoring is used to assess cardiac preload?

a. Systolic pressure
b. Diastolic pressure
c. Mean arterial pressure
d. Central venous pressure

85. When premeasuring an endotracheal tube, what landmarks should be used?

a. Larynx to the point of the shoulder
b. Muzzle to the point of the shoulder
c. Muzzle to the heart base
d. Muzzle to the larynx

86. A second lactation Jersey cow has recently freshened. Upon examination, the veterinarian determines that she has milk fever, also known as hypocalcemia. How should IV calcium be administered?

a. As fast as possible
b. With glucose for increased absorption
c. Very slowly
d. The rate of administration does not matter

87. What is the purpose of the regulator on the anesthesia circuit?

a. To indicate the rate of O_2 flow
b. To reduce the pressure from the O_2 tank to provide a safe, constant pressure
c. To provide a reserve of O_2 for the patient to breathe from
d. To monitor the pressure in cmH_2O within the circuit

88. Equines and, less frequently, ruminants require dental care to address pathology. The term used to refer to this process is called floating the teeth. What does this process involve?

a. Scaling the teeth to remove plaque and tartar
b. Filing the overgrown teeth to remove points that may cause intraoral trauma
c. Extracting overgrown teeth
d. Gingival probing to remove deep pockets of plaque and tartar

89. A 14-year-old spayed female domestic shorthair presents with an owner complaint of reluctance to jump off the counters. On physical exam, the patient displays muscle wasting of the rear limbs and sensitivity and decreased range of motion in the left hip. Radiographs show a non-healed fracture of the acetabulum. It is also noted that the patient showed hyperesthesia when the affected limb was touched, becoming fractious. What is likely the cause for the hyperesthesia?

a. Wind-up pain phenomenon secondary to chronic pain
b. Overstimulation due to multiple procedures
c. Normal response to chronic injury
d. Epinephrine stress response

90. Which of the following species have a dental pad in place of their upper incisors?

a. Canines and felines
b. Ruminants and camelids
c. Canines and equines
d. Equines and camelids

91. A 5-year-old female dachshund presents with suspected intervertebral disc compression of the spinal cord. She is experiencing paralysis of her rear limbs. Which of the following absences would carry the least desirable prognosis with regard to a return to function following spinal decompression surgery?

a. Loss of motor function
b. Loss of superficial pain response
c. Loss of deep pain response
d. Loss of bladder control

92. In addition to theobromine, what compound should be of concern with regard to chocolate toxicosis?

a. Caffeine
b. Xylitol
c. Ethylene glycol
d. Zinc toxicosis

93. You are attempting to perform radiography of a very energetic animal. Your first image is blurry, which you attribute to the increased motion. What setting(s) could you adjust to compensate for the movement and create the best image?

a. Increase the mA and shorten the time
b. Decrease the mA and shorten the time
c. Decrease the kV
d. Increase the kV

94. Which of the following group of suture gauges is listed in ascending order of size (smallest to largest)?

a. 3, 2, 1
b. 0, 2-0, 3-0
c. 2-0, 0, 0, 1, 2
d. 9-0, 10-0, 11-0

95. Antimicrobial residue can be inadvertently consumed by humans through the consumption of beef. Dairy and poultry products are an ongoing public health concern due to their risk for antimicrobial residue as well. Which of the following are used to mitigate residue risk?

a. Expiration dates
b. Withdrawal times
c. Administration holds
d. United States Department of Agriculture (USDA) certification

96. What analgesia technique is the only effective method of completely blocking pain?

a. Opioid at a constant rate infusion
b. Local nerve block
c. Nonsteroidal anti-inflammatory drugs given before a painful procedure
d. A combination of steroidal and nonsteroidal anti-inflammatory drugs

97. You have been advised to administer 30 mL of procaine penicillin G IM to a Jersey cow. What is the maximum volume that should be administered per injection site?

a. 5 mL
b. 10 mL
c. 20 mL
d. 30 mL

98. Which of the following terms refers to the density of urine when compared to water?

a. Osmolality
b. Specific gravity
c. Color
d. Clarity

99. Which radiographic setting has the highest influence on radiographic contrast?

a. Collimation
b. Kilovoltage
c. Distance
d. Filtration

100. What drug is the emetic of choice in canines?

a. Xylazine
b. Apomorphine
c. Hydrogen peroxide
d. Syrup of ipecac

101. The purpose of which system is to minimize exposure of personnel to exhaled waste anesthetic gas?

a. Rebreathing circuit
b. Vaporizer
c. Anesthetic mask
d. Scavenger

102. A 500 kg steer has been diagnosed with respiratory disease. The veterinarian instructs you to give 2.5 mg/kg SC of 100 mg/mL Baytril 100 (enrofloxacin). What volume will you administer?

a. 15 mL
b. 12.5 mL
c. 12.5 L
d. 12.5 mg

103. Guinea pigs are commonly used for animal research. What deficiency are they prone to that must have special care taken to avoid?

a. Hypovitaminosis D
b. Hypovitaminosis C
c. Hypocalcemia
d. Hypophosphatemia

104. What is the primary method of excretion for inhaled anesthetic agents, such as isoflurane or sevoflurane?

a. Liver
b. Kidneys
c. Lungs
d. Gastrointestinal tract

105. A 3-year-old intact male Australian shepherd weighing approximately 25 kg presents for suspected trauma due to excessive bruising along his abdomen and evidence of superficial abrasions (road rash). His mucous membranes are pale, he is hypotensive, and he is tachycardic. The veterinarian tells you to start a shock dose of crystalloid fluids. What initial volume should be given as a rapid bolus?

a. 2.25 L
b. 1.5 L
c. 750 mL
d. 500 mL

106. Gentamicin is an example of which antibiotic class known to have nephrotoxic and ototoxic potential, even at therapeutic levels?

a. Penicillins
b. Tetracyclines
c. Lincosamides
d. Aminoglycosides

107. Which of the following equine surgeries is typically performed standing?

a. Laparotomy
b. Arthroscopy
c. Enucleation
d. Cesarean section

108. A farmer calls and relays that she has a 3-year-old Holstein with a lacerated milk vein and significant hemorrhage. The incident happened within the past 5 minutes. How would you classify this situation, and what is the best course of action?

a. The situation is nonurgent because a cow is large enough to withstand some blood loss until a clot forms.
b. The situation is urgent because the location is concerning, but the cow can be seen by the end of the day.
c. The situation is emergent and this farmer will be moved to the next appointment slot.
d. The situation is life-threatening, so the farmer should be instructed to initiate compression methods by whatever means are available, and the veterinarian will arrive as soon as possible.

109. Which of the following opioids has an extremely short duration of action and must be administered as a constant rate infusion in order to maintain therapeutic levels?

a. Fentanyl
b. Morphine
c. Methadone
d. Buprenorphine

110. Which of the following items is included in an employee handbook?

1. Disciplinary procedures
2. Dress code
3. Social media policy
4. Job descriptions

a. 1, 2, 3, and 4
b. 1, 4
c. 2, 3, 4
d. 1, 2, 3

111. The amount of drug that is administered at one time is called the:

a. Dose
b. Interval
c. Route
d. Concentration

112. Which of the following is NOT a role of the veterinary technician with respect to pain management?

a. Patient assessments to determine pain
b. Prescribing specific pain medications
c. Logging controlled substances
d. Requesting adjustments to medications for proper pain control

113. Which type of scissors should never be used to cut drape material?

a. Metzenbaum
b. Mayo
c. Bandage
d. Suture

114. Which of the following opioid medications should not be administered with a full mu-agonist for concerns of reduced efficacy?

a. Hydromorphone
b. Butorphanol
c. Ketamine
d. Diazepam

115. Which of the following parameters defines a patient's ventilation ability?

a. SpO_2
b. CO_2
c. Mean arterial pressure
d. Respiratory rate

116. A 3-month-old intact female Lab puppy presents to the veterinarian with a history of purulent vaginal discharge and a history of difficulty becoming house trained. What sample should be evaluated before starting antibiotics?

a. Urinalysis obtained by free-catch collection
b. Urine culture and sensitivity obtained via cystocentesis
c. Urine culture and sensitivity obtained by free catch
d. Urinalysis obtained by catheterization

117. An 8-week-old puppy presents bright and alert with a history of soft stool. The veterinarian has you perform a fecal flotation. What is the identity of the following ova?

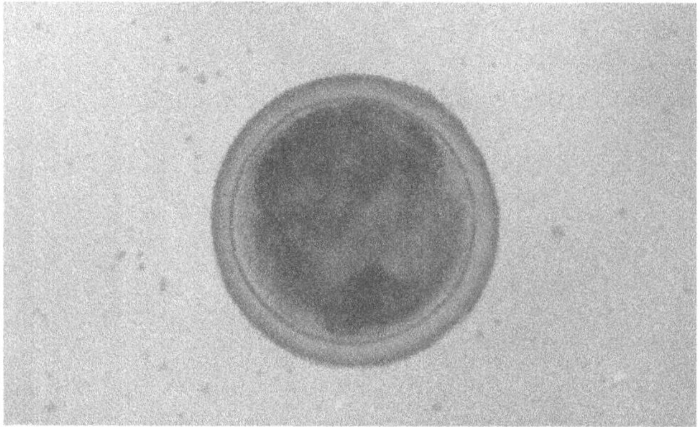

a. *Trichuris vulpis*
b. *Toxocara canis*
c. *Ancylostoma caninum*
d. *Giardia* spp.

118. Which of the following tests is used to identify an injury to the corneal epithelium?

a. Schirmer tear test
b. Fluorescein stain
c. Tonometry
d. Gonioscopy

119. You have been asked to evaluate a blood smear in order to perform a manual platelet count. What objective should you use, and what factor should you multiply each platelet observed in each field by to calculate the platelet amount manually?

a. 10×; 10,000
b. 40×; 10,000
c. 40×; 20,000
d. 100×; 20,000

120. A frantic owner calls to report worms in her dog's feces. You respond:

a. "That's an emergency. Bring your dog right in."
b. "Don't worry. Come in and pick up some medicine, I'll get it ready for you."
c. "Don't worry. Just keep your dog on monthly heartworm preventative."
d. "I'll schedule an appointment for you. Please bring a sample of feces with you for evaluation."

121. What is the appropriate method to administer chest compressions to small animals such as cats and small dogs?

a. With the patient in the dorsal recumbency position and pressing on the sternum
b. With the patient in the lateral recumbency position using one hand to "squeeze" the chest and using the other hand to support the back
c. With the patient in the lateral recumbency position with two-handed compressions over the largest part of the chest
d. With the patient in the lateral recumbency position with two-handed compressions directly over the heart

122. A neonatal puppy is found to be weak, minimally responsive, and hypothermic with a temperature of 85 °F. What should be the first step in resuscitating this patient?

a. Gradual rewarming
b. Rapid rewarming
c. Feeding via nasogastric tube
d. IV catheter placement

123. Which of the following urine specific gravity values would indicate hyposthenuria?

a. 1.005
b. 1.011
c. 1.020
d. 1.035

124. Which of the following local anesthetic blocks would provide anesthesia to the bone, teeth, and soft tissue rostral to the side on which the block is placed?

a. Maxillary infraorbital
b. Inferior alveolar
c. Middle mental
d. Caudal maxillary

125. When positioning a patient for a VD view of the thorax, how would you position the patient on the table with a fixed x-ray tube?

a. Sternal recumbency
b. Dorsal recumbency
c. Right lateral recumbency
d. Left lateral recumbency

126. A 2-year-old intact male cat presents for an annual exam. During the physical exam, the veterinarian notes severe inflammation of the entire oral cavity including the gums, tongue, and soft palate and diagnoses the patient with stomatitis. What is the most effective treatment option for long-term management of this condition?

a. Immunosuppressive doses of corticosteroids
b. Lifelong antibiotic therapy
c. Full-mouth tooth extractions
d. Dental cleaning with stringent at-home care

127. An 8-year-old spayed female papillon presents for GI upset with a 2-day history of vomiting, diarrhea, and lethargy. During the physical exam, a cardiac arrythmia is discovered and diagnosed as a second-degree AV block. An atropine challenge test is performed. What should the electrocardiogram show after atropine administration?

a. Bradycardia
b. Sinus tachycardia
c. Third-degree AV block
d. Ventricular tachycardia

128. A mutation of the multidrug resistance 1 (MDR1) gene has been shown to increase sensitivity to certain drug classes. Which breed classification is known to be at higher risk for carrying a mutation in this gene?

a. Toy breeds
b. Retrievers
c. Hounds
d. Herding breeds

129. Feline lower urinary tract disease is a common cause of cystitis and urinary obstruction. What is the most important treatment aspect that should be discussed with cat owners?

a. Antibiotic therapy
b. Environmental change to reduce stress
c. Prescription urinary diet
d. Pheromone therapy

130. A 3-year-old beagle presents with a history of polyuria, polydipsia, and anorexia. The patient has been vaccinated only against rabies. Laboratory work reveals acute kidney failure and elevated liver enzymes as well as the presence of glucosuria. The veterinarian begins treatment for leptospirosis. What unique concerns does leptospirosis present?

a. Zoonotic potential
b. Sepsis
c. Diabetes
d. Chronic hepatitis

131. A 4-year-old neutered male Great Dane presents with a gastric dilatation and volvulus requiring emergency surgery, including a splenectomy. What is the most common arrythmia following this procedure?

a. Atrioventricular (AV) block
b. Atrial fibrillation
c. Supraventricular tachycardia
d. Premature ventricular contractions

132. Which of the following is an appropriate method for performing a dental procedure in a small animal?

a. General anesthesia
b. Heavy sedation
c. Light sedation
d. No sedation

133. What is the maximum amount of blood that you should draw from an avian?

a. 1 mL
b. 5% of body weight
c. 5 mL
d. 1% of body weight

134. What is the main difference between a rebreathing and a nonrebreathing system?

a. Rebreathing refers to breathing a mixture of fresh and expired gases, whereas nonrebreathing means that all expired gases are scavenged.
b. Rebreathing refers to outside breathing via a mechanical ventilator or an individual providing breaths, whereas nonrebreathing depends on the patient's own respirations.
c. Rebreathing refers to room air combined with anesthetic gas, whereas nonrebreathing uses oxygen to deliver the anesthetic gas.
d. Rebreathing refers to a mask system used to deliver inhaled anesthetic gas, whereas nonrebreathing requires an endotracheal tube.

135. Which stage of anesthesia is characterized by excitement, delirium, and involuntary muscular movement?

a. Stage 1
b. Stage 2
c. Stage 3
d. Stage 4

136. Which type of blood product would be most indicated for a patient with thrombocytopenia?

a. Fresh whole blood
b. Packed red blood cells
c. Oxyglobin
d. Platelet-rich plasma

137. Which drug are ruminants extremely sensitive to, necessitating a dose that is approximately 10 times less than that used for equines?

a. Xylazine
b. Butorphanol
c. Lidocaine
d. Acepromazine

138. You have drawn a blood sample and performed centrifugation. The serum appears to be a shade of white above the clot. What is the classification of this serum sample?

a. Lipemic
b. Icteric
c. Hemolyzed
d. Hypoproteinemic

139. Which of the following is NOT a benefit of preanesthetic medications?

a. Reduction of anxiety
b. Facilitation of a smoother induction
c. Prevention of wind-up pain
d. Shortening of time to anesthetic induction

140. When injecting animals used for meat production, such as cows or pigs, what is the ideal location to administer the injection to avoid unnecessary damage to the meat?

a. Rear legs
b. Rump
c. Neck
d. Shoulder

141. When referring to ultrasound images, what does the term hyperechoic mean?

a. Lighter or whiter than the surrounding structures
b. Darker or blacker than the surrounding structures
c. The same darkness as the surrounding tissues
d. Completely black

142. Which of the following parameters would indicate an acceptable anesthetic depth for surgical procedures?

a. Tight jaw tone
b. Ventromedial eye position
c. Loss of corneal reflex
d. Central eye position

143. Identify the following abnormality:

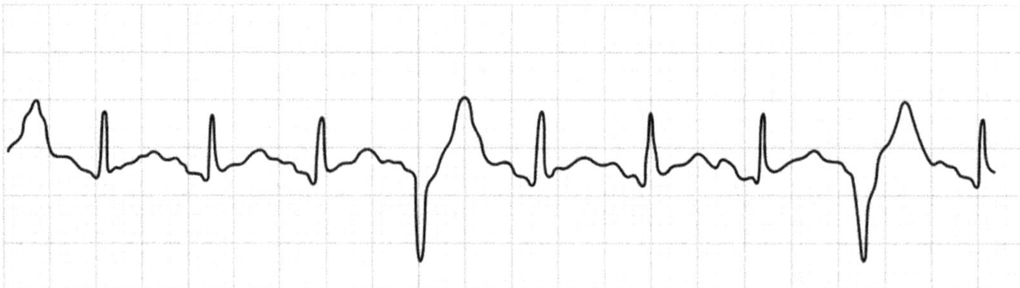

a. Atrial fibrillation
b. Premature ventricular contraction
c. AV block
d. Ventricular tachycardia

144. Which of the following routes of blood collection should only be used in a terminal blood draw in rodents?

a. Retro-orbital sinus
b. Saphenous
c. Cardiac
d. Tail nick

145. For how long do chemotherapeutic agents persist at high levels in bodily fluids?

a. 12 hours
b. 24 hours
c. 36 hours
d. 48 hours

146. A 4-year-old intact male coonhound presents with a fever, lameness, and a history of anorexia. The veterinarian is concerned about tick-borne disease and prescribes doxycycline and requests for the submission of whole blood for a comprehensive tick disease polymerase chain reaction panel. When should the sample be collected with regard to the antibiotic administration?

a. Prior to the antibiotic administration
b. 12 hours after the first antibiotic dose
c. 24 hours after the first antibiotic dose
d. Timing is not a concern with polymerase chain reaction testing

147. Which of the following equine vaccinations is strongly recommended for equines being fed from large, round hay bales?

a. Botulism
b. Rabies
c. West Nile
d. Tetanus

148. Which of the following accurately lists body tissues from the most radiopaque to the least radiopaque?

a. Bone – soft tissue – fat – air
b. Bone – fat – soft tissue – air
c. Bone – soft tissue – air – fat
d. Air – fat – soft tissue – bone

149. A dog breeder calls the clinic concerned that his female dog is experiencing difficulties whelping. She has had one puppy so far, but he states there have been at least five confirmed radiographically. In order to triage appropriately, you ask him how long it has been since the last puppy was delivered. What is the maximum amount of time that should lapse between delivery of each puppy given strong contractions?

a. 30–60 minutes
b. 2–3 hours
c. 3–4 hours
d. 4–5 hours

150. Which of the following criteria would indicate a dehydration status of approximately 5%?

a. Tachycardia
b. Severely dry mucous membranes
c. Enophthalmos
d. Minimal loss of skin turgor

151. An 8-year-old female pug presents as an ocular emergency after being attacked by a German shepherd. Her right eye is fully proptosed. What quick test can you perform to identify if the globe damage may be visual?

a. No such test exists; enucleation is the only option.
b. Pupillary light reflex – if the direct and consensual reflexes are intact, prognosis is favorable for the vision to be salvaged.
c. Intraocular pressure – if increased, there is little chance of the vision being salvaged.
d. Fluorescein staining – the presence of corneal ulcers may indicate the possibility of vision loss.

152. When assessing blood pressure via indirect monitoring (i.e., Doppler) the cuff width should be what percentage of the limb circumference?

a. 80–100%
b. 60–80%
c. 40–60%
d. 20–40%

153. What is the minimal amount of time of preoperative fasting required for equines?

a. 6 hours
b. 8 hours
c. 10 hours
d. 12 hours

154. Bite injuries are an occupational hazard when handling animals, especially sick or injured patients. Cat-induced bites are known to be exceptionally dangerous due to the presence of what oral bacteria?

a. *Salmonella* spp.
b. *Escherichia coli*
c. *Staphylococcus* spp.
d. *Pasteurella multocida*

155. Which of the following is the correct order when preparing instruments for the autoclave?

a. Rinse instruments with tap water, rinse in instrument milk, allow to dry, and wrap for sterilization.
b. Rinse instruments with tap water and instrument cleaner, clean in an ultrasonic cleaner, allow to dry, and wrap for sterilization.
c. Rinse instruments with distilled water, clean in an ultrasonic cleaner, allow to dry, and wrap for sterilization.
d. Rinse instruments in distilled water and instrument cleaner, clean in an ultrasonic cleaner, rinse in instrument milk, allow to dry, and wrap for sterilization.

156. Which of the following is/are the most common negative side effect(s) that canines experience when given NSAIDs?

a. Seizure
b. Liver dysfunction
c. Vomiting and diarrhea
d. Renal failure

157. A 6-month-old feedlot calf is suffering from recurrent bloat. What procedure refers to a long-term opening in the rumen to allow for release of gas?

a. Gastrotomy
b. Rumenotomy
c. Rumenostomy
d. Rumenectomy

158. A 2-year-old neutered male feline presents for urinary obstruction. What electrolyte abnormalities should you be most concerned for in a patient with urinary obstruction?

a. Elevated blood urea nitrogen
b. Elevated creatinine
c. Elevated phosphorus
d. Elevated potassium

159. The veterinarian has asked you for a #15 scalpel blade. Which of the following pictured blades would you select?

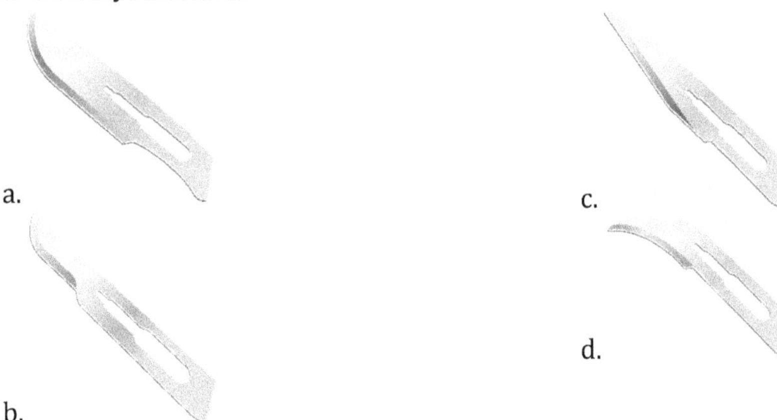

160. Which of the following statements is NOT true regarding jugular intravenous drug administration in horses?

a. The needle should be inserted caudally into the jugular vein in order to match the direction of blood flow.
b. The cranial third of the neck should be used to access the jugular vein to avoid accidental entry into the carotid artery.
c. The medication should be bolused as quickly as possible.
d. Arterial versus venous blood cannot be differentiated by color when drawn into a syringe filled with fluid.

161. A 4-year-old intact female husky presents with a distended abdomen and a history of diarrhea. Which of the following laboratory values would be expected for protein-losing enteropathy (PLE)?

a. Hypoalbuminemia
b. Hypoglobulinemia
c. Panhypoproteinemia
d. Anemia

162. When using an ultrasound machine, which of the following frequencies would provide the highest resolution, assuming that the velocity remains the same?

a. 3 MHz
b. 5 MHz
c. 10 MHz
d. 12 MHz

163. Which of the following pain management interventions would provide the most effective analgesia for a healthy 50-lb canine undergoing castration?

a. Administration of carprofen before surgery, neuroleptanalgesia, followed by carprofen daily for 5–7 days postoperatively
b. Neuroleptanalgesia followed by local testicular analgesia; carprofen is to be given if needed postoperatively
c. Administration of carprofen before surgery; no additional pain medication is necessary
d. Administration of carprofen before surgery, neuroleptanalgesia followed by intratesticular local anesthesia, followed by carprofen daily 5–7 days postoperatively

164. A 5-year-old Labrador presents with a 3-day history of excessive head shaking and dark discharge from the ears. The veterinarian asks you to review an ear cytology using the Diff-Quik stain, and you note the following structures. What is the identification of the pictured organisms?

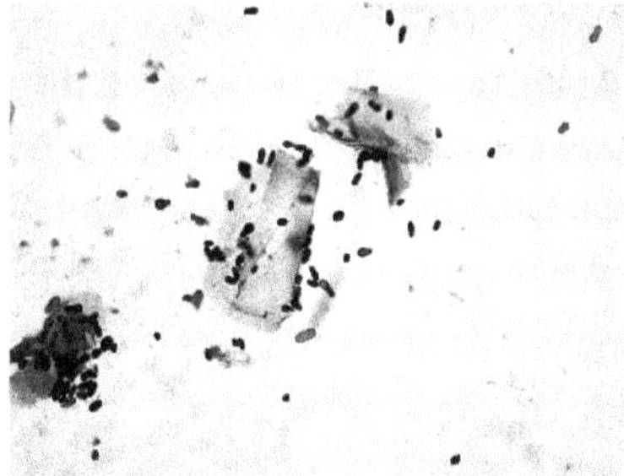

a. *Malassezia*
b. Cocci-shaped bacteria
c. Rod-shaped bacteria
d. Gram-positive bacteria

165. When counseling owners regarding assessing a patient's pain level, what parameter should not be used exclusively to determine the presence or absence of pain?

a. Disuse, such as of a limb
b. Elevated heart rate
c. Reluctance to move
d. Vocalization

166. Which of the following is the most appropriate method of euthanasia for an awake animal weighing less than one kilogram?

a. Intracardiac injection of barbiturates
b. IV injection of barbiturates
c. Intraperitoneal injection of barbiturates
d. Enclosed chamber with carbon dioxide

167. Hyperexcitement, nystagmus, and ataxia are common side effects seen with which classification of anesthetic agent?

a. Benzodiazepines, such as diazepam
b. Dissociative anesthetics, such as ketamine
c. Nonbarbiturate anesthetics, such as propofol
d. Inhalant anesthetics, such as isoflurane

168. When assisting ventilation by giving a breath by squeezing the reservoir bag, what is the maximum pressure you should provide?

a. 10 cmH_2O
b. 20 cmH_2O
c. 30 cmH_2O
d. 40 cmH_2O

169. A 6-year-old neutered male cat presents for a routine dental procedure during which multiple teeth are extracted. He is given a long-acting buprenorphine that is FDA approved for use in cats to help control postoperative pain. Later in the day, he is found to have pale mucous membranes and is nonresponsive. The veterinarian administers an opioid reversal, which resolves the signs. To which of the following agencies would it be appropriate to report an adverse drug event?

a. Drug Enforcement Agency (DEA)
b. United States Department of Agriculture (USDA)
c. Food and Drug Administration (FDA)
d. American Veterinary Medical Association (AVMA)

170. Before starting anesthetic procedures, what should be done to the anesthesia machine?

a. It should be thoroughly cleaned.
b. The soda lime canister should be changed.
c. The unilateral flutter valves should be cleaned.
d. It should be checked for pressure leaks.

Answer Key and Explanations for Test #1

1. A: Triage is the process of assessing a patient quickly and determining the degree of urgency with which the patient needs to be assessed and when intervention should take place. A pet owner's ability to perform triage is often unreliable, and it is the technician's role to ask the appropriate questions to obtain an accurate history and description of their concerns, starting with the initial phone call. Many different triage acuity scales are used, so it is important that the staff within a clinic are operating within the same parameters. These scales typically classify a patient's condition (in descending order of severity) as life threatening, emergent, urgent, or nonurgent.

2. A: The patient is showing signs of hyperadrenocorticism. Hyperadrenocorticism is also known as Cushing's disease when it is caused by an overproduction of glucocorticoids. Because this patient's hyperadrenocorticism is secondary to doctor-prescribed medication administration, this is a case of iatrogenic hyperadrenocorticism.

3. D: Aerosolized bacteria will form a cloud within 6 feet of the dental scaler. Anyone within this distance should be diligent about donning personal protective equipment (PPE) including a surgical cap and mask, protective eyewear, and gloves. The introduction of these bacteria to mucous membranes could cause infection.

4. A: Increased, or "bounding," distal digital pulses in equines are an important early indicator of laminitis or inflammation of the hoof wall. Horses that have undergone colic surgery are predisposed to this due to systemic inflammation. Fecal output, packed cell volume, and the presence of gastric reflux are important postoperative parameters for colic patients, but they are not direct indicators of laminitis.

5. C: Packed cell volume is a quick, patient-side test that involves centrifugation of a whole blood sample in a microhematocrit tube and then allows one to measure the percentage of red blood cells within the sample. It is often faster and more cost effective than running a complete blood count when the parameter of interest is the red blood cell quantity only. A value of 20% indicates a moderate anemia. The packed cell volume is analogous to a hematocrit level obtained via complete blood count.

6. C: Parenteral drug administration refers to a method of delivery that bypasses the gastrointestinal (GI) tract. This includes medications administered intravenously (IV), subcutaneously (abbreviated SC or SQ), and intramuscular (IM). Per os (PO) means by mouth. Medications administered PO are swallowed and absorbed by the GI system.

7. D: Calcium oxalate **monohydrate** urolithiasis is a common occurrence in animals that have ingested antifreeze (ethylene glycol). It occurs as a result of ethylene glycol metabolism in the liver, the end products of which are several potentially lethal toxic metabolites, one of which is oxalate. These metabolites direct their toxic effects on the kidneys by destroying renal epithelial cells as well as by obstructing the renal tubules, which ultimately results in acute renal failure.

8. C: Patients in status epilepticus that are refractory to treatment with benzodiazepines, such as midazolam, should be started on a propofol constant rate infusion IV for a minimum of 6 hours and up to 24 hours. During that time, the patient will be anesthetized and should be intubated and closely monitored. Ketamine should be used with caution, especially in patients with increased intracranial pressure. There is research currently underway investigating the efficacy of ketamine in combination with dexdomitor, but it is not yet standard practice. Isoflurane is not known to be effective at treating status epilepticus.

9. A: The transfer of globulins (specifically IgG) is critical for the establishment of immune function in ruminants and foals. Because the majority of the protein measured in the blood is composed of albumin and globulins, FPT will be reflected in a low total protein. A total protein level less than 5.5 g/dL is supportive of this diagnosis. IgG ELISA tests are also available but are significantly more costly. FPT may be concurrently hypoglycemic as a consequence of inadequate feeding, but this is not as consistent if the patient ate but had low-quality colostrum.

10. A: The P wave is the electrical indication of atrial depolarization. Ventricular depolarization is denoted by the entire QRS complex, and the T wave indicates ventricular repolarization. Atrial repolarization is obscured by ventricular depolarization but occurs during the QRS complex.

11. C: Opioids are considered controlled substances, and separate administration logs are required in addition to the prescription instructions. Although some anticonvulsants are considered controlled substances and need to be recorded, this is not an exclusive characteristic of the class. Antibiotics are not considered controlled substances.

12. A: Tetanus is caused by *Clostridium tetani*, a bacterium that is ubiquitous in the soil. Ruminants such as calves and goat kids are more susceptible than other species, and cases of tetanus are most commonly linked to wounds, such as surgical wounds. This can be prevented by the administration of tetanus toxoid at the time of the procedure. Botulism and listeria are diseases caused by ingestion of the infectious agent, and rabies is transmitted via the saliva of an infected animal.

13. C: Diluted povidone iodine (Betadine) solution is the preferred antiseptic for surgical procedures involving the ocular area because it is the gentlest antiseptic to use on the delicate conjunctiva. Chlorhexidine preparations are standard for skin preparation for all other surgeries. Alcohol and peroxide should not be used because they are irritating to the mucous membranes.

14. D: The urinary reagent strip indicating the presence of blood in urine is sensitive to myoglobin, free hemoglobin, and intact red blood cells (erythrocytes). Leukocytes (white blood cells) have a separate indicator strip; this strip tends to be inaccurate for dogs and cats.

15. B: The anatomical structure that holds the tooth to the alveolar bone and radiographically appears as a radiolucent line between the two structures is the periodontal ligament. Because the structure is composed primarily of collagen, it appears as a radiolucent line between the radiopaque tooth root and the alveolar bone. The apex refers to the very tip of the tooth root below the gumline, whereas the crown is the portion of the tooth above the gumline. The cementoenamel junction is the junction between the root and the crown.

16. B: Organophosphate toxicity leads to the stimulation of the parasympathetic nervous system, resulting in the "rest and digest" mechanism. This includes miosis (constriction of the pupils); clinically, the degree of constriction is extreme and the pupils are referred to as pinpoint. Parasympathetic stimulation also results in increased production of secretions (tears, saliva) and a decreased heart rate.

17. C: For specific chemicals, the facility should have on hand and have the ability to immediately consult the Safety Data Sheet (SDS), which lists all of the major chemicals and toxins and how to appropriately handle spills and exposures. The Occupational Safety and Health Administration (OSHA) does provide guidance for general handling of anesthetic gases. The Environmental Protection Agency (EPA) would regulate the disposal of certain chemicals that may contain hazardous materials, such as chloroform. The Food and Drug Administration (FDA) provides guidance on prescribing medications and drug effects.

18. A: Feline herpesvirus is one infectious agent implicated in upper respiratory disease. It is ubiquitous in the cat population with estimates being greater than 80% of cats having been exposed and/or carrying the virus. The virus may not be completely eliminated from the body and will recrudesce under times of stress, such as overcrowding in a shelter situation. Vaccination is important for prevention of disease but is a long-term solution. Antibiotics are not effective against a viral disease. Lysine supplementation was previously thought to help through inhibition of viral replication, but recent studies have found that the effect is minimal.

19. A: Olsen-Hegar needle drivers have scissors located behind the forceps portion to allow the user to cut sutures without a separate pair of scissors. This is preferred for a surgeon without an assistant rather than having to switch instruments in order to cut sutures. Mayo-Hegar needle drivers do not contain scissors and require separate scissors for cutting sutures. Allis and mosquito are types of hemostatic forceps, not needle drivers.

20. C: Orthogonal view is the term used for two radiographs that are taken at 90° angles to each other. The most common examples are a lateral view and a ventral-dorsal view. Orthogonal views are imperative to highlight a disease process that may be obscured in one of the views. A third view decreases the opportunity for overlay even further, such as a right and left lateral as well as a ventral-dorsal.

21. A: The shark fin appearance indicates an obstruction of the endotracheal tube. Mucous plugs or a kink of the endotracheal tube are the most common causes, but this can also occur with bronchoconstriction. If this waveform is seen, intervention must occur or else the patient is at risk of becoming hypoxemic or hypercapnic.

22. A: Weight reduction is a critical component to managing osteoarthritis by removing extra weight and resulting stress from the affected joints. Weight loss can be difficult to achieve with severe mobility impairment. Nutraceutical supplementation, such as with glucosamine and chondroitin, may be helpful as an adjunct, but its efficacy is variable. A grain-free diet is not recommended as a complete diet and can have negative side effects. Finally, cage rest may be helpful with acute injuries but is not helpful with chronic conditions and may add to weight gain.

23. C: Practices with a team philosophy and efficient work habits cross-train staff. Each staff member learns the responsibilities of his or her own position as well as responsibilities of staff members in other roles. A kennel worker, for example, is trained to restrain animals and set up laboratory samples. A technician learns receptionist duties including handling payment at discharge.

24. C: Securing the end of the tail to prevent inadvertent contamination of the surgery site is very important; however, care must be taken when doing so to avoid trauma to the tail. The best way to do this is to secure it to the cow's leg, typically the contralateral leg to which surgery is being performed. Securing the tail to an object such as a gate, post, or the ground could cause amputation if she would swing away from the object.

25. A: Thoracic radiographs should be taken at peak inspiration to maximally inflate the lungs. This creates the most accurate representation of the lung field and cardiac silhouette and minimizes artifacts caused by partially inflated lungs. In contrast, the abdomen should be imaged at end expiration.

26. C: True animal hoarding is a type of mental illness. Hoarders attempt to maintain far more animals than they can adequately care for. Hoarders are often experienced at hiding signs of this behavior. Some tip-offs that a patient lives with a hoarder or that a client is a hoarder are:

- Inconsistent or unidentified number of pets in the home
- Interest in further animal acquisition
- Inconsistent care of individual patients, but many visits with different patients
- Attempting to obtain medications for unseen animals
- Bringing in one or more poorly conditioned animals claiming stray status

Not every client with multiple pets, or a higher than average number of pets is a hoarder. An owner taking proper care of all pets is not likely to be a hoarder.

27. B: TID (Latin: *ter in die*) is the abbreviation for three times a day. SID (Latin: *semel in die*) is used exclusively in veterinary medicine to refer to once a day. BID (Latin: *bis in die*) refers to twice a day, and QID (Latin: *quater in die*) refers to four times a day.

28. A: A medicated water supply is a common and accepted method of distributing a medication (and sometimes vaccinations) to these two species in a production setting. Individual oral administration and injections are very labor intensive because each animal must be handled by at least one person. Topical preparations have very limited scope and availability.

29. D: Hypothermia is a very common cause of delayed anesthetic recovery, especially from a prolonged dental procedure in which the patient typically may become wet due to the use of water-spraying tools. Hypothermia is a consequence of nearly any anesthetic procedures, and appropriate heat-conserving methods should be implemented. If the patient becomes hypothermic, providing safe external heat sources such as warm blankets, circulating hot water blankets, or hot air blankets is preferred to the use of heating pads. Deep anesthesia could result in a delayed recovery as well, but the plane of anesthesia should be monitored throughout the process. Pain may result in a dysphoric recovery but will not delay it. Anemia after a dental procedure would be very rare.

30. D: E-collars prevent the patient (dogs and cats) from chewing at the suture site and subsequently causing an opening of the incision. In the instance of an ovariohysterectomy in which the incision is full thickness through the abdominal wall, dehiscence would result from an opening that allows the internal organs to move outside the body. This is a medical emergency, and, if the organs become bruised or contaminated, the mortality rate is very high. To a lesser degree, an E-collar will also prevent postop incisional infection and hemorrhage from the animal licking the incision site. E-collars do not affect an animal's activity level.

31. D: Aspirating air through a tube with the intent to be placed in the stomach could indicate placement through the trachea rather than the esophagus. Liquid should absolutely not be administered at this time because of the risk of drowning the patient. If placed properly, the nasogastric tube can be visualized passing through the esophagus lateral to the trachea externally or palpated as a distinct structure. You may also be able to auscultate the introduction of air into the stomach.

32. B: Multimodal analgesia refers to the synergistic effect that occurs when pain medications of different classes are used in conjunction with each other. For example, using an NSAID with an opioid results in better pain management than using each one separately. Matching analgesia is a term used to describe the idea of providing analgesia for the type of procedure and the subsequent pain that will occur. Preemptive analgesia is introducing analgesics before pain is experienced in an effort to prevent it. Local anesthesia is a pain management technique.

33. B: The tail vein (ventral coccygeal) provides an easy site for blood collection, especially in the restraint system described and the large volume of animals to be tested. The jugular is a common location for a blood draw on a single animal; the subcutaneous abdominal vein should never be used because of the significant risk of hematoma and vascular compromise. The auricular vein can be useful for access in calves and small ruminants, but its access requires a halter restraint.

34. D: This foal is suffering from a condition called strangles, or infection with *Streptococcus equi* subspecies *equi*. This condition causes caseous lymphadenitis resulting in extreme enlargement of the submandibular lymph nodes resulting in upper airway obstruction. Tracheostomy tube placement is necessary to allow proper oxygenation, and antibiotic therapy is instituted. Endotracheal intubation is not practical long term for equine patients, the nasal canula would not provide the degree of oxygenation necessary, and thoracocentesis is not indicated because there is not fluid compressing the lung cavity. Additionally, this bacterium is extremely contagious and strict isolation protocols should be followed when handling any equine with strangles.

35. D: Chloramphenicol is prohibited for use in food-producing animals. There is a risk of chloramphenicol-containing meat/milk causing aplastic anemia in humans if consumed. Dogs, cats, and horses are all considered companion animals in the United States, and they can therefore be safely treated with chloramphenicol. However, in countries where horses are considered food animals, chloramphenicol use should be discouraged.

Florfenicol is a newer antibiotic related to chloramphenicol that is approved for use in some food animal subgroups.

36. C: An accumulation of CO_2 via altered respiratory excretion (i.e., not "blowing off" enough CO_2) will result in hypercapnia. Because of the acidic nature of CO_2, its excess will shift the blood pH lower, resulting in acidosis. Excessive depth of anesthesia, airway obstruction, and pulmonary disease are some conditions that could result in respiratory acidosis. Respiratory alkalosis would result from blowing off excessive CO_2 (hyperventilation). Metabolic changes are dictated by blood bicarbonate levels, which are regulated by the kidneys and are measured via blood gas analysis.

37. D: If a drug's half-life is 2 hours, that means that after 2 hours there will be only 50% of the drug remaining in circulation. In another 2 hours, 50% of the remaining half of the drug left in circulation would remain, resulting in 25% of the original amount of the drug remaining in the system.

38. A: The technician should administer the injection in a front leg in order to avoid the renal portal system in the caudal half of the body. The renal portal system is a complex of blood vessels associated with the kidneys. Injections given in the caudal half of the body could potentially be carried to the kidneys before entering the systemic circulation. As a result, the drug may not reach therapeutic levels because a portion may be excreted prematurely. Renal damage could also occur since the drug has not had an opportunity to be metabolized by the body.

39. B: The left paralumbar fossa area should be clipped in preparation for a standing procedure. Standing C-sections in cattle are typically done from the left side in a standing animal because the large rumen will act as a natural retractor and will prevent the small intestines from entering the surgical field, which is more likely to happen on the right side. The ventral midline and paramedian approaches refer to the cow being placed in dorsal recumbency. This is to be avoided, if possible, in ruminants especially in a field situation because the added weight/pressure that it puts on the lung field can lead to complications.

40. D: If an FDA-approved product is available to treat the specific condition, cost is not considered to be an acceptable reason to prescribe a compounded alternative. Compounding can cause changes in a drug's actions and efficacy. Acceptable circumstances in which prescribing a compounded medication would be acceptable include if the currently available dosage is inappropriate (e.g., too high for a very small patient), if the route available is impeding compliance (e.g., converting an oral medication for a cat into a transdermal application), or if there is not an approved product to treat the specific condition.

41. C: Proud flesh is the layman's term for excessive granulation tissue production in the bed of the wound. This highly vascular tissue prevents epithelialization and healing of the wound, resulting in a chronic wound. Horses are extremely prone to proud flesh, especially on the distal limbs.

42. C: DTM is a type of media designed to grow dermatophytes and turn the media red, typically within 3 to 4 days. The DTM fungal culture would be advised to test for ringworm in this patient. Wood's lamp evaluation is a positive indicator in only 50% of feline dermatophyte infections. Skin scrapes and hair plucks without special staining do not identify dermatophytes. Another diagnostic tool is a dermatophyte polymerase chain reaction assay that would require laboratory submission and is faster for identification of dermatophyte infections.

43. C: A PET scan uses a radiopharmaceutical intervention alone or in combination with CT to highlight tissues of interest. The radioactive substance will result in "tagged" areas of interest that exhibit increased uptake and are used to plan surgery, chemotherapy, or targeted radiation. Appropriate PPE must be used when handling any animal receiving a radiopharmaceutical treatment until they have reached an acceptable level for discharge.

44. B: Lidocaine has historically been used for local anesthesia, such as nerve blocks, but research has shown significant success in treating pain when administered systemically, especially neuropathic pain. This route is typically used in conjunction with other IV medications, such as morphine and ketamine, and given as a constant rate infusion.

45. A: Cystocentesis should be avoided in patients that may have bladder neoplasia. If performed, this procedure could result in translocation of neoplastic cells from the lumen of the bladder through the abdomen via the track of the needle. Urinary catheterization would be an alternative if a culture was required.

46. C: The carnassial tooth (fourth upper premolar) is the most common tooth to experience fracturing and subsequent root abscess. Tooth fractures that expose the pulp cavity allow for passage of oral bacteria to the root, and this can result in abscess formation. Tooth fractures are common in dogs that chew on hard objects, such as rocks. Abscess of any root is possible, but the anatomy of the carnassial tooth results in abscess noted ventral to the orbit of the affected side. The anatomical locations of the roots of the canine and first premolar would be more rostral, whereas the first molar would result in a more caudal presentation.

47. D: Medicated shampoos should be allowed to have 10–20 minutes of contact time before being rinsed with lukewarm water. Complete rinsing is important to avoid skin irritation when residues are left. If the animal has excessive dirt/debris on their haircoat, they should be washed with a gentle all-purpose shampoo before the medicated shampoo is used.

48. B: Hydromorphone, like other opioids, has been implicated in lowering the seizure threshold in patients with a history of seizures. Opioids are not known to cause seizures in animals without any history of seizures. Acepromazine, a phenothiazine tranquilizer that is commonly used for large- and small-animal sedation, was long thought to have a similar effect, but recent studies have cast doubt on this notion. Diazepam and propofol generally raise the seizure threshold and are often used to stop active seizures.

49. C: Tooth overgrowth is the most common dental problem for lagomorphs, such as rabbits, because their teeth grow continually and require wear through chewing. Inappropriate diets that do not provide enough abrasion contribute to overgrowth, as does malocclusion. Treatment includes either extraction, in the case of malocclusion, or using a Dremel tool to mechanically file down the affected teeth and changing husbandry practices.

50. C: Hypsodont teeth are those in which the crown grows continually throughout the animal's lifetime and must be worn down to avoid overgrowth. In addition to equine and bovine, some small mammals such as rabbits also have hypsodont teeth. Diphyodont refers to mammals that have two sets of teeth, deciduous and permanent. Hypsodonts may also have some diphyodont teeth.

51. B: Centrifugation techniques concentrate the ova in feces and give a more accurate reading than flotation-only techniques. Sheather's sugar has a specific gravity higher than the ova of interest, which enables them to float to the top. Gross exam and direct smears are not effective at identifying parasite ova. Flotation with sodium nitrate is a common in-house technique used due to its ease of use; however, this method has a high rate of false-negative results.

52. B: Rabies virus is almost 100% fatal if contracted by humans or animals and can be passed from infected animals to humans through contact with saliva. Distemper is not zoonotic (transmissible to humans from animals). West Nile virus and Eastern equine encephalitis can be passed through humans via vector transmission, but they are not 100% fatal. Extreme care must be taken when handling any animal displaying neurological symptoms.

53. B: Polishing is the important final step in a dental cleaning. The polishing head and abrasive paste act to smooth any microcracks in the enamel that would act as a nidus for plaque accumulation. Ultrasonic scaling or hand scaling should be completed before the polishing step because it routinely causes these microcracks. Gingival probing is important for identifying deep gingival pockets but is diagnostic only.

54. D: These tissue forceps are Adson-Brown thumb forceps. Rat-toothed thumb forceps have fewer, larger teeth that interdigit when opposed. Olsen-Hegar and Kelly hemostatic forceps both have box locks that allow them stay locked in position.

55. B: Normal saline is the preferred IV fluid choice for an Addisonian crisis. Given that this patient is hypoglycemic, a diluted bolus of glucose may be indicated. Glucocorticoid administration of dexamethasone will not interfere with the results of an adrenocorticotropic hormone stimulation test to confirm the diagnosis. Lactated Ringer's and Normosol-R are common crystalloid replacement therapies and would be the second choice if normal saline was not available. Hypertonic saline is indicated for rapid intravascular volume expansion in conjunction with isotonic crystalloids.

56. C: In cases of poison ingestion, it is critical that the owner provides the packaging information that lists the ingredients (active and inactive) for the ingested substance. The mechanism of action for different types of poisons determines the appropriate treatment; for example, a vitamin K antagonist, such as warfarin, has a different treatment than a vitamin D analog. Vaccine records and previous history are helpful for routine wellness but are unlikely to have a significant impact on the treatment for this incident. Insurance information would not have an influence on the treatment decisions.

57. A: Increased respiratory rate and effort combined with additional indications of severe parenchymal disease (dyspnea, hypoxia, and labored breathing) should give immediate concern for oxygenation ability. Obtaining an SpO_2 reading should occur before attempting diagnostics, such as radiographs. An animal in respiratory distress could decompensate quickly when placed in certain positions, such as on their back for ventral-dorsal radiographs. The patient should be stabilized with oxygen therapy and venous access should be achieved before confirming a presumptive diagnosis of pneumonia.

58. B: Procedures that require entry into the GI tract are classified as clean-contaminated as long as they are performed in a controlled nature without any spillage of the intestinal contents. Clean procedures do not involve entry into the respiratory, GI, or genitourinary systems. A contaminated procedure would involve spillage of GI contents or urine, and a dirty procedure involves purulent discharge or significant contamination, such as an intestinal perforation.

59. A: A rabies pole may be used to restrain fractious and aggressive dogs but should never be used to restrain a cat. There is a significant risk of injury/death with this type of device when used with a cat. A properly applied cat-specific muzzle, a towel wrap or "burrito," or an E-collar are all acceptable devices to assist in the restraint of fractious felines.

60. C: Propofol is an anesthetic agent that is titrated to the desired effect via IV administration. It commonly produces apnea and, if administered too rapidly or in large volumes, may produce respiratory arrest. A similar GABA agonist called alfaxalone may produce less apnea; however, it may be cost prohibitive, especially in larger animals.

61. A: Hair covers, masks, and shoe covers are essential for all occupants of the surgical suite. Gloves are typically not required unless the individual is participating in the procedure as the surgeon or as an assistant. In addition to the previously listed items, scrubs are required attire and street clothes should not be worn.

62. A: The calculation for this question is as follows:

$$55 \text{ lb} \div 2.2 \text{ lb/kg} = 25 \text{ kg}$$

$$25 \text{ kg} \times 2 \text{ mg/kg} = 50 \text{ mg}$$

$$50 \text{ mg} \times \frac{1 \text{ dose}}{12 \text{ hrs}} \times 24 \text{ hours} = 100 \text{ mg}$$

63. B: Platelets are prone to forming larger conglomerates or clumping together, which decreases the platelet count. This is exacerbated by prolonged blood draws. A decreased automated platelet count should always be followed by a manual evaluation of a blood smear to identify the presence of large platelet clumps. Neutrophils, monocytes, and red blood cells are not prone to clumping.

64. C: A sternal restraint can often be used to restrain a fractious animal for minor procedures such as a nail trim, injections, or blood draws. In a larger breed such as a German shepherd, two people are usually required – one to control the head and front legs and a second to restrain the rear limbs. If an animal is still resistant to the procedure, it may be appropriate to discontinue it and proceed at a later time when sedation/antianxiety medication may be given.

65. B: This is an example of allowing the wound to heal from the inside out, or second-intention healing. Second-intention healing is commonly used for infected or old wounds. First-intention healing refers to the surgical closure of wounds or small/recent lacerations. Third-intention healing allows for initial healing of a wound by second intention followed by surgical closure (delayed primary closure). Debridement is the process of removing necrotic tissue to facilitate healing by first-, second-, or third-intention healing.

66. D: Basic CPR, also known as basic life support, includes chest compressions, airway management, and ventilation. The remaining choices would fall under advanced CPR, or advanced life support, and would also include postresuscitation management. Chest compressions may alternate with abdominal contractions to aid in venous return to the heart. CPR has a very low success rate in animals, reportedly between 6% and 7%.

67. D: The gold standard for radiograph use in extractions is to take full-mouth films to asses root and alveolar bone health before extraction followed by postextraction films of individual teeth. This allows the veterinarian to determine if there is evidence of root resorption and other disease processes of the root before attempting extractions. Postextraction films are recommended to ensure that full root extraction has been accomplished.

68. B: The Triadan system divides the oral cavity into quadrants and issues each tooth a three-digit number. It starts with the upper right quadrant and associated teeth as the 100s and moving clockwise to the 200s for the upper left quadrant, the 300s for the lower left quadrant, and the 400s for the lower right quadrant. The fourth tooth moving clockwise from the first medial incisor is the canine, 204. The canines serve as landmarks because they always end in 4 across small mammal species. Deciduous teeth follow the same pattern but start with 5, 6, 7, or 8.

69. C: Sinus tachycardia is an increase in heart rate that can occur due to a variety of physiologic (e.g., exercise, pain, fear), pharmacologic (drugs such as atropine, epinephrine, acepromazine), or pathologic influences (e.g., anemia, heart failure, shock). The heart remains under the control of a normal SA node and the P-QRS-T complexes appear normal.

70. C: Jugular veins are preferred for blood draws in a patient also requiring IV catheter placement in order to preserve the peripheral veins (saphenous and cephalic) for catheter placement. Jugular vein samples may give a more accurate platelet count as well, due to the ability to use a larger needle and obtain a cleaner sample. Cephalic veins are the most common for catheter placement. Saphenous veins may be accessed but can be easily occluded if an animal is not recumbent.

71. C: Potassium is an intracellular electrolyte. When hemolysis occurs, intracellular potassium is released and can result in the appearance of hyperkalemia. Glucose levels are not significantly elevated with hemolysis; however, they can be falsely lowered if there is a delay in separating the red blood cells from the serum. Creatine is a by-product of muscle metabolism that is cleared through the kidneys and is not affected by hemolysis. Albumin is a freely circulating plasma protein that is also not affected by hemolysis.

72. D: The ability for the patient to protect its airway is the determining factor for readiness to remove of the endotracheal tube. This is indicated by a strong swallow reflex. Typically, the patient should be able to swallow two to three times consecutively before removing the endotracheal tube. If extubation occurs prior to evidence of an intact swallow reflex, the patient is at risk for aspiration, and if it is delayed, the patient may inadvertently chew the end of the tube.

73. B: Patients that are unresponsive to normal environmental stimuli but respond to pain are classified as stuporous. Normal mentation is considered alert. Comatose animals will not respond to painful stimuli. Animals experiencing delirium will respond inappropriately to stimuli, such as displaying an exaggerated response to a normal noise. This classification provides a quick assessment of the patient's central nervous system.

74. B: Polyglactin 910 (Vicryl) is the only suture material listed that is able to be broken down by the body, or absorbed. Nylon, polyester, and silk are nonabsorbable and need to be manually removed.

75. C: IV catheter placement is essential in hyperthermia cases to begin the administration of cool fluids. Blood work may be required for organ assessment but can be done after catheter placement. Submersion in cold water is not recommended because it has been shown to have reflex peripheral vasoconstriction and is an ineffective method of cooling. A better option would be to put alcohol on the paw pads for evaporative cooling and to put cool towels on hairless areas such as the ventral abdomen.

76. B: Iodine-131 treatment is a type of nuclear medicine that is used for patients with an overproduction of thyroid hormone. The active tissue takes up the radioactive isotope resulting in tissue destruction and subsequent loss of function. The advantage is that this treatment usually is curative and will destroy active glandular tissue located away from the thyroid gland. For many clients, the procedure is cost prohibitive and, in some instances, may need to be repeated.

77. A: Furosemide is a loop diuretic that promotes water excretion through the kidneys through an active transport system in the distal convoluted tubule that exchanges sodium for potassium, resulting in the increased excretion of potassium. For this reason, the patient's potassium levels should be monitored regularly due to the risk of hypokalemia.

78. B: The secondary bandage layer is typically composed of an absorbent material such as gauze or, in the case of excessively productive wounds, cotton may be used. The primary layer is the layer in contact with the wound, and the tertiary layer is the outermost layer. A fortified bandage provides rigidity such as in the case of a splint. The layer in which this is placed is determined by the type of material used (i.e., cast vs. splint).

79. B: For a young, healthy animal with no history of cardiovascular concerns, the most effective short-acting sedation protocol for this patient would be dexmedetomidine and butorphanol in combination IV. The combination of the two drugs provides a synergistic effect and allows for a lower dose of each. The combination will provide sufficient sedation and analgesia for a moderately painful procedure such as porcupine quill extraction. Telazol is a combination of tiletamine and diltiazem more commonly used as an induction agent—this degree of anesthesia is unnecessary given the small number of porcupine quills. Propofol similarly will provide anesthesia rather than sedation. Acepromazine and hydromorphone is a common preanesthetic combination but will not provide sufficient sedation to safely remove intraoral quills.

80. C: Two indicator strips are the minimum requirement to ensure pack sterility. The outermost indicator tape will show if the autoclave reached temperature, and the innermost indicator will show that the temperature was achieved inside the packs. The internal indicator strip should never be placed directly on top of the instruments.

81. D: Lymphocytes are more abundant than other white blood cells (leukocytes) in cattle, whereas neutrophils are the most common in other mammals. Monocytes are white blood cells that may be increased in the presence of inflammation. Erythrocytes are red blood cells.

82. C: The pubic symphysis of guinea pigs fuses together between 7 and 8 months of age and is normally not an issue with nonbreeding females. Guinea pigs that are acquired for breeding purposes, however, and are bred after 6 months of age will experience difficult labor and possibly dystocia if they are unable to separate the symphysis during parturition.

83. A: The lungs are the most common organ to experience metastasis from a primary tumor due to their high level of blood flow, which provides a translocation opportunity for neoplastic cells. This would be the first location to radiograph; however, not all neoplastic cells will metastasize. Metastasis to the lungs would be a contraindication for anesthesia, and referral to an oncologist would be recommended.

84. D: The central venous pressure measurement estimates the pressure in the right atrium and assesses cardiac preload. This is done via a central catheter placed in the patient's right jugular vein and either a water manometer or an electronic pressure transducer to take multiple measurements and demonstrate trends. An excessive central venous pressure reading would indicate fluid overload, whereas a low reading would indicate hypovolemia.

85. B: The endotracheal tube should extend from slightly past the rostral aspect of the muzzle to the point of the shoulder, but not past it. Measuring from the larynx to the point of the shoulder would result in an intraoral connection to the anesthetic machine, which is undesirable, whereas measuring from the muzzle to the larynx would be too short to adequately protect the airway. If the tube extends to the heart base, there is a significant risk of bronchial intubation.

86. C: Rapid IV administration of calcium-containing solutions causes profound bradycardia. For that reason, IV calcium should be given very slowly and signs of bradycardia (slowing of the heart) should be monitored. Glucose-containing solutions are typically avoided in the absence of hypoglycemia, but, when they are given, the rate must also be monitored to avoid bradycardia.

87. B: The O_2 supply is stored in compressed medical gas cylinders. Because the gas is under such high pressure, the regulator reduces the pressure to a safe and constant rate to be delivered to the patient. This is not the same as the check valve located on the actual cylinder. The flow meter indicates the rate of O_2 flow being delivered to the patient (in L/min), the reservoir bag provides a reserve of O_2 that the patient can easily draw from, and the manometer is the monitor that measures the pressure within the circuit.

88. B: Filing the overgrown parts of the crown is referred to as floating the teeth. Because these teeth continually grow, abnormal wear can result in sharp points that cause significant intraoral trauma; common signs are difficulty chewing or dropping feed. Scaling and gingival probing are not commonly done because these animals are less prone to calculus accumulation. Extraction of equine teeth may be performed, but it is typically only done under field conditions when the tooth is extremely mobile.

89. A: Wind-up pain is a phenomenon in which untreated pain leads to increasing pain. This is seen as hyperesthesia and as an exaggerated response with respect to the degree of manipulation. Feline pain management is difficult because there is often a delay in diagnosis and pharmacological limitations with approved pain medications. Many geriatric felines have concurrent systemic illness such as chronic renal disease, which can further reduce safe options for pain medication. Behavioral responses can be difficult to differentiate from true medical conditions, but one should assume that pain is present rather than let it go untreated.

90. B: Ruminants and camelids (pseudoruminants) do not have upper incisors. In place of these teeth, they have a dental pad, which consists of gingiva overlaying their rostral maxilla. Canines, felines, and equines all have upper incisors.

91. C: Loss of deep pain response carries the least favorable prognosis with regard to likelihood to return to function following spinal decompression surgery. The nerve fibers that transmit deep pain (tested by extreme pressure across a bone such as a toe) lie deep in the spinal cord with respect to the superficial pain fibers. The nerves that are responsible for motor responses are the most superficial. These sensations are lost from the superficial to the deep nerves, and they return in the opposite manner with a compressive lesion such as disc protrusion into the spinal canal. It is highly discouraged to test for the presence of pain responses in a patient that has intact motor responses.

92. A: Caffeine (a methylxanthine) toxicosis can occur in conjunction with theobromine toxicosis because the cocoa bean contains both of these compounds. Doses of more than 20 mg/kg are known to have excitatory central nervous system and cardiac effects, and doses of more than 60 mg/kg are known to induce seizures. Xylitol, ethylene glycol, and zinc are known to have toxicity risks; however, none of them are directly associated with chocolate.

93. A: Although increasing the milliamperes (mA) and shortening the time, and decreasing the mA and shortening the time will result in a shorter exposure time, the former is recommended for decreasing blurriness that results from movement during an x-ray. The shortened time allows for less time for the patient to move, whereas the increased milliamperes allows for more current and therefore more detail in the image. Increasing the mA to a longer exposure time would increase motion artifact. Adjustments with kV will affect the contrast, not the exposure time.

94. C: Suture size, or diameter, is given in the USP (United States Pharmacopeia) system by a number. "Thick" sutures are given a single number greater than zero. The thicker the suture, the bigger the number: 2 is bigger than 1, which is bigger than 0. "Thin" sutures are even thinner than 0. Their numbers are written with a dash and a zero, like 2-0. The zero is pronounced "ought," so 2-0 suture is called "two-ought." The bigger the number in front of the "ought," the smaller the suture: 3-0 is smaller than 2-0. One way to think of this is like a number line, where the numbers with an "ought" are to the left of 0 (the negative side). The bigger the number in front of the "ought," the further the size is from 0, and since they are to the negative side, the smaller the suture. Another way to think of it is that the number in front of the "ought" is the number of zeroes in the size, so 3-0 would be 000 and 2-0 would be 00; this means that 1-0 is the same as 0, which is why no one ever mentions 1-0 suture. All of the suture sizes in the answer choices, listed smallest to largest, are: 11-0, 10-0, 9-0, 3-0, 2-0, 0, 1, 2, 3.

95. B: All drugs labeled for use in food animals have a labeled time in which the products from that animal, such as milk, must be discarded, referred to as withdrawal times. These times reflect the time it takes for the drug level in the animal (and their by-products) to decrease to a safe level. Off-label use of drugs is prohibited in food-producing animals. Expiration dates refer to the time in which food may no longer be safe to eat due to decomposition. USDA certification allows food to be certified to the consumer as organic.

96. B: Local anesthesia (commonly referred to as a nerve block) is the only effective method of blocking pain. These sodium channel blockers impair the propagation of pain signals along nerves. They are useful adjuncts to most surgical procedures, such as amputations, dental extractions, or even skin incisions. Local anesthetics have a wide variety of duration from 1 hour (lidocaine) to 10 hours (bupivacaine).

97. B: A total of 10 mL of medication or less is acceptable for each IM injection in a Jersey cow. In a situation in which the total volume exceeds this limit, multiple injections may be necessary. It would be appropriate to administer each aliquot in the same injection area.

98. B: Urine specific gravity refers to the density of urine when compared to water, with normal typically being 1.015–1.045 in dogs and 1.035–1.065 in cats. The higher the specific gravity, the more concentrated the urine is, which reflects the animal's hydration status. Osmolality is the concentrations of solutes in a solution and is not routinely measured in urinalysis. Color refers to the color of the urine (i.e., yellow, brown, or red), and clarity refers to how cloudy the urine appears.

99. B: Kilovoltage (kV) represents the tissue-penetrating power produced during an x-ray, with a higher kV penetrating more tissue than a lower kV. The higher kV will also produce more scatter radiation, which results in a gray overlay of the entire image (appearing shadowed). Therefore, increasing the kV will directly decrease the subject contrast. Collimation reduces beam scatter and exposure time, increasing safety for the patient and the operator. Distance will slightly affect the beam penetration but not as significantly as the kV. Filtration is an added measure of protection from radiation produced by the x-ray beam. Filtration blocks the alpha and beta rays from penetrating the patient's body tissues, allowing only the image-producing radiation to reach the patient.

100. B: Apomorphine is the most reliable and effective drug for the induction of emesis in canines. When administered intravenously or intramuscularly, apomorphine can produce emesis in a matter of minutes. It is also available in a tablet form that can be crushed and a small amount placed in the conjunctival sac.

Xylazine is an effective and fast-acting (1–2 minutes) emetic in cats. Hydrogen peroxide can induce vomiting in dogs by irritating the gastric mucosa. Results, however, are often not immediate and may not occur at all. Syrup of ipecac can also induce vomiting in dogs, but only after 15–30 minutes following administration. It must reach the intestine before it exerts is effects.

101. D: The scavenger system serves to remove exhaled waste gases. It may be active, which requires a vacuum pump or fan, or passive, which directs waste to a special canister to absorb the gases. These are used with rebreathing and nonrebreathing circuits. The vaporizer houses the anesthetic liquid that is converted into gas form. Anesthetic masks expose personnel to an increased amount of waste gas when compared to an endotracheal tube and should be used as little as possible.

102. B: The calculation for this problem is as follows:

$$500 \text{ kg} \times 2.5 \ \frac{\text{mg}}{\text{kg}} = 1{,}250 \text{ mg}$$

$$1{,}250 \text{ mg} \div 100 \ \frac{\text{mg}}{\text{mL}} = 12.5 \text{ mL}$$

103. B: Hypovitaminosis C, also known as scurvy, is a common nutritional deficiency of guinea pigs; special care must be taken to meet their nutritional requirements. Untreated, this condition results in lethargy, weakness, anorexia, diarrhea, and changes in the haircoat. Vitamin C deteriorates in feed quickly, and a new bag of pelleted feed should be opened every 90 days to avoid this deterioration. Additionally, plenty of fresh vegetables rich in vitamin C should be offered. The remaining nutrients are adequately provided in a balanced diet and are not susceptible to the rapid breakdown as seen with vitamin C.

104. C: Inhalant anesthetics are primarily excreted through the lungs through exhaling, although small amounts are metabolized and excreted via the liver, kidneys, and GI tract. Because these drugs are excreted quickly through the lungs, recovery is fairly rapid once the gas is removed.

105. C: The shock dose of resuscitation fluids is 90 mL/kg (this is higher than the maintenance dose, which is between 40 and 60 (mL/kg)/hr), and one-third of the total volume is given as a bolus to expand the intravascular volume rapidly. In this case, 25 kg × 90 mL/kg = 2,250 mL. Then, 2,250 mL ÷ 3 = 750 mL is given as a rapid bolus. After this bolus, the animal should be reassessed.

106. D: Gentamicin is an aminoglycoside. Aminoglycosides are known to have nephrotoxic and ototoxic potential even at therapeutic doses. Careful monitoring of renal values is important during administration of this class of antibiotics. Penicillins and tetracyclines have a similar toxicity spectrum with the most common concerns being allergic reactions or GI upset. The most common negative effects for lincosamides are severe vomiting and diarrhea from overgrowth of pathogenic bacteria.

107. C: Enucleations are performed on a standing animal with local sedation with or without standing sedation. General anesthesia is a higher risk for equine and bovine patients due to their large size and the risk of respiratory depression. When general anesthesia is required, specialized facilities are needed.

108. D: A laceration of the milk vein is a life-threatening condition because the cow could exsanguinate rapidly from blood loss. Having the farmer start interventions while the veterinarian is en route is very important.

Pressure could be applied, or, if clamps are available, the farmer could place one clamp on either side of the injury. Superficial lacerations do not constitute this degree of urgency.

109. A: Fentanyl is rapidly eliminated from the body due to extensive first-pass metabolism; the therapeutic effects last approximately 30 minutes. For this reason, for fentanyl to be maintained at a therapeutic level, it must be administered as a constant rate infusion. Morphine and methadone provide therapeutic benefits for approximately 4 hours and buprenorphine for 6 hours.

110. D: Employee handbooks can be extensive summaries of a practices rules and policies. An employee handbook includes information on the practice and the type of employment, general employment information including ADA and EEO information, attendance policies, work safety issues, reimbursement policies, compensation and benefits information, time off work, performance evaluation procedures, complaint procedures, and workplace monitoring. It does not include job descriptions.

111. A: The amount of drug administered at one time is called the dose. The interval is the time between the dose administrations and is therefore incorrect. The route is the method of administration (such as intramuscularly [IM] or by mouth), and the concentration is the amount of drug per unit of volume when in solution.

112. B: Veterinary technicians have a crucial role in pain management because they are typically performing monitoring during and after painful procedures. They may assess pain using various parameters or formal surveys, log controlled drugs as required, and work closely with the veterinarian to make recommendations regarding adjustments to the pain protocol. They may not prescribe specific medications because this is outside the parameters of their licensure. Although they may add valuable input, ultimately, the veterinarian issues any prescriptions.

113. A: Metzenbaum scissors are extremely delicate and should only be used for sharp dissection of tissue. When they are used to cut drape material, they can become dull or damaged very easily. Mayo scissors are typically included in a sterile pack for this purpose. When cutting drape material in a nonsterile manner, bandage scissors are acceptable to use. Suture scissors are impractical (but not strictly prohibited) to cut drape material given their small size and specialized shape.

114. B: Butorphanol is a mixed agonist–antagonist; therefore, it can act as a mu-antagonist and will reverse the effects of mu-agonists, such as hydromorphone and morphine. Ketamine is an N-nitrosodimethylamine (NDMA) receptor agonist, and it therefore does not affect the mu-receptor at all, whereas diazepam is a gamma aminobutyric acid (GABA) receptor agonist.

115. B: The patient's level of CO_2 indicates their ventilation status, with an increase in CO_2 caused by hypoventilation (retained CO_2) and a decrease in CO_2 indicating hyperventilation (breathing off excessive CO_2). The SpO_2 value measures a patient's oxygenating ability. Mean arterial pressure is an indicator of tissue perfusion. The respiratory rate will affect the CO_2 and SpO_2 values and should be monitored throughout the anesthetic procedure.

116. B: Urine culture and sensitivity should be performed if there is suspicion of a urinary tract infection before the administration of antibiotics. Cystocentesis is a method in which urine is drawn directly out of the bladder with a needle and syringe and is the preferred sample for the urine culture and sensitivity in order to avoid contamination from the external urogenital tract. Urinalysis is helpful for evaluating the composition of urine, but it is not always definitive for identifying infection and is unable to determine antimicrobial sensitivity.

117. B: This is an ovum from *T. canis*, commonly known as the roundworm. They have a characteristic dark-brown, thick-walled egg. *T. vulpis* (whipworm) has a barrel-shaped egg with bipolar plugs. *A. caninum* (hookworm) is clear, smooth, and thin-walled. Species of the genus *Giardia* are protozoans with clear cysts that are much smaller than the listed ova.

118. B: Fluorescein stain will glow green under blacklight conditions when in contact with a defect in the corneal epithelium and can be used to identify corneal ulcers. The stain will also indicate the patency of the nasolacrimal duct by appearing on the external nares if patent. The Schirmer tear test assesses tear production, tonometry measures intraocular pressure, and gonioscopy is a method to examine the iris angle and anterior chamber of the eye.

119. D: Manual platelet counts are important tools for identifying thrombocytopenia (decreased platelets). Manual platelet counts should be performed under a 100× (oil immersion) objective. A minimum of 10 fields should be examined, and the number of platelets per high-powered field is multiplied by 20,000 to give an accurate count. Values of less than 100,000 are considered significant in mammals.

120. D: While worms in the feces are not an emergency, they are of great concern and must be addressed. Dogs may be infected with multiple intestinal parasites, and should not be diagnosed or treated solely on the basis of visible worms. Medication should not be dispensed without a valid doctor-client-patient relationship and a doctor's prescription. The dog should be evaluated for signs of disease. The dog's feces should be evaluated for other parasites. The client should be educated on treatment and limiting the likelihood of further infection.

121. B: Most CPR on dogs and cats should be performed with the patient in lateral recumbency, although there are a few exceptions. Small dogs and cats should receive circumferential compressions (using one hand to squeeze the chest directly over the heart) rather than lateral two-handed compressions. The point of the elbow is a reference landmark for the heart location. Keel-chested dogs should receive compressions at the widest part of their chest (choice C), whereas for barrel-chested dogs, compressions should be at the point of the heart.

122. A: Hypothermic neonates must be rewarmed gradually at no more than 2 °F per hour. The best source of heat is warm ambient temperatures, such as an incubator, rather than a heating pad or similar because a debilitated animal will not be able to move away from a direct heat source. This can result in burns. Rapid rewarming can result in shock. Feeding should not take place until the neonate is normothermic because gut motility is compromised during hypothermia. Catheter placement (either IV or interosseous) may be considered if there is a dehydration component, and warm fluid therapy may be instituted as part of a gradual rewarming process, but this would not be the first step in resuscitating this patient.

123. A: Urine specific gravity is used to assess the concentrating ability of the renal tubules with respect to that of plasma. Isosthenuria would be indicated in a urine specific gravity sample with the density the same as plasma (1.008 to 1.012). Hyposthenuria would be a value more dilute than water, typically less than 1.008. Hypersthenuria indicates that the urine is more concentrated than plasma, and species-specific ranges have been quantified to determine acceptable urine concentration values.

124. A: The maxillary infraorbital anesthetic block interrupts pain signals of the structures rostral (toward the nose) of the third premolar on the side it is placed. The inferior alveolar anesthetic block interrupts pain signals from all structures of the affected mandible and is accessed intraorally. The middle mental anesthetic block interrupts pain signals from rostral to the mandibular second premolar, and the caudal maxillary anesthetic block interrupts pain signals from the cranial structures to the maxillary molar.

125. B: VD is the abbreviation for ventrodorsal because radiograph views are named for the part of the body that the beam enters followed by where it exits. VD means that the beam should enter the ventral aspect of the animal and exit dorsally. For most small-animal patients, this will mean laying on their backs (dorsal recumbency) with the x-ray tube shooting from above. The remaining positions could accomplish this view with a mobile tube.

126. C: Feline gingivostomatitis is a severe disease in which medical management routinely fails and full-mouth extractions are necessary for long-term management. The etiology is thought to be due to an immune hypersensitivity to oral bacteria that exists in tartar and plaque formation. Cases may initially be treated with steroids and antibiotics, followed by dental cleaning and at-home care, but the disease process often becomes refractory to this treatment. Full-mouth tooth extraction is the most effective long-term treatment for this condition.

127. B: A patient with a normal AV node should respond positively to atropine with sinus tachycardia (a normal heart rhythm with a heart rate greater than 140 beats per minute). If bradycardia persists or if the arrhythmia progresses to third-degree AV block, the AV node is diseased and a pacemaker would be necessary. Ventricular tachycardia independent of atrial activity is not a normal response to an atropine challenge test.

128. D: Herding breeds, such as border collies and Australian shepherds, are shown to have a higher chance of mutation at the MDR1 gene. Deficiency in this gene has shown to compromise the integrity of the blood–brain barrier, allowing drugs to access the brain that normally wouldn't, such as ivermectin. Other drugs known to have neurologic effects may be more pronounced, such as sedatives and chemotherapeutic agents.

129. B: Although all of the listed modalities are implemented in managing feline lower urinary tract disease, decreasing stressors is the single most significant factor in reducing clinical signs. Antibiotics are only indicated in the presence of bacteria. Prescription diets have been shown to decrease the likelihood of urinary blockage by facilitating a more dilute urine, and pheromones such as Feliway have also been shown to be beneficial.

130. A: *Leptospira* spp. may be shed in the urine of infected animals and can be transmitted to humans through contamination of mucous membranes or ingestion. Disease transmission from animals to humans is classified as a zoonotic infection. A leptospirosis suspect should be placed in isolation, and full PPE should be used for anyone handling the patient until the diagnosis has been confirmed and treatment is completed. Many mammals may transmit *Leptospira* spp., including small rodents and wildlife. Immunocompromised individuals are considered to be at high risk.

131. D: Premature ventricular contractions are the most common post-gastric dilatation and volvulus arrythmia. They classically respond well to medical management with antiarrythmics such as lidocaine, but, left untreated, they may be life-threatening by causing interrupted cardiac output.

132. A: All dental procedures should be carried out under general anesthesia. This includes cleanings, radiographs, and any intervention that may be necessary. Placing an endotracheal tube is essential to protect the airway in order to effectively scale and polish the teeth. Anesthesia-free dentistry is heavily discouraged because it is ineffective and could pose a significant risk to the patient.

133. D: Blood collection in an avian should be based on weight and should never exceed 1% of the bird's total weight in milliliters (mL). For example, when drawing blood on an 80 g bird, one should not draw more than 0.8 mL:

$$80 \text{ g} \times 0.01 = 0.8 \text{ mL}$$

134. A: A rebreathing circuit is one in which the patient will inhale a mixture of expired and fresh gases, while a portion of the expired gases are diverted to the scavenger. This is advantageous for large patients because it reduces the amount of oxygen and anesthetic agent that are used. The expired gases also help to warm and humidify the incoming gases. Ventilation can be assisted through a ventilator or a person using a rebreathing or a nonrebreathing system, and all systems require endotracheal intubation. All systems require oxygenation to vaporize the anesthetic, and room air is not used.

135. B: Stage 2 of anesthesia exhibits the signs of excitement, delirium, and involuntary muscular movement, and it is typically unpleasant to observe. However, with proper preanesthetic and induction agents, this phase can be minimized or eliminated. Stage 1 is the induction stage with beginning loss of consciousness. Stage 3 is the stage of surgical anesthesia and is divided into phases 1–4 depending on anesthetic depth. Stage 4 is extremely deep anesthesia in which there is a risk of death from cardiac arrest.

136. D: Platelet-rich plasma would be indicated if the only hematologic abnormality was thrombocytopenia (low platelets). Fresh whole blood may be used if plasma is not available; however, it could potentially cause polycythemia (elevated red blood cell count). Packed red blood cells are indicated for treatment of anemia, whereas oxyglobin is an alternative to packed red blood cells.

137. A: Ruminants such as cattle, sheep, and goats are extremely sensitive to the sedative effects of xylazine. This low-toxicity dose is not observed in other alpha-2 agonists, but xylazine is labeled for use in cattle and thus is the one that is most commonly used. An important requirement when administering xylazine is to have an alpha-2 antagonist readily available to reverse the negative effects of xylazine.

138. A: The white appearance to serum is an indication of lipemia, or increased fat in the bloodstream. This can be secondary to a recent meal, hypertriglyceridemia, or pancreatitis. Lipemic samples may affect the accuracy of readings for serum values, such as cholesterol. Icteric samples appear yellow, whereas hemolyzed samples are pink or shades of red. Hypoproteinemia (low blood protein) cannot be visualized in a centrifuged sample and requires analysis.

139. D: Preanesthetic medications are typically a combination of analgesics and sedatives such as acepromazine with hydromorphone. Administration of premedication will reduce anxiety, prevent wind-up pain, and facilitate a smoother anesthetic induction (and recovery), but it will increase the interval to induction. This delay is minimal, typically 20 minutes with medications that are administered subcutaneously. This delay can be minimized with either IM or IV administration and should not be a reason to forgo premedication.

140. C: For cattle, the ideal location for injections is the lateral cervical muscles of the neck. These muscles form a triangle, bordered by the cranial aspect of the shoulder, ventrally by the cervical spine, and dorsally by the nuchal ligament. In pigs, the dorsolateral cervical muscles are used. Rear legs, rump, and shoulders should be avoided because any injection has the potential to create scar tissue, which will result in condemnation when the animals reach the slaughter inspection. Dairy cattle are more likely to have had injections in the rear legs during their production years for ease of administration; however, this should be avoided if at all possible.

141. A: Hyperechoic means a structure is lighter or whiter than the surrounding tissues, or whiter than the structure should be normally. Darker or blacker would be called hypoechoic, the same contrast as the surrounding structures would be called isoechoic, and completely black would be called anechoic.

142. B: Ventromedial eye position indicates stage 3, plane 2 anesthetic depth, which is the ideal surgical plane. The presence of jaw tone indicates a light surgical plane and may be acceptable for nonpainful procedures, such as radiographs. Loss of corneal reflex occurs at plane 4, which is extremely deep anesthesia and precedes respiratory and cardiac arrest. Central eye position is observed at plane 1 anesthesia and again at plane 4.

143. B: The presence of a wide and bizarre QRS complex lacking an associated P wave amidst a normal sinus rhythm is a premature ventricular contraction. If these complexes become frequent, they may affect the animal's cardiac output and require treatment. They are the most common arrythmia seen following splenectomy.

144. C: Cardiac blood draw is considered a terminal process and should only be used under deep anesthetic. For routine blood collections, the other collection routes (retro-orbital sinus, saphenous vein, and the tail vein nick procedure) would be appropriate. These routes may be done in restrained, awake animals.

145. D: Chemotherapeutic agents that are used to kill neoplastic cells have many side effects for the patient receiving them and potentially for the individuals that handle them. Because the drugs attack any rapidly dividing cells, such as bone marrow cells and intestinal cells, humans that come in contact with contaminated body fluids (vomitus, feces, urine, etc.) should consider these fluids to be hazardous waste. The waste is the most harmful for 48 hours after administration. Owners should be counseled on the proper handling and disposal of such waste.

146. A: Ideally, the blood sample would be drawn before antibiotic administration to allow the most accurate result. Antibiotic therapy can quickly decrease the load of infectious organisms, and submission after antibiotic therapy could give a false-negative result. A gold standard of practice is to draw sufficient samples before therapy is administered in the event that the diagnostic plan could change.

147. A: Botulism is most commonly seen through ingestion of feed contaminated with deceased rodents. This more commonly occurs in large, round hay bales due to their immense size and the method in which they are fed free choice with little inspection of the interior. Rabies and tetanus are considered core vaccines regardless of diet. West Nile virus, which is transmitted by infected mosquitoes, has a risk-based vaccine strategy.

148. A: Radiopaque refers to an object's ability to block x-rays and prevent them from exposing the underlying film. The more radiopaque a tissue is, the whiter an image will appear. Bone is the most radiopaque followed by soft tissue, then fat, and, finally, air, which is not radiopaque. Water has the same radiopacity as soft tissue.

149. A: Given strong contractions, it should take no longer than 30–60 minutes between each puppy. Criteria for dystocia indications include more than 2 hours lapsing between puppies with infrequent contractions or longer than 4 hours with weak contractions. In the event of suspected dystocia, early intervention is more likely to lead to a successful outcome resulting in live puppies and a live bitch.

150. D: Tachycardia and severely dry mucous membranes are seen in 10% dehydration and enophthalmos (sunken eyes) begins with 8% dehydration. A 5% degree of dehydration is minimal, so the signs will be mild, such as minimal loss of skin turgor and semidry mucous membranes. The most severe signs of dehydration include hypotension, tachycardia, weak pulse, and altered consciousness.

151. B: Proptosis of the eye occurs when the globe is fully dislodged from the socket. This occurs fairly easily in short-faced breeds with shallow sockets, such as pugs. In addition to trauma, occasionally, an aggressive neck restraint can also provide enough pressure to result in proptosis. The presence of a direct and consensual pupillary light reflex indicates that the optic nerve is intact, and there is a greater chance of salvaging vision than if one is not present. Intraocular pressure is not accurate before replacement of the eye in its socket, and glaucoma can occur as a sequela to injury. Fluorescein staining may be helpful once the globe is replaced to identify corneal ulcers and guide treatment but will not predict the viability of vision resulting from the proptosis.

152. C: The blood pressure cuff width should be approximately 40%–60% of the circumference of the appendage that it is being applied on. A cuff that is too large or too small will give inaccurate blood pressure readings, which may lead to unnecessary interventions or may deter an intervention when it might be needed. Direct blood pressure monitoring involves placement of a specialized arterial line and is not commonly used in general practice.

153. D: A 12 hour preoperative fasting period is recommended for equine patients with the exception of in the case of an emergency surgery. In the event of an emergency, withholding food may not be required. Water is typically allowed for hydration.

154. D: *P. multocida* is a commensal bacterium of the feline oral cavity. This bacterium is known to cause severe infections of the surrounding tissue if not treated appropriately and quickly after contamination. Consultation with a physician after any cat bite that breaks the skin is strongly recommended. This bacterium is also found in the oral cavity of large cats, such as mountain lions, as well as domestic house cats.

155. D: Distilled water and approved instrument cleaner should be the first to be used in removing gross debris; tap water should not be used because mineral deposits may be left on the instruments. Instrument milk is important for lubrication and inhibiting rust formation, a step that is missing in answer C.

156. C: Canines most frequently show gastrointestinal (GI) signs as a negative side effect of NSAIDs even if approved for the species. The most common side effects are mild, such as vomiting and diarrhea, and they resolve when the medication is discontinued. However, severe adverse effects such as GI bleeding or perforations can occur, especially when NSAIDs are administered inappropriately. Liver dysfunction is a rare side effect, and renal failure is the main negative side effect seen in felines. Seizures are not known to be caused by NSAIDs.

157. C: Rumenostomy is a term for a semipermanent opening from the rumen to the skin. A rumenotomy would involve closure of the rumen, whereas a rumenectomy would suggest full removal of the organ. Gastrotomy is an inappropriate term when referring to ruminants; the gastric organ is called the abomasum.

158. D: While the changes listed are all concerns regarding a urinary obstruction, the electrolyte abnormality that is the most concerning would be elevated potassium (hyperkalemia). Potassium is secreted in the urine, and prolonged obstruction results in significant elevation, which can have profound cardiac effects by causing bradycardia.

159. B: The #15 scalpel blade is used for precise cuts and small incisions. (A) is an example of a #10, which is the most common basic blade for incising skin (in large animals, a #20 is commonly used, which is a larger version of a #10). (C) illustrates a #11 blade, which is used to sever ligaments or is commonly used for dental procedures. (D) shows a #12 blade, which may be used when lancing a pocket of fluid.

160. C: Caution must always be exercised when performing an intravenous (IV) injection in the jugular vein of horses because the carotid artery lies in close proximity to the jugular vein, and can therefore be mistakenly accessed even by the most experienced technicians. Steps to help minimize this error include utilizing the cranial third of the neck for venipuncture. This is because the artery does not lie in such close proximity to the vein as it does in the more caudal aspect of the neck.

Another tactic would be to insert a large bore needle first and watch the blood as it exits the hub. If it is a gentle drip, then the needle is in the vein. If it is a steady, pulsating stream, the needle is in the artery and needs to be readjusted. Once the needle is in the vein, the drug should be administered slowly in order to give the technician or veterinarian ample time to stop the injection in the event of an adverse reaction. For example, sometimes horses move during an injection and cause the needle to be redirected into the carotid artery. If medication is injected into the carotid artery, it travels straight to the brain where it can cause potentially lethal consequences. Thus, it is extremely important not to be overconfident with these injections, and always use good judgment and safe techniques.

161. C: PLEs result in the loss of albumin and globulins resulting in panhypoproteinemia (low total protein). Clinical signs such as third-spacing of fluid (ascites, in this case) results from the decreased intravascular hydrostatic pressures from the loss of the albumin component. Panhypoproteinemia is more specifically indicative of PLE as opposed to hypoalbuminemia, which has multiple etiologies.

162. D: A higher frequency (measured in megahertz [MHz]) results in a shorter wavelength when maintaining a consistent velocity (velocity = wavelength × frequency), which in turn provides greater resolution. The negative aspect of high frequency is that the shorter wavelengths have less tissue penetration, which limits their ability to reach deeper structures. It is important that a frequency is selected that will be able to penetrate the tissue to the appropriate depth based on the structure/organ that requires imaging.

163. D: Presurgical administration of a nonsteroidal anti-inflammatory drug (NSAID) such as carprofen is effective at decreasing surgical pain and should be continued postoperatively for this healthy patient. Neuroleptanalgesia is a preanesthetic combination of an opioid and a sedative—opioids are excellent analgesics and should be part of any surgical procedure. Intratesticular local anesthesia will provide an added level of comfort in the perioperative period.

164. A: This is a classic example of *Malassezia*, a type of yeast commonly implicated in canine and feline otitis externa. They are characterized by their "snowman" or "footprint" shape, and they stain dark purple for most in-house differential stains. These are not bacteria, and this type of stain does not allow for Gram classification.

165. D: Vocalization is an unreliable indicator of pain, especially the assumption that the absence of vocalization indicates that the animal must not be feeling pain. Pain signs can be subtle and sometimes subjective; however, disuse, reluctance to move, and an elevated heart rate are consistent parameters of pain. These parameters are helpful when used together. Owners must be strongly advised that an animal does not have to vocalize constantly to indicate that it is in pain.

166. C: Intraperitoneal injection of barbiturates is the preferred method of euthanasia for an animal of this size. IV injection would be difficult due to the small size and risk of extravascular administration. Intracardiac injection would only be acceptable with deep anesthesia. Enclosed chambers with carbon dioxide are not typically used for the euthanasia of a single animal.

167. B: Dissociative anesthetics, such as ketamine, produce a cataleptic state through central nervous system excitement, rather than depression. Hyperexcitement, ataxia, and nystagmus are seen when using these medications; however, the effects can be minimalized through using appropriate premedication and appropriate doses of dissociative anesthetics. It is common to administer dissociative anesthetics in combination with other drugs, such as benzodiazepines or alpha-2 agonists, such as dexmedetomidine. These adjuncts may also be administered during recovery to provide sedation if these side effects persist.

168. B: When ventilating a patient, you should not exceed 20 cmH_2O of pressure. Exceeding this amount can result in damage to the pulmonary alveoli and subsequent pneumomediastinum (free air in the mediastinum) or pneumothorax (free air in the pleural space). Either of these complications can lead to respiratory complications and hypoxia. A common cause of increased pulmonary pressure is failure to release the pop-off valve during ventilation. It is critical that this valve is never left closed.

169. C: The FDA is responsible for processing all reports of adverse reactions related to veterinary medication. The USDA would process concerns regarding biologics, such as vaccines. The DEA is responsible for monitoring drug compliance, such as for the proper handling of controlled substances. AVMA is not a regulatory body.

170. D: Before daily use, the anesthesia machine should be pressure checked to ensure that there are no leaks within the circuit. Leaks will prevent the right mixture of oxygen and anesthesia to be delivered to the patient, as well as expose humans to potentially harmful gases. Cleaning of the system should be done regularly, including the valves being cleaned periodically to prevent them from becoming stuck, but cleaning is not typically done immediately before use. The soda lime canister should be changed as needed.

VTNE Practice Tests #2 and #3

To take these additional VTNE practice tests, visit our online resources page:
mometrix.com/resources719/vtne

How to Overcome Test Anxiety

Just the thought of taking a test is enough to make most people a little nervous. A test is an important event that can have a long-term impact on your future, so it's important to take it seriously and it's natural to feel anxious about performing well. But just because anxiety is normal, that doesn't mean that it's helpful in test taking, or that you should simply accept it as part of your life. Anxiety can have a variety of effects. These effects can be mild, like making you feel slightly nervous, or severe, like blocking your ability to focus or remember even a simple detail.

If you experience test anxiety—whether severe or mild—it's important to know how to beat it. To discover this, first you need to understand what causes test anxiety.

Causes of Test Anxiety

While we often think of anxiety as an uncontrollable emotional state, it can actually be caused by simple, practical things. One of the most common causes of test anxiety is that a person does not feel adequately prepared for their test. This feeling can be the result of many different issues such as poor study habits or lack of organization, but the most common culprit is time management. Starting to study too late, failing to organize your study time to cover all of the material, or being distracted while you study will mean that you're not well prepared for the test. This may lead to cramming the night before, which will cause you to be physically and mentally exhausted for the test. Poor time management also contributes to feelings of stress, fear, and hopelessness as you realize you are not well prepared but don't know what to do about it.

Other times, test anxiety is not related to your preparation for the test but comes from unresolved fear. This may be a past failure on a test, or poor performance on tests in general. It may come from comparing yourself to others who seem to be performing better or from the stress of living up to expectations. Anxiety may be driven by fears of the future—how failure on this test would affect your educational and career goals. These fears are often completely irrational, but they can still negatively impact your test performance.

Elements of Test Anxiety

As mentioned earlier, test anxiety is considered to be an emotional state, but it has physical and mental components as well. Sometimes you may not even realize that you are suffering from test anxiety until you notice the physical symptoms. These can include trembling hands, rapid heartbeat, sweating, nausea, and tense muscles. Extreme anxiety may lead to fainting or vomiting. Obviously, any of these symptoms can have a negative impact on testing. It is important to recognize them as soon as they begin to occur so that you can address the problem before it damages your performance.

The mental components of test anxiety include trouble focusing and inability to remember learned information. During a test, your mind is on high alert, which can help you recall information and stay focused for an extended period of time. However, anxiety interferes with your mind's natural processes, causing you to blank out, even on the questions you know well. The strain of testing during anxiety makes it difficult to stay focused, especially on a test that may take several hours. Extreme anxiety can take a huge mental toll, making it difficult not only to recall test information but even to understand the test questions or pull your thoughts together.

Effects of Test Anxiety

Test anxiety is like a disease—if left untreated, it will get progressively worse. Anxiety leads to poor performance, and this reinforces the feelings of fear and failure, which in turn lead to poor performances on subsequent tests. It can grow from a mild nervousness to a crippling condition. If allowed to progress, test anxiety can have a big impact on your schooling, and consequently on your future.

Test anxiety can spread to other parts of your life. Anxiety on tests can become anxiety in any stressful situation, and blanking on a test can turn into panicking in a job situation. But fortunately, you don't have to let anxiety rule your testing and determine your grades. There are a number of relatively simple steps you can take to move past anxiety and function normally on a test and in the rest of life.

Physical Steps for Beating Test Anxiety

While test anxiety is a serious problem, the good news is that it can be overcome. It doesn't have to control your ability to think and remember information. While it may take time, you can begin taking steps today to beat anxiety.

Just as your first hint that you may be struggling with anxiety comes from the physical symptoms, the first step to treating it is also physical. Rest is crucial for having a clear, strong mind. If you are tired, it is much easier to give in to anxiety. But if you establish good sleep habits, your body and mind will be ready to perform optimally, without the strain of exhaustion. Additionally, sleeping well helps you to retain information better, so you're more likely to recall the answers when you see the test questions.

Getting good sleep means more than going to bed on time. It's important to allow your brain time to relax. Take study breaks from time to time so it doesn't get overworked, and don't study right before bed. Take time to rest your mind before trying to rest your body, or you may find it difficult to fall asleep.

Along with sleep, other aspects of physical health are important in preparing for a test. Good nutrition is vital for good brain function. Sugary foods and drinks may give a burst of energy but this burst is followed by a crash, both physically and emotionally. Instead, fuel your body with protein and vitamin-rich foods.

Also, drink plenty of water. Dehydration can lead to headaches and exhaustion, especially if your brain is already under stress from the rigors of the test. Particularly if your test is a long one, drink water during the breaks. And if possible, take an energy-boosting snack to eat between sections.

Along with sleep and diet, a third important part of physical health is exercise. Maintaining a steady workout schedule is helpful, but even taking 5-minute study breaks to walk can help get your blood pumping faster and clear your head. Exercise also releases endorphins, which contribute to a positive feeling and can help combat test anxiety.

When you nurture your physical health, you are also contributing to your mental health. If your body is healthy, your mind is much more likely to be healthy as well. So take time to rest, nourish your body with healthy food and water, and get moving as much as possible. Taking these physical steps will make you stronger and more able to take the mental steps necessary to overcome test anxiety.

Mental Steps for Beating Test Anxiety

Working on the mental side of test anxiety can be more challenging, but as with the physical side, there are clear steps you can take to overcome it. As mentioned earlier, test anxiety often stems from lack of preparation, so the obvious solution is to prepare for the test. Effective studying may be the most important weapon you have for beating test anxiety, but you can and should employ several other mental tools to combat fear.

First, boost your confidence by reminding yourself of past success—tests or projects that you aced. If you're putting as much effort into preparing for this test as you did for those, there's no reason you should expect to fail here. Work hard to prepare; then trust your preparation.

Second, surround yourself with encouraging people. It can be helpful to find a study group, but be sure that the people you're around will encourage a positive attitude. If you spend time with others who are anxious or cynical, this will only contribute to your own anxiety. Look for others who are motivated to study hard from a desire to succeed, not from a fear of failure.

Third, reward yourself. A test is physically and mentally tiring, even without anxiety, and it can be helpful to have something to look forward to. Plan an activity following the test, regardless of the outcome, such as going to a movie or getting ice cream.

When you are taking the test, if you find yourself beginning to feel anxious, remind yourself that you know the material. Visualize successfully completing the test. Then take a few deep, relaxing breaths and return to it. Work through the questions carefully but with confidence, knowing that you are capable of succeeding.

Developing a healthy mental approach to test taking will also aid in other areas of life. Test anxiety affects more than just the actual test—it can be damaging to your mental health and even contribute to depression. It's important to beat test anxiety before it becomes a problem for more than testing.

Study Strategy

Being prepared for the test is necessary to combat anxiety, but what does being prepared look like? You may study for hours on end and still not feel prepared. What you need is a strategy for test prep. The next few pages outline our recommended steps to help you plan out and conquer the challenge of preparation.

Step 1: Scope Out the Test

Learn everything you can about the format (multiple choice, essay, etc.) and what will be on the test. Gather any study materials, course outlines, or sample exams that may be available. Not only will this help you to prepare, but knowing what to expect can help to alleviate test anxiety.

Step 2: Map Out the Material

Look through the textbook or study guide and make note of how many chapters or sections it has. Then divide these over the time you have. For example, if a book has 15 chapters and you have five days to study, you need to cover three chapters each day. Even better, if you have the time, leave an extra day at the end for overall review after you have gone through the material in depth.

If time is limited, you may need to prioritize the material. Look through it and make note of which sections you think you already have a good grasp on, and which need review. While you are studying, skim quickly through the familiar sections and take more time on the challenging parts. Write out your plan so you don't get lost as you go. Having a written plan also helps you feel more in control of the study, so anxiety is less likely to arise from feeling overwhelmed at the amount to cover.

Step 3: Gather Your Tools

Decide what study method works best for you. Do you prefer to highlight in the book as you study and then go back over the highlighted portions? Or do you type out notes of the important information? Or is it helpful to make flashcards that you can carry with you? Assemble the pens, index cards, highlighters, post-it notes, and any other materials you may need so you won't be distracted by getting up to find things while you study.

If you're having a hard time retaining the information or organizing your notes, experiment with different methods. For example, try color-coding by subject with colored pens, highlighters, or post-it notes. If you learn better by hearing, try recording yourself reading your notes so you can listen while in the car, working out, or simply sitting at your desk. Ask a friend to quiz you from your flashcards, or try teaching someone the material to solidify it in your mind.

Step 4: Create Your Environment

It's important to avoid distractions while you study. This includes both the obvious distractions like visitors and the subtle distractions like an uncomfortable chair (or a too-comfortable couch that makes you want to fall asleep). Set up the best study environment possible: good lighting and a comfortable work area. If background music helps you focus, you may want to turn it on, but otherwise keep the room quiet. If you are using a computer to take notes, be sure you don't have any other windows open, especially applications like social media, games, or anything else that could distract you. Silence your phone and turn off notifications. Be sure to keep water close by so you stay hydrated while you study (but avoid unhealthy drinks and snacks).

Also, take into account the best time of day to study. Are you freshest first thing in the morning? Try to set aside some time then to work through the material. Is your mind clearer in the afternoon or evening? Schedule your study session then. Another method is to study at the same time of day that you will take the test, so that your brain gets used to working on the material at that time and will be ready to focus at test time.

Step 5: Study!

Once you have done all the study preparation, it's time to settle into the actual studying. Sit down, take a few moments to settle your mind so you can focus, and begin to follow your study plan. Don't give in to distractions or let yourself procrastinate. This is your time to prepare so you'll be ready to fearlessly approach the test. Make the most of the time and stay focused.

Of course, you don't want to burn out. If you study too long you may find that you're not retaining the information very well. Take regular study breaks. For example, taking five minutes out of every hour to walk briskly, breathing deeply and swinging your arms, can help your mind stay fresh.

As you get to the end of each chapter or section, it's a good idea to do a quick review. Remind yourself of what you learned and work on any difficult parts. When you feel that you've mastered the material, move on to the next part. At the end of your study session, briefly skim through your notes again.

But while review is helpful, cramming last minute is NOT. If at all possible, work ahead so that you won't need to fit all your study into the last day. Cramming overloads your brain with more information than it can process and retain, and your tired mind may struggle to recall even previously learned information when it is overwhelmed with last-minute study. Also, the urgent nature of cramming and the stress placed on your brain contribute to anxiety. You'll be more likely to go to the test feeling unprepared and having trouble thinking clearly.

So don't cram, and don't stay up late before the test, even just to review your notes at a leisurely pace. Your brain needs rest more than it needs to go over the information again. In fact, plan to finish your studies by noon or early afternoon the day before the test. Give your brain the rest of the day to relax or focus on other things, and get a good night's sleep. Then you will be fresh for the test and better able to recall what you've studied.

STEP 6: TAKE A PRACTICE TEST

Many courses offer sample tests, either online or in the study materials. This is an excellent resource to check whether you have mastered the material, as well as to prepare for the test format and environment.

Check the test format ahead of time: the number of questions, the type (multiple choice, free response, etc.), and the time limit. Then create a plan for working through them. For example, if you have 30 minutes to take a 60-question test, your limit is 30 seconds per question. Spend less time on the questions you know well so that you can take more time on the difficult ones.

If you have time to take several practice tests, take the first one open book, with no time limit. Work through the questions at your own pace and make sure you fully understand them. Gradually work up to taking a test under test conditions: sit at a desk with all study materials put away and set a timer. Pace yourself to make sure you finish the test with time to spare and go back to check your answers if you have time.

After each test, check your answers. On the questions you missed, be sure you understand why you missed them. Did you misread the question (tests can use tricky wording)? Did you forget the information? Or was it something you hadn't learned? Go back and study any shaky areas that the practice tests reveal.

Taking these tests not only helps with your grade, but also aids in combating test anxiety. If you're already used to the test conditions, you're less likely to worry about it, and working through tests until you're scoring well gives you a confidence boost. Go through the practice tests until you feel comfortable, and then you can go into the test knowing that you're ready for it.

Test Tips

On test day, you should be confident, knowing that you've prepared well and are ready to answer the questions. But aside from preparation, there are several test day strategies you can employ to maximize your performance.

First, as stated before, get a good night's sleep the night before the test (and for several nights before that, if possible). Go into the test with a fresh, alert mind rather than staying up late to study.

Try not to change too much about your normal routine on the day of the test. It's important to eat a nutritious breakfast, but if you normally don't eat breakfast at all, consider eating just a protein bar. If you're a coffee drinker, go ahead and have your normal coffee. Just make sure you time it so that the caffeine doesn't wear off right in the middle of your test. Avoid sugary beverages, and drink enough water to stay hydrated but not so much that you need a restroom break 10 minutes into the test. If your test isn't first thing in the morning, consider going for a walk or doing a light workout before the test to get your blood flowing.

Allow yourself enough time to get ready, and leave for the test with plenty of time to spare so you won't have the anxiety of scrambling to arrive in time. Another reason to be early is to select a good seat. It's helpful to sit away from doors and windows, which can be distracting. Find a good seat, get out your supplies, and settle your mind before the test begins.

When the test begins, start by going over the instructions carefully, even if you already know what to expect. Make sure you avoid any careless mistakes by following the directions.

Then begin working through the questions, pacing yourself as you've practiced. If you're not sure on an answer, don't spend too much time on it, and don't let it shake your confidence. Either skip it and come back later, or eliminate as many wrong answers as possible and guess among the remaining ones. Don't dwell on these questions as you continue—put them out of your mind and focus on what lies ahead.

Be sure to read all of the answer choices, even if you're sure the first one is the right answer. Sometimes you'll find a better one if you keep reading. But don't second-guess yourself if you do immediately know the answer. Your gut instinct is usually right. Don't let test anxiety rob you of the information you know.

If you have time at the end of the test (and if the test format allows), go back and review your answers. Be cautious about changing any, since your first instinct tends to be correct, but make sure you didn't misread any of the questions or accidentally mark the wrong answer choice. Look over any you skipped and make an educated guess.

At the end, leave the test feeling confident. You've done your best, so don't waste time worrying about your performance or wishing you could change anything. Instead, celebrate the successful completion of this test. And finally, use this test to learn how to deal with anxiety even better next time.

Review Video: Test Anxiety
Visit mometrix.com/academy and enter code: 100340

Important Qualification

Not all anxiety is created equal. If your test anxiety is causing major issues in your life beyond the classroom or testing center, or if you are experiencing troubling physical symptoms related to your anxiety, it may be a sign of a serious physiological or psychological condition. If this sounds like your situation, we strongly encourage you to seek professional help.

Online Resources

Due to our efforts to try to keep this book to a manageable length, we've created a link that will give you access to all of your online resources:

mometrix.com/resources719/vtne

It's Your Moment, Let's Celebrate It!

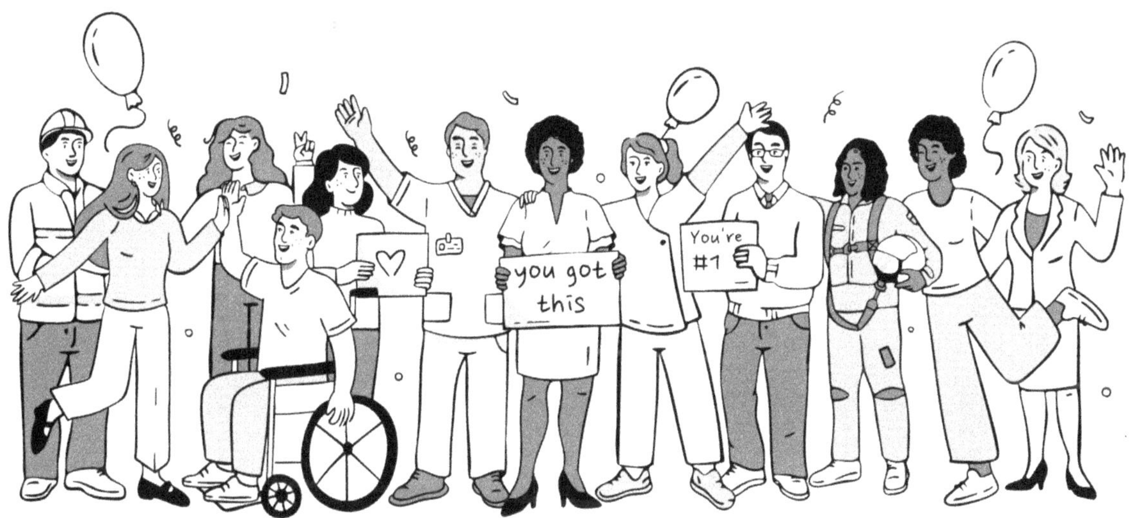

Share your story @mometrixtestpreparation

www.ingramcontent.com/pod-product-compliance
Lightning Source LLC
Chambersburg PA
CBHW061323190326
41458CB00011B/3873
* 9 7 8 1 5 1 6 7 0 5 6 7 2 *